DESIGN AND ANALYSIS OF ANIMAL STUDIES IN PHARMACEUTICAL DEVELOPMENT

Biostatistics: A Series of References and Textbooks

Series Editor
Shein-Chung Chow
Covance, Inc., Princeton, New Jersey, and
Temple University, Philadelphia, Pennsylvania

1. *Design and Analysis of Animal Studies in Pharmaceutical Development,* edited by Shein-Chung Chow and Jen-pei Liu

ADDITIONAL VOLUMES IN PREPARATION

DESIGN AND ANALYSIS OF ANIMAL STUDIES IN PHARMACEUTICAL DEVELOPMENT

EDITED BY

Shein-Chung Chow
Covance, Inc.
Princeton, New Jersey

Jen-pei Liu
National Cheng-Kung University
Tainan, Taiwan

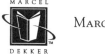
MARCEL DEKKER, INC.   NEW YORK · BASEL · HONG KONG

ISBN: 0-8247-0130-5

The publisher offers discounts on this book when ordered in bulk quantities. For more information, write to Special Sales/Professional Marketing at the address below.

This book is printed on acid-free paper.

MARCEL DEKKER, INC.
270 Madison Avenue, New York, New York 10016
http://www.dekker.com

Current printing (last digit):
10 9 8 7 6 5 4 3 2 1

PRINTED IN THE UNITED STATES OF AMERICA

Series Introduction

The primary objectives of the Biostatistics book series are to provide useful reference books for researchers and scientists in academia, industry, and government, and also to offer textbooks for undergraduate and/or graduate courses in the area of biostatistics. This book series will provide comprehensive and unified presentations of statistical designs and analyses of important applications in biostatistics, such as those in biopharmaceuticals. A well-balanced summary will be given of current and recently developed statistical methods and interpretations for both statisticians and researchers/scientists with minimal statistical knowledge who are engaged in applied biostatistics. The series is committed to providing easy-to-understand state-of-the-art references and textbooks. In each volume, statistical concepts and methodologies will be illustrated through real examples.

As detailed in *Design and Analysis of Animal Studies in Pharmaceutical Development*, the development of a new product is a lengthy and costly process that involves a number of critical stages such as discovery and formulation. Also involved is laboratory development, such as assay method development and validation, preclinical animal studies, clinical development including Phases I–IV clinical investigations, manufacturing process validation, control and assurance, and postmarketing activities. Among these critical stages, preclinical animal studies are often conducted to assess the toxicity of the study drug. With the assumption that the results from animal studies can predict results in humans, preclinical animal testing for toxicity provides valuable information regarding the safety of the study drug. To accurately and precisely assess the toxicity of the study drug, valid statistical design and analysis are necessarily employed.

Shein-Chung Chow

Preface

During drug development, certain toxicities of a product, such as impairment of fertility, mutagenicity, and carcinogenicity, cannot ethically be investigated in humans. Therefore, the toxicity of the drug product is usually assessed in either in vitro assays or animal models during preclinical drug development. In vitro assay and animal testing are often considered as surrogate for human testing, with the assumption that they can predict results in humans. Thus, it is important to provide a fair and unbiased assessment for toxicity before the drug can be used for clinical development. The success of preclinical assessment is the key to the success of clinical development and, consequently, the key to the success of the entire drug development procedure.

The goal of this book is to provide a comprehensive and unified presentation of statistical designs and methods for all aspects of animal studies in pharmaceutical research and development through real examples. It is our goal to provide a useful reference book for pharmaceutical scientists, toxicologists, and biostatisticians in the pharmaceutical industry, regulatory agencies, and academia. This book can also serve as a textbook for graduate courses in the areas of pharmaceutical development, toxicology, and biostatistics.

The scope of this book is restricted to statistical designs and analyses in in vitro assays and animal studies for assessment of drug safety in preclinical development prior to the investigational new drug application (IND). Chapter 1 provides an overview of pre-clinical assessment for toxicity in drug development. Also included in this chapter are regulatory requirements for submission of new drug application (NDA). In Chapter 2, some key principles in experimental design for animal studies are discussed. Chapter 3 covers statistical methods for determination of median lethal dose or median effective dose. Some principles in statistical testing in randomized toxicological studies are given in Chapter 4. Chapter 5 provides a comprehensive review of statistical design and analysis for subacute toxicity studies. In Chapter 6, we provide a statistical view of the proof of safety versus proof of hazard for safety assessment of toxicology studies. Chapters 7 and 8 cover the design and analysis of long-term carcinogenicity studies, respectively. The design and analysis of reproductive studies are discussed in Chapters 9 and 10. For in vitro assays, Ames tests for genotoxicity and CHO/HGPRT mutagenesis studies are given in Chapters 11 and 12, respectively.

Each chapter, whenever possible, provides real examples to illustrate the concepts and appropriate applications of statistical methods. Comparisons of relative merits and disadvantages of these methods are also discussed. Topics for possible future research development are also provided.

From Marcel Dekker, Inc., we would like to thank Graham Garratt, Executive Vice President and Publisher, for providing us with the opportunity to work on this book, and Maria Allegra, Acquisitions Editor and Manager, for her outstanding efforts in preparing this book for publication. Dr. Chow is deeply indebted to the Bristol-Myers Squibb Company, Covance, Inc., and to Temple University for their support, and in particular, to S. A. Henry and T. Newman. We are grateful to all the authors for their support and contributions toward this book volume. We also wish to thank E. Nordbrock, A. P. Pong, and M. L. Ting for their constant support and encouragement. Dr. Chow also wishes to express his appreciation to his wife, Yueh-Ji, and two daughters, Emily and Lilly, for their patience and understanding during the preparation of this book.

Shein-Chung Chow
Jen-pei Liu

Contents

Contributors

Hongshik Ahn Department of Applied Mathematics and Statistics, State University of New York at Stony Brook, Stony Brook, New York

A. John Bailer Department of Mathematics and Statistics, Miami University, Oxford, Ohio

Steven Bailey Biometrics Department, Wyeth-Ayerst Research Laboratories, Chazy, New York

Marshall N. Brunden Department of Research Support Biostatistics, Pharmacia & Upjohn, Inc., Kalamazoo, Michigan (Retired)

James J. Chen Division of Biometry and Risk Assessment, National Center for Toxicological Research, Food and Drug Administration, Jefferson, Arkansas

Shein-Chung Chow Department of Biostatistics and Data Management, Covance, Inc., Princeton, New Jersey

Dieter Hauschke Department of Preclinical Biometry, Byk Gulden Pharmaceuticals, Konstanz, Germany

Wherly P. Hoffman   Department of Mathematical and Statistical Sciences, Eli Lilly and Company, Greenfield, Indiana

Ludwig A. Hothorn   Department of Bioinformatics, University of Hannover, Hannover, Germany

Ralph L. Kodell   Division of Biometry and Risk Assessment, National Center for Toxicological Research, Food and Drug Administration, Jefferson, Arkansas

Jen-pei Liu   Department of Statistics, National Cheng-Kung University, Tainan, Taiwan

Walter W. Piegorsch   Department of Statistics, University of South Carolina, Columbia, South Carolina

Keith A. Soper   Department of Biometrics Research, Merck Research Laboratories, West Point, Pennsylvania

R. John Weaver   Department of Research Support Biostatistics, Pharmacia & Upjohn, Inc., Kalamazoo, Michigan

1

Introduction

SHEIN-CHUNG CHOW
Covance, Inc., Princeton, New Jersey

JEN-PEI LIU
National Cheng-Kung University, Tainan, Taiwan

I. INTRODUCTION

In the pharmaceutical industry, drug development is a lengthy process that involves drug discovery, preclinical development, clinical development, regulatory registration, manufacturing, and postmarketing safety monitoring. The purpose of this lengthy process is to not only ensure the effectiveness and safety of the drug product, but also to assure that the drug product possesses some good characteristics, such as identity, strength, quality, purity, and stability of the drug product, as specified in the *United States Pharmacopeia* (*USP*). A drug product will not be approved by a regulatory agent unless the sponsor provides substantial evidence of the effectiveness and safety of the drug product. In this book, our emphasis will be placed on the discussion of issues on design and analysis of studies that are commonly conducted during preclinical drug development before the filing of an Investigational New Drug Application (IND). In other words, we will focus on in vitro assays and animal studies for evaluation of safety, rather than efficacy at preclinical development. For issues on design and analysis that are commonly encountered at various stages of drug development, comprehensive review and discussion can be found in Chow and Liu (1992) for bioavailability and bioequivalence studies; Chow and Liu (1995) for assay validation, process controls, and stability, and Chow and Liu (1998) for clinical development.

The primary focus of preclinical drug development is to evaluate the safety of the drug product through in vitro assays and animal studies. In vitro assay and animal testing are often considered as surrogate for human testing, under the assumption that they can be predictive of results in humans. Basically, preclinical drug development includes the stages of chemical synthesis, screening for activities, and preclinical testing. At preclinical drug development, the mess compounds are necessarily screened to distinguish those that are active from those that are not. The purpose of drug screening is to identify a stable and reproducible compound with fewer false-negative and false-positive results. For this purpose, a multiple stage screening procedure is usually employed. A compound must pass all stages to be active. The commonly encountered problem in drug screening for activity is the choice of dose. In practice, the dose is often chosen too low to show activity or too high to exhibit a toxic effect. Drug screening for activities could be a general screening, based on pharmacological activities in animal or in vitro assays, or a targeted screening based on specific activities, such as an enzyme. *Pharmacological activity* is usually referred to as selective biological activity of chemical substances on living matter. A chemical substance is called a *drug* if it has selective activity with medical value in treatment of disease.

Preclinical testing involves dose selection, toxicological testing for toxicity and carcinogenicity, and animal pharmacokinetics. For selection of an appropriate dose, dose-response (dose-ranging) studies in animals are usually conducted to determine the effective dose, such as the median effective dose (ED_{50}). In addition, drug interactions, such as potentiation, inhibition, similar joint action, synergism, and antagonism, are also studied. For these studies, the determination of drug potency is crucial. Drug potency in animals is usually determined by *bioassay*, which is an analytical method used to estimate and compare potency according to some reference standards as specified in the *USP*. Bioassay plays an important role in preclinical drug development by studying dose–response for effective dose and drug interaction. In drug development, because certain toxicities, such as impairment of fertility, teratology, mutagenicity, and overdosage, cannot be investigated ethically in humans, the toxicity of the drug product is usually assessed in either in vitro assays or animal models. The objective of toxicological testing in animal studies is then to explore not only realistic safety extrapolation, but also to evaluate new methods to test for toxicity. In addition, such studies emphasize meaningful interpretation of results and encourages more mechanistic approach to toxicology.

In general, in vitro assays or animal toxicity studies are intended to alert the clinical investigators to the potential toxic effects associated with the investigational drugs so that those effects may be watched for during the clinical investigations. In most circumstances, acute and subacute toxicity studies are typically conducted in rodent and nonrodent mammalian species. Segments I, II, and III reproductive toxicity studies, various in vitro clastogenic and mutagenic studies, and chronic and carcinogenic studies are necessarily conducted to provide a complete spectrum of toxicological effects an investigational drug can elicit. In addition, absorption, distribution, metabolism, and excretion (ADME) studies for the investigational drug in animal species should be performed to identify those pharmacokinetic parameters that are similar to those in humans and to verify the applicability of the animal species used in the toxicological tests. Note that regulatory agencies also require that the routes of drug administration in animal studies should mimic the intended clinical route(s), and the duration of animal testing should be equal to or exceed that in the anticipated clinical trials.

In the pharmaceutical industry, although significant volume of capital is invested in standard toxicological testing, problems encountered are not usually solved or explained by routine or standardized toxicological testing. The standardized testing for toxicity is usually designed based on a fixed protocol that is not designed for problem solving. In addition, it is neither innovative nor mechanistic. The reasons for carrying out toxicological testing are to exclude unacceptable toxic effects, to warn of possible acceptable toxicity, and the presence of effects in humans that are not detected in the laboratory could be considered as the failure of toxicological testing. An ideal testing of toxicity should include the following characteristics: (a) problem oriented, (b) providing mechanism, (c) requiring originality, and (d) discovery of toxicology within the planned time frame and with reasonable costs. However, in practice, it is not possible to attain a situation of no risk. Therefore, it is necessary to define acceptable risk. This could be either the best available practical option, or a risk that is as low as is reasonably possible.

In the next section, we provide an overview of regulatory requirements for toxicological testing in animal studies. The objectives and scopes of various animal studies, such as reproductive and carcinogenic-ity studies, are outlines in Section III. Some statistical considerations that are commonly encountered during various animal studies are dis-cussed in Section IV. The aims and the remaining structure of the book is given in Section V.

II. REGULATORY REQUIREMENTS

For regulatory review and approval of an investigational drug, as de-scribed in Part 21 of Codes of Federal Regulations (CFR) Section 314.50 (d), the US Food and Drug Administration (FDA) requires that a section of nonclinical pharmacology and toxicology be included in the technical section of the New Drug Application (NDA) submission for the investi-gational drug. The section of nonclinical pharmacology and toxicology should include studies of the pharmacological actions of the drug in relation to its proposed therapeutic indication, and studies of the toxico-logical effects of the drug as they relate to the drugs intended clinical use. Toxicological studies include studies, as appropriate, for assessing the drug's acute, subacute, and chronic toxicity and carcinogenicity, and studies of toxicities related to the drug's particular mode of administra-tion of conditions of use. In addition, the FDA also requires that studies, as appropriate, of the effects of the drug on reproduction and on the developing fetus, and any studies of the absorption, distribution, metab-olism, and excretion of the drug in animals be included in the section.

The FDA emphasizes that each nonclinical laboratory study is sub-ject to the good laboratory practice (GLP) regulations under 21 CFR 58. If the study was not conducted in compliance with those regulations, a brief statement of the reason for the noncompliance should be given.

A. General Principles

Under 21 CFR 10.90, the FDA issues a *Guideline for the Format and Content of the Nonclinical Pharmacology/Toxicology Section of an Ap-plication* to assist the sponsor organizing and presenting the pharmaco-logical and toxicological data required under 21 CFR 314.50 (d)(2) in the nonclinical section of the application. The guideline provides several general principles that may be applied to the submission of all toxicologi-cal studies, regardless of the characteristics of a particular study. Some of these key general principles include the availability of data, tables and graphs, the animals used for study, the route and mode of administration, the study doses, and laboratory determinations. For the availability of data, the guideline not only addresses typical circumstances of data review, but also requires that the database should be edited, quality controlled, and kept available for all relevant observations such as toxic signs, clinical pathology, tumor palpation, sacrifice or death, and necropsy results for each animal so that the reviewer may be rapidly supplied with requested data in the form needed. In addition, the guideline also states some specific requirements for the format of tables and graphs. It is recommended that graphs be used as a supplement to, not a replacement for, data tables. Whenever possible, summary tables should permit comparison of selected results from all dosage groups and relevant controls on the same page. When more than one animal species is used in a particular type of test or study, it is suggested that the data be reported or tabulated in the relative order of mouse, rat, hamster, other rodent(s), rabbit, dog, monkey, other nonrodent mammals and nonmammals; males preceding females; and adult animals preceding infant, geriatric, or disease model animals. The FDA also indicates that it is important to include age and weight ranges, strains, and animal suppliers for each study.

For the dose, route, and mode of administration, the guideline also has specific requirements. For example, the FDA prefers that multidose data be displayed from the lowest to the highest dose. In addition, within each multigroup study, it is suggested that the results in all tables should be presented in order or increasing dosage, such as untreated control, vehicle control, low-dose, middle-dose(s), high-dose, and positive or comparative control(s). Dose should be based on the active moiety component if the drug is a salt or other dissociable derivative, which should be expressed on a body weight basis (e.g., milligrams per kilogram; mg/kg). For route and mode administration, studies for each species within each type of study should first represent the intended route of human use, followed by data for other routes in the relative order of oral, intravenous, intramuscular, intraperitoneal, subcutaneous, inhalation, topical, other in vivo and in vitro. For laboratory determinations, the guideline requires that all biological tests and statistical methods be described in the study report. It is suggested that the variability or group mean values be presented by approximately labeled standard errors, standard deviations, or confidence limits for assessment of accuracy and reliability. The guideline also requires that studies with a radioactive drug should indicate the molecular location of the radioisotope and its specific activity.

B. Format and Content

For the format and content of the submission of an application, in addition to requirements for a table of contents, cross-references, and summary discussions, the guideline also requires that all studies in the submission be presented in a specific order. A submission based on the chronologic sequence of dates of conduct or previous submission of studies to the IND is not considered acceptable. The following order is recommended for submission of various studies, as appropriate to a particular application:

1. Pharmacology studies
2. Acute toxicity studies
3. Multidose toxicity studies (e.g., subchronic, chronic, and carcinogenicity)
4. Special toxicity studies
5. Reproduction studies
6. Mutagenicity studies
7. Absorption, distribution, metabolism, and excretion studies

In addition, the guideline also provide specific requirements for the format and content of individual study types. For example, for acute toxicity studies, the guideline requires that pretest conditioning and age of animals, dosing procedure, vehicles used, and dosage volumes be specified for each study. The types of severity of toxic signs and their onset and progression or reversal in relation to dosage and time after dosing should also be described for each species. The guideline also suggests that lethal dose data should be tabulated for interstudy or interspecies comparison.

For multidose toxicity studies, it is suggested that studies and respective study reports be grouped by species in order of increasing duration or by route of administration. Summary discussions of notable findings in all studies in each species should emphasize relations to dose and duration of treatment. For each study, some descriptive information, such as species, strain, source, age of initiation of dosing, number of males and females per group at the beginning and end of the study, route and mode of administration, doses and rationale for doses selection, interim sacrifice (if any), duration of treatment and study, and drug batch or lot number, should be included. In addition, within each individual study, the information of observed effects; mortality; body weight; food and water consumption; physical examinations; hematology, bone marrow and coagulation; blood chemistry, urinalysis and ADME data; organ weights; gross pathology; and histopathology should also be provided. The guideline also suggests that group mean tabulations and individual animal tabulations should be presented to allow comparison among individuals, among several related determinations, or among patterns of responses over time. Mean values and standard deviations should be included for intercolumn or intergroup comparison.

The guideline suggests that in vivo results from special toxicity studies be tabulated to show group comparison and time-related or progressive effects within each group. The in vitro results should also be tabulated to indicate the type of test or test system, dose range in increasing order, and effects related to dose. Note that as indicated in the guideline, special toxicity studies may include parental or topical irritation studies, in vitro hemolysis, or studies with a particular animal model relevant to the human disease or age.

For reproductive studies, the guideline requires that all studies be summarized followed multidose toxicity studies in the order of segments I (i.e., fertility and reproductive performance), II (teratology), III (perinatal and postnatal), and other studies such as multigeneration. Observations and their incidence in relation to dosage or time should be presented in the order of maternal effects and day of parturition or necropsy (and paternal effects in segment I study), maternal necropsy (e.g., corpora lutea, uterine contents, implantations, dead fetuses), fetuses grouped by litter (e.g., sex ratio, weight, viability, gross observations, visceral abnormalities, and skeletal abnormalities), and neonates to weaning (e.g., sex ratio, viability, growth, behavior and performance, and anatomical abnormalities).

For the mutagenicity studies, the results of available studies should be tabulated to indicate type of study, methods used, dose range in increasing order, and effect at each dose. In addition, the guideline suggests the studies be presented in the order of in vitro nonmammalian cell system, in vitro mammalian cell system, in vivo mammalian system, and in vivo nonmammalian system. For ADME studies in animals, for each species or strain, absorption, pharmacokinetics, serum half-life, protein binding, tissue distribution and accumulation, enzyme induction or inhibition, metabolism characteristics and metabolites, and excretion pattern should be reported. In addition, study descriptions should clearly state the dose(s) used in each study.

III. TOXICOLOGICAL TESTING

Basically, the role of toxicology in preclinical drug development before an IND is filed is threefold. First, it provides a toxicity background series or therapeutic agents in the area at the time of lead compound declaration. Second, it reviews the reactions observed in pharmacological screens. Finally, it studies the hazard risk of the drug product through acute toxicological testing, the toxicity of a targeted organ through subacute toxicological testing, and the tolerance through chronic toxicological testing. In addition, it also examines dose ranging to identify major toxicity. This information is valuable and useful in clinical development. As a result, toxicological testing in animal studies is to support not only the immediate clinical development, but also to study new molecules that have never before been tested. Moreover, toxicological testing provides extrapolations for evaluation of safety margins.

A minimum group of toxicological studies typically include bacterial mutagenicity (Ames); acute (single) toxicity, subacute (repeated dose) toxicity, systemic toxicity, and reproductive toxicity, including segments I, II, and III; and carcinogenicity studies. Because the design and analysis of these studies are similar, in what follows, we will focus only on reproductive studies and carcinogenicity studies. Detailed discussions of these studies will be given in the subsequent chapters of this book.

A. Reproductive Studies

Basically, reproductive toxicity studies can be divided into three categories; namely, segments I, II, and III, based on the time of dosing in relation to the expected timing of organogenesis. These categories are summarized in Table 1. As indicated in this table, the study type of segment I studies are usually fertility and reproduction. For segment I studies, dosing occurs before and during organogenesis. The rat is the species of interest. The F_0 generation males or females, or both, are dosed before and throughout the mating period. Segment II studies are commonly referred to as teratology studies. Dosing occurs during organogenesis. The rat and rabbit are the primary species of interest. The mouse usually serves as an alterative species for the rat. Note that dose-

TABLE 1   Reproductive Toxicity Studies

Segment	Study type	Species	F_0 sex doses	Timing and dosing
I	Reproduction	Rat	Males, females, both	Before and during organogenesis
II	Teratology	Rat, rabbit, (mouse, monkey, dog)	Females	During organogenesis
III	Late gestation and lactation	Rat	Females	After organogenesis

ranging studies in nonpregnant rabbits and pregnant rats and rabbits are often included in segment II studies that are run before the teratology studies to determine appropriate dose levels. Segment III studies are also known as late gestation and lactation studies. Dosing occurs after organogenesis from day 15 of pregnancy through day 21 postpartum in pregnant F_0 generation rats.

Segments I, II, and III studies generally have a common design theme. Usually, for each species to be tested, there are four equally sized dose groups to which F_0 generation animals are allocated at random. The first dose group is either a negative or a vehicle control and the remaining three groups receive graded doses of the compound. Following the initiation of the treatment to the F_0 generation animals and subsequent mating, various response parameters are recorded for the F_0 and the resulting F_1 generation animals. The F_0 generation parameters are evaluation of gonadal function, mating behavior, conception rates, parturition, lactation, and maternal care, whereas the F_1 parameters investigate survival, growth, reflexes, behavior, internal and external morphology; prenatal, postnatal, and late fetal development; and pre- and postweaning fetal development (Bradstreet and Clark, 1987). As an example, Table 2 provides a partial list of some commonly considered primary parameters for these studies: some of the parameters are common to more than one of the three categories of studies, whereas others will be category-specific.

Bradstreet and Clark (1987) provided the segments I, II, and III study procedures that are reproduced in Figs. 1–4. Figure 1 illustrates a segment I general study procedure for a combined reproduction study.

TABLE 2   Examples of Reproductive Study Parameters

Dam food and water consumption
Dam and pup weight over time
Number of days to mating
Dam and fetal survival rates
Number of implants per pregnant dam
Percentage pre- and postimplantation loss
Fertility, fecundity, and gestation indices
Length of gestation
Litter size, sex ratio of the litter
Percentage fetal anomalies per litter
Fetal anogenital distance
Proportion of pups responding positively for auditory startle, free-fall righting,
    testes descent, vaginal canalization
Number of swims for pups to escape successfully three consecutive times
    from a single-T swim maze
Number of fetal pellets dropped and number of light beams broken by pups
    during open-field testing
Fetal anogenital distance

Those corresponding to a male reproduction study are shown in Fig. 2. Note that a female reproduction study is conducted similar to the combined reproduction study except that the F_0 generation male animal remains untreated. Figure 3 displays the segment II dosing periods of the three most commonly used species, and segment III study procedures are illustrated in Fig. 4.

B. Carcinogenicity Studies

The purpose of carcinogenicity studies is to determine whether the substances under study are carcinogenic in particular strains of laboratory animals. The challenge is to better understand the biology of the response and the animal models currently employed to determine the carcinogenic potential of the substance under study. Two species that are routinely used in carcinogenicity studies are the rat and mouse. For the rat, the strains most commonly used are Sprague–Dawley derived, with some use of the F344 rat. For mice, the CD-1 strain is most commonly used, with some use of the B6C3F1 mouse (PMA, 1988). For carcinoge-

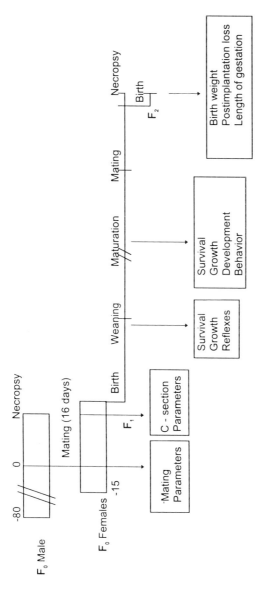

FIGURE 1   Segment I: combined reproduction study.

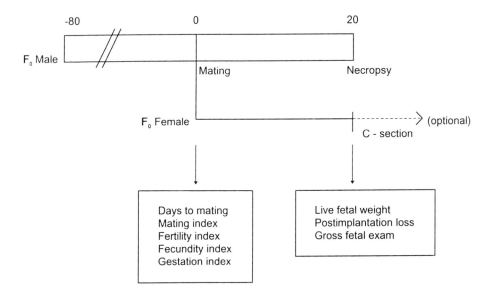

FIGURE 2   Segment I: male reproduction study.

nicity studies with rats or mice, three dose levels, with a dual or double-sized control, with the minimum group size of 50 per sex per group are usually considered. The targeted study duration is usually for at least 24 months. In most rat and mouse studies for carcinogenicity, the mode of drug administration is often by dietary admix. However, in some pharmaceutical companies, the predominate mode is gavage. It is suggested that a combination of gavage and dietary admix be considered based on what is most appropriate for a given compound.

For dose selection, the high dose is usually the dose considered to be the maximum-tolerated dose, whereas the low dose is a small multiple of the human-use dose. The middose is usually placed at the geometric mean between the high and low dose. Note that, according to a survey by the Drug Safety Subsection of the Research and Development Section of the Pharmaceutical Manufacturers Association (PMA), the factors most commonly considered as appropriate for the maximum-tolerated dose usually include no adverse effect on survival, up to a 10% decrement in body weight, some, but minimal, overt signs of toxicity or target organ toxicity (PMA, 1988). The survey also indicated that before FDA approval, carcinogenicity studies are not usually sought. However, ma-

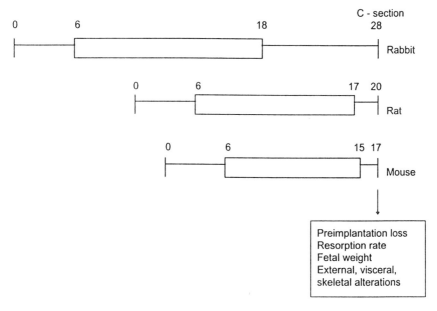

FIGURE 3   Segment II: teratology study.

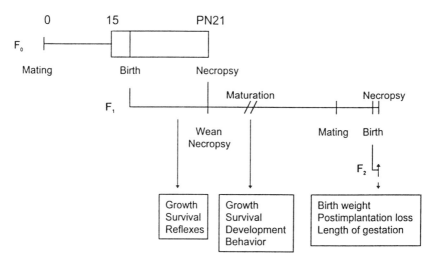

FIGURE 4   Segment III: late gestation and lactation study.

jor issues that need to be addressed are the definition of the maximum-tolerated dose for dose selection and the interpretation of the results of the bioassay.

In practice, it should be noted that low survival may cause the rejection of the study by regulatory agencies. Low survival (control and treatment groups) would require the study to be repeated. Other examples that may cause regulatory problems owing to low survival include (a) number of survivors deemed inadequate to make a valid assessment; (b) an increased mortality at high dose resulted in inadequate animals to validly assess, because the increase in tumor that was not statistically significant might have been significant if survival had been higher; (c) high mortality caused by drug-induced renal disease (for rat). In addition, the acceptance of a rat carcinogenicity study with poor survival may be withheld pending completion and review of other carcinogenicity studies with alternative species, such as the mouse.

In carcinogenicity studies, it is important to distinguish various tumor types. An observed tumor does not always reflect the true carcinogenic effect. It may occur by a secondary mechanism, such as a physiological perturbation, or by an exaggeration of a pharmacological effect. The International Agency for Research on Cancer (IARC) classifies the tumors as incidental, fetal, and mortality-independent, according to the context of observation within which the tumors arose. The PMA survey reveals that the most frequently observed tumor type by target organ was rat and mouse hepatic. For endocrine tumors, rats appear to have a much higher percentage than mice. Among the endocrine tumors, the most frequently observed tumor sites were mammary, thyroid, and pituitary; followed by adrenal, testicular, uterine, or ovarian. On the other hand, less frequently observed tumor sites in rats include gastrointestinal tract, kidney, urinary, bladder, brain, and pancreas.

IV. STATISTICAL CONSIDERATIONS

At preclinical assessment for toxicity of the drug product under investigation, the most commonly encountered practical issues that are worthy of statistical consideration are probably experimental unit, multiplicity, and dose selection. These issues will affect not only the selection of appropriate statistical methods for data analysis, but will also have a significant influence on the interpretation of the results. Therefore, it is suggested that these issues be taken into account when planning a toxicological study to assess an agent's toxicity.

A. Experimental Unit

Since the early 1970s, whether the litter or the fetus constitutes the proper experimental unit has become one of many important statistical considerations in toxicological studies (see, e.g., Weil, 1970; Kalter, 1974; Palmer, 1975; Haseman and Hogan, 1976). The experimental unit has an effect on the validity of statistical tests employed for assessment of toxicological studies involving reproduction, teratogenesis, or carcinogenesis. In the past several decades, several approaches have been proposed by considering either that the experimental unit is fetus or that the experimental unit is litter. We will refer to these two approaches as the per-fetus approach and the per-litter approach, respectively.

Some considerations for the per-fetus approach include (a) all of the fetuses in a litter do not receive identical blood supplies and, therefore, may be receiving different amounts of drug, and (b) there is evidence of joint maternal and fetal contribution in the production of malformations. On the other hand, the most important justification for the per-litter approach is that all statistical tests commonly used in the analysis of reproductive toxicity data require that the sampling units be independent of one another. In most reproductive toxicity studies, the fetuses, however, do not respond independently because maternal influence and other environmental factors will generally cause littermates to be more alike in weight, mortality, and anomalies than fetuses from different litters. If the effect of the drug is not equally distributed among litters, it is suggested that the effect is probably on the maternal organism and the sample size to be used for statistical testing should equal the number of litters. On the other hand, if the effect is uniformly distributed among litters, the suggestion is that the effect is probably associated with the fetuses. Therefore, the fetus should be used as the sample unit for statistical testing.

In summary, a per-fetus test is valid only if there is no litter effect. Type I error rates are usually inflated using the per-fetus approach. The litter should be viewed as the appropriate unit unless it can be undeniably demonstrated that there is nonmaternal influence on the fetal response. The per-litter analyses are always valid. Note that the within-litter information can be reflected in a composite score. Heyse (1987) indicated that it is important to incorporate litter size in the analysis of fetal malformation data. The interpretation of theses data is very difficult when litter size differs between treatment groups, regardless of the method used.

B. Multiplicity

In toxicological studies, multiplicity often occurs that depends on the objective of the intended trials, the nature of the design, and the statistical analysis. The causes of multiplicity are mainly the formulation of statistical hypotheses and the experimentwise false-positive rates in subsequent analyses of the data. As a result, statistical results should be carefully interpreted, because false-positive findings in number may increase as the number of significance tests performed increases. Heyse (1987) suggested the following adjustment. Let P_1 be the most extreme P-value observed among a class of K response variables. Heyse (1987) considered adjustment procedures of the form

$$P = 1 - (1 - P_1)^{K_1}$$

where K_1 depends on the class of variables being considered. When variables are independent, we may consider an extreme choice of $K_1 = K$. On the other hand, we may choose $K_1 = 1$ when variables are highly correlated. A compromise choice of $K_1 = K^{1/2}$ can be selected to account for some unknown amount of correlation.

Basically, multiplicity in toxicology studies can be classified as multiple comparisons, multiple response variables, and subgroup analyses. More details can be found in Tukey et al. (1985), Heyse and Rom (1988), and Morganthein et al. (1987). Questions of multiplicity of statistical tests need to be addressed when interpreting data from reproductive toxicological studies, in particular, and safety assessment screening studies, in general.

C. Dose Selection

Dose selection is one of the most important variables in the design of a toxicological study. Most toxicological studies employ at least three graded dose levels, with four dose groups, in addition to the controls. Dose selection is a prospective exercise of scientific judgment for prediction of the effects that will be produced in animals over a time period of exposure that can only be assessed retrospectively. Selection of doses too high may result in (a) compromising the survivability of the animal, (b) producing confounding effects, and (c) toxicity that makes interpretation of the results difficult.

Although the information used for dose selection most often comes from subchronic toxicity studies, information on the pharmacological and biochemical effects of a drug and information on pharmacokinetics and drug metabolism are often taken into account. The dose considered to represent the maximum-tolerated dose (MTD) is selected for the high-dose group. The low dose is usually selected as a small multiple (e.g., one to five times) of the clinical-use dose, and the middose is usually chosen as the geometric mean between the high and low doses. In practice, MTD is not a dose that can be precisely defined. It is commonly considered as the maximum dose that can be administered for a time period that will not compromise the survival of test animals by factors other than carcinogenicity. Some factors that are frequently considered appropriate for selection of the MTD are no adverse effects on survival, up to a 10% decrement in body weight, some but minimal overt signs of toxicity or target organ toxicity. Effects considered inappropriate for the MTD included increased mortality, body weight decrement in excess of 10%, marked pharmacological signs, marked signs of toxicity, or target organ toxicity.

D. Statistical Methods

For reproductive or teratology toxicity studies, the primary objectives are (a) to describe the response variables, (b) to assess treatment effects, and (c) to detect a potential pattern or trend in no-observable-effect levels (NOEL) in response to the three or four graded doses of the test drug in question. For this purpose, several methods for data analysis are available, which include parametric models, jackknife (e.g., Gladen, 1979), and split-started fractions (e.g., Ciminera et al., 1989). The response variables can be expressed by (a) parametric models (e.g., Rai and Van Ryzin, 1985), (b) empirical methods (e.g., Paul and Mantel, 1987), and (c) composite scores (e.g., Morganthein et al., 1987). For assessing treatment effects, commonly considered methods include (a) pairwise comparisons (e.g., Dunnett, 1964), (b) trend analysis (e.g., Tukey et al., 1985), (c) ordered alternatives (e.g., Williams, 1971, 1972) and (d) dose response (e.g., Rai and Van Ryzin, 1985; Kupper et al., 1986). The assessment of no-observable-effect levels are usually performed by a trend testing called no statistical significance of trend (NOSTASOT) sequential trend analysis approach proposed by Tukey et al. (1985). The

dose–response in this situation may be analyzed by the methods proposed by Rai and Van Ryzin (1985) and Kupper et al. (1986). Note that
the NOSTASOT analysis approach is also useful in detecting treatment
effects by a nonzero trend that is not only a more balanced, but also a
more powerful, procedure than others.

For analysis of tumor data from carcinogenicity studies, the IARC
suggests some considerations be taken into account. First, it is suggested
that separate analyses of the effects of treatment on each separate type
of tumor be performed. This is because carcinogenic treatments usually
seem to affect one or a few particular tumor types quite strongly,
whereas they hardly affect any other tumor types. Second, under the
consideration of tumor multiplicity within one organ (e.g., one mouse
may develop several hepatomas), it is preferred to analyze the number of
animals with a particular tumor type, rather than the total number or
average number of such tumors per animal. The disadvantages for using
the average number of tumors per animal are multifold. The average
number of tumors per animal cannot reflect the situation for which a
few animals are so prone that they spontaneously develop a dozen or
more such tumors, whereas many other animals in the same treatment
develop none. If animals usually develop several noninvasive, nonfetal
tumors spontaneously as they become older and a treatment is given that
causes such tumors to progress, then the average number of tumors
found in each animal would be reduced in that treatment group. In
addition, when one or a few tumors have grown large in an organ, it may
be impracticable at necropsy to accurately count the total number of
tumors originating in that organ. As a result, it would be more sensitive
to examine the carcinogenic effects by the total number of animals that
develop a tumor of the type to be studied, rather than the total number
of such tumors. Finally, because the effects of differences in longevity
on numbers of tumor-bearing animals can be very substantial, they
should be routinely corrected for when presenting experimental results.
For example, the death rate method is appropriate for fetal tumors, a
slight modification of it which yields the onset rate method is appropriate
for tumors observed in a mortality-independent context. For incidental
tumors, a completely different prevalence method is appropriate.

The most commonly employed statistical method for analysis of
tumor data is the Peto trend test, with adjustment for mortality of life
table methodology. When analyzing tumor data from carcinogenicity,
trend analysis is typically performed based on one-sided test. The next
most frequently used methods include Fisher's exact or chi-square (χ^2)

TABLE 3 Statistical Analysis Methods
Relatively Used for Tumor Data

---

1. Trends tests, mortality adjusted
   - a. Life table based methods
   - b. Peto/IARC style tests
2. Trend tests, unadjusted
3. Trend tests, no adjustment information
4. Nontrend tests, mortality adjusted
5. Nontrend tests, unadjusted
6. Nontrend tests, no adjustment information
7. No trend information, mortality adjusted
   - a. Life table methods
   - b. Method not indicated
8. Other methods, too general to classify

Source: PMA, 1988.

analysis. Table 3 lists statistical analytical methods that are routinely used for tumor data. Note that a nonsignificant p-value does not prove a lack of carcinogenic effect, nor is a barely significant p-value usually sufficient proof of carcinogenicity. It is suggested that the p-value should be combined with an equal amount of other relevant information for a scientific evaluation of the carcinogenic effect of the compound under study. Relevant information may include (a) results with the same test agent in other experiments, (b) historical experience on the likely background frequency of the tumor type of interest among control animals of the strain under approximately the same experimental conditions, (c) biological knowledge of whether the agent is known to cause precancerous or other lesions in the putative target organ, (d) knowledge of the activity or otherwise of the test agent in various short-term tests, and (e) structural considerations.

V. AIMS AND STRUCTURE OF THE BOOK

The goal of this book is to provide a comprehensive and unified presentation of statistical designs and methods of analysis for all aspects of animal studies in pharmaceutical research and development through real examples. It is our goal to provide a useful reference book for pharmaceutical scientists, toxicologists, and biostatisticians in the pharmaceutical industry, regulatory agencies, and academia. This book can also serve as a textbook for graduate courses in the areas of pharmaceutical development, toxicology, and biostatistics.

The scope of this book is restricted to statistical designs and analyses in in vitro assays and animal studies for assessment of drug safety in preclinical development before the IND application. In the next chapter, some key principles in experimental design for animal studies will be discussed. Also included in this chapter is dose selection in animal studies, including nonlinear dose response; maximum tolerated dose in chronic exposure studies; sequential dosing; and joint action. Chapter 3 covers statistical methods for determination of median lethal dose (LD_{50}) or median effective dose (ED_{50}). Some principles in statistical testing in randomized toxicological studies are discussed in Chapter 4. Chapter 5 provides a comprehensive review of statistical design and analysis for subacute toxicity studies. In Chapter 6, we provide statistical view for the proof of safety versus the proof of hazard, for safety assessment of toxicology studies. Chapters 7 and 8 cover the design and analysis of long-term carcinogenicity studies, respectively, and the design and analysis of reproductive studies are discussed in Chapters 9 and 10, respectively. For in vitro assays, Ames tests for genotoxicity and CHO/HGPRT mutagenesis studies are given in Chapters 11 and 12, respectively.

For each chapter, whenever possible, real examples are given to illustrate the concepts and appropriate applications of statistical methods. Comparisons of relative merits and disadvantages of these statistical methods are also discussed. When applicable, topics for possible future research development are provided.

REFERENCES

Bradstreet TE, Clark RL. The statistical evaluation of reproductive toxicity studies. Presented at the 1987 Annual Meeting of the Biostatistics Section of Pharmaceutical manufacturer's Association, San Diego, California, 1987.

Chow SC, Liu JP. Design and Analysis of Bioavailability and Bioequivalence Studies. New York: Marcel Dekker, 1992.

Chow SC, Liu JP. Statistical Design and Analysis in Pharmaceutical Science. New York: Marcel Dekker, 1995.

Chow SC, Liu JP. Design and Analysis of Clinical Trials. New York: John Wiley & Sons, 1998.

Ciminera JL, Heyse JF, Tukey, JW. (1989). Techniques for the graphical analysis of possibly skewed measurements. Journal of Quality Technology, 21, 223–231.

Dunnet CW. New tables for multiple comparisons with a control. Biometrics 20: 482–491, 1964.

Gladen B. The use of the jackknife to estimate proportions from toxicological data in the presence of litter effects. 74:278–283, 1979.

Haseman JK, Hogan MD. Selection of the experimental unit in teratology studies. Teratology 12:165–172, 1976.

Heyse JF. Technical issues in the design and analysis of teratology/reproduction studies. Presented at the 1987 Annual Meeting of the Biostatistics Subsection of the Pharmaceutical Manufacturer's Association, San Diego, CA, 1987.

Heyse JF, Rom D. Adjusting for multiplicity of statistical tests in the analysis of carcinogenicity studies. Biometrical Journal 30:883–896, 1988.

International Agency for Research on Cancer (IARC). Long-term and short-term screening assays for carcinogens: a critical appraisal. IAR Monogr Suppl 2. Author, Lyon: World Health Organization, 1980.

Kupper L, Portier C, Hogan M, Yamamoto E. The impact of litter effects of dose–response modeling in teratology. Biometrics 42:85–98, 1986.

Morgenthien EA, Free SM, Tingey HB. An alternative method for analyzing qualitative data in teratology studies in rodents. Presented at the Annual Meetings of the American Statistical Association, San Francisco, CA, 1987.

Palmer AK. Statistical analysis and choice of sample units. Teratology 10:301–302, 1975.

Paul SR, Mantel N. More comprehensive analysis of litter depletion data: I. Model-free approach. Technical report, Department of Mathematics, Statistics, and Computer Science. Bethesda, MD: American University, 1987.

Pharmaceutical Manufacturers Association (PMA). Results of a questionnaire involving the design of and experience with carcinogenicity studies. Author, 1988.

Rai K, Van Ryzin J. A dose–response model for teratological experiments involving quantal responses. Biometrics 41:1–9, 1985.

Tukey JW, Ciminera JL, Heyse JF, Testing the statistical certainty of a response to increasing doses of a drug. Biometrics 41:295–301, 1985.

Weil CS, Selection of the valid number of sampling units and a consideration of their combination in toxicological studies involving reproduction, teratogenesis or carcinogenesis. Food Cosmet Toxicol 8:177–182, 1970.

Williams DA. A test for differences between treatment means when several dose levels are compared with a zero dose control. Biometrics 27:103–117, 1971.

Williams DA. The comparison of several dose levels with a zero dose control. Biometrics 28:519–531, 1972.

2

Experimental Design Principles for Animal Studies in Pharmaceutical Development

WALTER W. PIEGORSCH
University of South Carolina, Columbia, South Carolina

A. JOHN BAILER
Miami University, Oxford, Ohio

I. BASIC TERMINOLOGY IN STUDY DESIGN

Whether conducting a laboratory experiment, an observational study, or some other kind of pharmacological study, the scientist must recognize and accord proper consideration to issues of study design. Design is a critical step in the formulation of any pharmacological investigation, and many modern texts are available that describe in detail important forms, structures, and facets of proper experiment design. Our goal is not to replicate these readily available details; rather, we will introduce basic design terminology and discuss briefly some of the fundamental aspects of experiment design that arise in pharmacological studies. For a good introduction to experiment design, we refer the reader to Moore and McCabe (1). For technical discussions on design issues, see Hinkelmann and Kempthorne (2), Kuehl (3), or the classic text by Cochran and Cox (4). Articles targeted to pharmacological study design include Al-Banna et al. (5), Powers (6), or Ette et al. (7).

We begin with a review of basic design terminology. An *experiment* is a controlled application or introduction of some external stimulus (or an intervention of the stimulus) to a set of individual sampling units. The sampling units are the basic material of the design: individual animals or human subjects; containers of cellular, microbial, or genetic material; and such. We often distinguish a controlled experiment from an *observational study*; the latter is a directed examination — possibly retrospective — of the effects of some stimulus on a group of subjects, but does not share the element of control that we assume is intrinsic to a true experiment.

We will assume that the sampling units are derived from a larger, possibly infinite *population* of subjects. It is to this population that all statistical inferences are directed. This is an important characterization: proper identification of the study population is the first essential step in any scientific investigation. The investigator must ask: to or for whom do I wish to describe pharmacological effects and draw inferences?

Example 1. Chromosomal Damage.   Laboratory studies of potential chromosomal damage of a pharmaceutical agent often employ in vitro cellular cultures. The damage is identified after exposing the cells to the agent and examining their chromosomes for aberrations or other detrimental effects. A common material for such a study is Chinese hamster ovary cells (8,9). Technically, the population in such a study is that of all Chinese hamster ovary cells that can be cultured, and all inferences are directed solely to this population. If inferences are to be made to cells from a different species, or to cells in vivo or in another study condition, then the experiment must employ material from those different species, different conditions, and so on.

Attempting to make inferences about toxic in vivo chromosomal response based on data from in vitro cell cultures is a form of *extrapolation* from one study population to another. In general, simple extrapolation is a weak basis for scientific inquiry, and the current example illustrates this: few would expect the chromosomal response of hamsters cells in culture to predict accurately the complex in vivo response of cells and their chromosomes inside the hamster body or, for that matter, inside the human body. There are, however, strategies available for using experimental data from one population or species to make useful scientific inferences to a more complex population or species. These are methods for addressing species extrapolation commonly encountered in *quantitative risk assessment* (10).

A. Local Control

Virtually all experiments or observational studies direct attention to some introduction or intervention of external stimuli on a population's members. Typically, we refer to the particular stimulus of interest as the *treatment*.

The goal of a proper experimental design is to eliminate any external variables unrelated to the treatment that may systematically or deterministically affect the experimental outcome(s). Common sense provides guidance for many of the strategies used in eliminating external variables. Kuehl (3) refers to this elimination as an attempt to achieve *local control* to increase the sensitivity of an experiment and better detect systematic, treatment-related effects.

The basic principle underlying local control is that the experimental units should be as similar as possible before treatment intervention. For example, tests on species that are sampled from the same strain and at the same age (roughly), help provide assurance that the animals are from the same population, with similar metabolisms, and are physiologically similar (for similarly aged animals from the same strain may have similar physiological features: similar fat content, muscle mass, and such). One must also closely monitor the experimental conditions and specimen preparation. Proper local control requires that all experimental conditions must be as similar as possible, to avoid *confounding* the inferences by factors, such as temperature, humidity, or other external influences.

Another important aspect of local control is consistency in the data-recording process. That is, the process of measuring responses in the experimental units should be performed using the same chemical preparations, measurement devices, and background conditions. And, the investigators themselves must be careful not to bias measurements as they record them. This latter point may seem obvious and simple to attain; it is, in fact, overlooked in many pharmacological studies. For instance, suppose pathologists are recording the results from a study of tumor onset after laboratory animals are exposed to a carcinogen. The pathologists read tissue sections on slides from animals in each of the dose groups. Suppose an individual pathologist believes a priori that increased exposures to the carcinogen are likely to be related with increased tumorigenicity. Although perhaps reasonable, this belief should be established from the experimental data and not vice versa. Nonetheless, the pathologist may examine slides from animals exposed to higher doses of the carcinogen with greater attention than those from animals exposed to lower doses, and possibly report greater frequencies of cancer in the high-dose groups, wholly as a result of increased attention to those groups. This is not necessarily a conscious attempt to bias the observations, but it can still lead to serious biases in the recorded data and, hence, spurious statistical conclusions.

A simple remedy is available for the problem of investigator bias: *blinding* or *masking* the information on exposure or treatment levels during data recording. There are various possible levels of this blinding. In a *single-blind study*, the experimental unit does not know which treatment it receives. (This level of blinding is more relevant in human clinical trials than in, say, preclinical and drug development experiments.) In a *double-blind study*, the single-blind conditions are extended so that the investigator or data recorder does not know which subjects (slides, in the foregoing pathology example) came from which treatment group. The data are coded so that treatment information is not immediately obvious. Lastly, *triple-blind studies* extend double-blinding to the data analyst. That is, double-blind data are analyzed using the codes from the double-blind readings (or, even using new codes). The results are then decoded by an unbiased supervisor to yield appropriate inferences about the treatment. [Triple-blinding is not practical, however, if the treatment represents some quantitative variable, such as dose of a drug. If the quantitative features of the variable are to be employed in the statistical analysis (e.g., in regression modeling; 11), the analyst must be aware of this.] In essence, blinding attempts to shield the observation process from biases that may be introduced by human predispositions. Although blinding is more common in clinical trials research, its implementation is just as relevant in pharmacological studies.

B. Control Groups for Comparison

When external, systematic components known to influence the experimental subjects or material cannot be eliminated by local control efforts, they must be controlled by incorporation into the study design. For instance, when the experiment has a comparative nature, it often important to record or observe responses from a group of subjects that have received no treatment or intervention. We call this a concurrent *control group*. Any experiment intended to make inferences about a compound's effect on a population of interest should always include a concurrent control. This group serves as a basis or foundation from which to make descriptive and inferential comparisons.

Although not always possible to achieve, the goal in control group specification is for the corresponding treatment group(s) to differ in only one critical aspect from the control group: that being the exposure, treatment, intervention or other. Comparisons between the treatment group and the control group then represent as purely as possible the treatment's effect on the experimental material.

There are several different ways to construct a control group. The simplest is to leave a group of subjects completely untreated and unaffected: an *untreated control*. This is perhaps the most common form of control group in pharmacological studies. For example, in preclinical toxicity-screening studies various gradations of a drug constitute the "treatment" groups, whereas the comparison or control group corresponds to no-administered drug.

Three other forms of control groups are possible in pharmacological studies. In the first form, the control group may reflect a well-established standard. Comparisons made to a *standard control group* are common with biological organisms, for which use of an untreated group is not ethical, given the availability of an efficacious alternative. (This is common in biomedical studies of pharmaceutical preparations when a proved therapeutic compound is already commercially available.)

A second form of control group is a *positive control*, which provides a condition that is expected to elicit as strong a response as possible. Use of a positive control may seem counterintuitive, but it has an important consequence: it can identify whether a complex experimental system or device is operating properly. For instance, is a mass spectrometer measuring correct chemical responses of the experimental material, or does it require recalibration? The positive control group provides a performance check on the experimental mechanisms and components expected not to vary from study to study.

A third form of control group is used when comparisons are made among treated subjects handled in a consistent, systematic fashion (except for exposure to the actual stimulus or intervention). In this case, a control group may receive the same vehicle used to administer the treatment, or receive the same intervention without an active ingredient. We call this group the *sham control, placebo control*, or *vehicle control*, depending on the experimental context. Vehicle or sham controls are especially important when even the action of administering a chemical stimulus to the subject (without toxic exposure) may induce a response. The vehicle control group helps in this case to identify and adjust for such nonexposure-related effects.

Example 2. Control Groups in Laboratory Animal Experiments.
In laboratory experiments with animal subjects, chronic exposure regimens are employed to study the long-term exposure effects of chemicals on mammalian tissues (12,13). Different routes of exposure are applied for different chemicals, depending on the expected context of human ingestion or exposure to the compound. For exposures through feed, water, or inhalation, it is appropriate to employ an untreated control group. In some experiments, however, it is important to control precisely the amount of chemical the animal receives. Under these circumstances, the chemical is often delivered by esophageal gavage, in a corn oil suspension.

Consider specification of the control group in a laboratory study using gavage exposures. Here, an untreated control group differs from the treatment group not only in the presence or absence of the treatment, but also in the presence or absence of the corn oil medium. Such a comparison confounds the question of whether the corn oil, the chemical under study, or even the process of handling the animals for gavage is the source of any observed increase in carcinogenicity in the treatment group. Indeed, evidence has appeared that suggests corn oil may cause pseudocarcinogenic responses in certain animals (14). This does not invalidate the material for use, but it does require the investigator to carefully design the type of control group(s) used for comparison with the treatment group(s).

We say the corn oil gavage is the "vehicle" here: the vehicle control group animals receive the corn oil gavage without any added chemical. The base comparison group on which to gauge chemical effects is this concurrent vehicle control, because it represents animals exposed to the same systematic experimental conditions as those in the treatment group, sans the exposure. Any significant differences observed between the two groups are then attributable ostensibly to the chemical.

It is also possible to employ multiple control groups [e.g., an untreated and a vehicle control in an experimental study (15,16), or even in observational studies]. Rosenbaum (17) gives a greater discussion on the use of multiple control groups.

C. Treatments, Factors, and Levels

When there is no true treatment applied to the population under study, the term *treatment* is used in a generic sense to indicate the stimulus or exposure regimen. (For example, a treatment level in an observational study may simply correspond to a different population under study.) A more general term for any well-defined, designed source of explainable variability is to call the source an experimental *factor*. We say a factor is composed of individual *levels*. A factor for which levels differ only in a nominal fashion is called a *qualitative factor*, whereas a factor, the levels of which differ in quantitatively meaningful ways, is called a *quantitative factor* or, in some settings, a *covariate* or *explanatory variable*.

For our purposes, we assume almost exclusively that factor levels correspond exactly to the levels of scientific interest. The factors are then viewed as *fixed effects*. An alternative to fixed-effect factors, which we will discuss only in passing, views a factor's levels as a sample of all possible levels for that particular factor. This is called a *random effect* (18). For instance, in some pharmaceutical experiments it is common to view the individual animals as "random." This fixed-versus-random distinction must be made clear at the beginning of the study, for it can have great implications on the statistical analysis (e.g., when multiple measurements are made on each experimental unit, such as with serial sampling of serum levels drawn from the same animal).

In a simple, fixed-effects, exposure-versus-control experiment, the factor is the presence or absence of the exposure, and we say it has two levels: one level is the presence, and the other level is the absence of the exposure. In a multiple level experiment of some chemical stimulus, the factor is the particular stimulus, and the levels are the various quantified doses of that stimulus, including a zero-dose control.

Multifactor experiments can involve complicated designs in which the individual factors are *crossed*, so that each level of one factor is observed at all levels of the other factor(s). This produces a *factorial design*, and it is often of interest to study complex, multiple interactions between the various factors in such studies [see, e.g., the general discussions in Neter et al. (18) or Steinberg and Hunter (19)]. In factorial experiments, a treatment received by an individual experimental unit corresponds to a combination of levels of various factors.

D. Blocking

In many experimental and observational settings, it is known that a specific factor will affect the population in a specific, deterministic manner. There is no interest in studying the effects of this factor, but because it is a known source of variability in the experiment, it must be controlled. In this case, we call the known source of variability a *blocking factor*, or simply a *block*. When left unrecognized, a blocking factor contributes in a systematic fashion to experimental error in the observations. By recognizing and incorporating blocking factors into the design, we improve the efficiency and sensitivity of the experiment to detect true differences among the treatment effects (18,20). In essence, a design with blocking requires one to first divide the experimental units into homogeneous groups over the levels of the blocking factor. Treatments are then assigned randomly to experimental units within each block. In its simplest form, the design and analysis of an experiment that includes one or more blocks can proceed in a fashion roughly similar to that of any multifactor experiment, but very complex block designs are also possible (21). For a greater exposition on blocking factors, factorial designs, and other associated issues, see the texts by Cochran and Cox (4) or Hinkelmann and Kempthorne (2).

II. THE EXPERIMENTAL UNIT

We now introduce an important definition. For any study or experiment, the *experimental units* are the largest self-contained sampling units to which the external treatment or stimulus is applied. When experimental units are humans or other animals, these study units are frequently called *subjects*. (Notice that we have used these terms throughout the previous section.)

Statistical analyses are generally based on the information provided by the experimental unit, and it is the population from which these units are drawn to which inferences are directed. The identification of experimental units is related to the concept of deriving information from independently responding units. This distinction may seem obvious, but it often slips by unwary investigators. Here is a classic example arising in teratology.

Example 3. Litter Effects.   In laboratory studies of the effects of pharmaceutical agents, a common endpoint of interest is the damaging effect of the agent on developing conceptuses of an exposed parent. The induction of damage to the developing conceptus is called *teratogenesis*. When induced chemically, this is a form of *developmental toxicology* (22). In a typical teratogenesis study, pregnant female rodents (or *dams*) are administered the agent of interest during gestation. The animals are later sacrificed and examined to determine whether or not they exhibit toxicity-related effects on a conceptual endpoint of interest, such as

losses in uterine implantation, or increases in mortality or malformations. Although the toxin is administered to the adult animal, the primary variables of interest involve conceptual response. Thus, the question arises: What is the appropriate experimental unit on which to base
the statistical analysis?

The experimental unit is the largest sampling unit to which the
treatment is applied. For the developmental toxicity paradigm described
here, the pregnant dam is exposed to the toxin. Hence, the dam is seen
as the experimental unit. In this case, conceptuses sampled from an
individual dam represent multiple observations on a single experimental
unit, and it is likely that the per-conceptus responses will be correlated
(23). If, for example, the observations are simple dichotomous outcomes, say, whether each conceptus died or not in utero, the per-
conceptus responses represent *correlated binary data.* The associated
intralitter correlation — a form of *intralevel* or *intraclass correlation* —
adds excess variability to the per-conceptus observations; this is known
as a *litter effect.* The resulting increase in variability is a form of excess
variation, often called *overdispersion.* Failure to recognize overdispersion can cause undesirable behavior in many statistical procedures (24) —
for example, inflated false-positive error rates are common when over-
dispersed litter data are analyzed without taking the excess variation into
account.

In many experiments, the experimental unit is straightforward to
characterize and identify. As the litter effect example shows, however,
investigators must avoid cavalier specification of the experimental unit.
Here is another example:

Example 4. Salmonella *mutagenesis.* Consider again the laboratory determination of genotoxicity. Now, however, suppose interest concerns genetic damage in the form of DNA mutation. Study of toxicity-
related *mutagenesis* possesses numerous similarities to the study of
toxicity-related teratogenesis, as in Example 3, but also possesses some
inherent differences.

Perhaps the most common mutagenesis experiment involves the
Salmonella mutagenicity assay (25), employing the bacteria *S. typhimurium* to identify damage to DNA after exposure to chemical stimuli.
Bacterial or microbial systems such as the *Salmonella* assay combine ease
of use and lower costs (26) with shorter time scales for study; for example, bacteria reproduce rapidly, providing information on toxic response
over a period of days or weeks, rather than months or years for multicel-
lular animals.

The *Salmonella* assay proceeds by seeding a million or more bacteria on or into a microenvironment, such as a Petri plate. The bacteria are exposed to the toxin to study their mutagenic response. Here, again, specification of the experimental unit requires careful consideration: the largest sampling unit to which the treatment is applied is the Petri plate, *not* the individual bacterial cells. Hence, the plate is the experimental unit, and the observed mutant counts or mutant frequencies are taken at a per-plate level.

III. RANDOM SAMPLING AND RANDOMIZATION

Two essential ingredients of a properly conducted experiment are the use of a representative sample of experimental units from a particular population of interest and the careful allocation of these units to the various levels of the treatments or factors. The first ingredient requires consideration of simple random sampling, and the second ingredient requires consideration of the randomization of experimental units to treatment conditions. We explain both these features in this section.

Usually, it is impossible or prohibitive to observe responses from every member of a population under study, so instead we *sample* experimental units from the population. As suggested at the start of this chapter, the obtained sample should represent the study population of interest, and it is important not to overlook this fundamental feature of study design. In the worst case, haphazard sampling can introduce severe biases, limiting the scope of statistical inferences an experiment can provide. To avoid these sorts of systematic biases in the sampling process, one must sample the units randomly (i.e., collect a *random sample* of experimental units from an appropriate target population).

In its simplest form, we say a random sample is a sampling of experimental units from a larger population in which each unit has an equally likely chance of being selected. This is a *simple random sample.* Simple random sampling carries two important repercussions. First, knowledge of the probability of inclusion into a sample provides the foundation for inferences back to the population. Second, if members of a population are being selected totally at random with equal probability, then we expect each sampled unit not to affect or influence any other sampled unit's observed response to the treatment or intervention. This is a form of statistical *independence* among the observations. Details for selecting simple random samples, as well as more complicated sampling strategies, can be found in texts devoted to sample survey methods (e.g., Scheaffer et al.; 27).

In previous sections of this chapter, we discussed the imposition of local control techniques to avoid the influence of extraneous factors, blinding to avoid potential investigator bias, and blocking to control known sources of variability. Unfortunately, even with all of this care and effort, control of all possible extraneous factors often cannot be achieved. Simply put: Experimental units will differ. The mechanism we employ to balance out uncontrolled systematic effects in the experiment is called *randomization*, the random assignment of experimental units to treatment conditions. The concept is simple; before imposition of some treatment or intervention, the experimental units are allocated to different treatment levels so that each experimental unit has the same chance of being assigned to each treatment level. This process is appropriate for any designed experiment, such as a laboratory study of a compound's effect in some organism.

In general, to achieve a random sample one must assign experimental units to the different treatment levels (and, if a blocking factor is also considered, to the block levels) using a random device, such as a random number table. Random number tables are available in a variety of sources (1,28,29). From these one assigns labels or identifiers to each experimental unit, and uses these labels to assign each unit randomly to a treatment group. Greater detail on randomization is available in numerous sources (e.g., in Moore and McCabe; 1).

IV. SAMPLE SIZES AND OPTIMAL ANIMAL ALLOCATION

When designing pharmacological studies, it is a basic experimental precept that one pre-select whenever possible the number of experimental units to be allocated to the treatment groups, to minimize resource requirements. The use of multiple, independent experimental units in each treatment group is a form of *replication*, and the independent experimental units are called *replicates*. This is yet another critical principle in experiment design: by employing a large enough set of replicates in each treatment or study group and allocating them randomly to the treatment groups, any random differences that exist among the similarly treated experimental units in each group are, in effect, averaged out, increasing the statistical sensitivity to detect any systematic treatment effects.

The assignment of the same number of experimental units to each factor level is a special form of replication, called *equireplication*. Equireplication *balances* the experimental resource among all the treatment levels, and this balance can lead to simplifications in the statistical analysis. We often design studies to exhibit balance.

We call the total number of experimental units employed in the study the *sample size*. It is often desired to determine sample size requirements for the study before generating the random sample(s). Too small a sample size can lower the experiment's sensitivity to identify significant differences among the treatment groups, whereas too large a sample size wastes resources that may be applied in another study or for some other important pharmacological endpoint. Indeed, if the study involves exposure to a toxin, a secondary benefit of a priori sample size determination is the exposure of as few subjects or animals as possible to the potentially damaging effects of the toxin (30).

An additional concern in some pharmacological studies is the loss of experimental units because of external factors: *dropouts*. These are not uncommon in observational studies with human subjects or when data are taken in the field, but they can be controlled to some extent in laboratory experiments. Nonetheless, organisms can die before the end of a study, or Petri plates can be dropped inadvertently, and some consideration to account for dropouts may be necessary when selecting sample sizes. In addition, if the dropout is related mechanistically to the response (e.g., an animal dies from overt toxicity to a pharmacological agent before it can develop a cancer) then some adjustment is necessary in the statistical analysis.

The probability of detecting treatment differences when such differences exist may be used to quantify the sensitivity of a statistical test procedure. This probability is called the statistical *power* of a test procedure. Power is a function of the sample size: a properly constructed statistical test will increase in its power as sample sizes increase. By reversing this relation, one can ask what sample size specification is required to generate a preselected level of power.

Besides power, sample size is a function of the size of the treatment difference that we wish to detect. (The desired treatment difference is often expressed as a difference in mean response, relative to the anticipated standard deviation.) Not surprisingly, large differences between treatments are easier to detect than smaller differences. Hence, at a fixed level of power, the sample size decreases as the size of the desired detectable treatment effect increases. Sample size is also a function of the false positive (type I) error rate, α. (A false-positive error occurs when we conclude that a difference between treatment groups exists, when, in fact, it does not.) As α is lowered, the sample size required to detect a specified treatment effect increases.

Combining these three components—desired power, detectable treatment difference(s), and α—we can calculate an optimum sample size for the experiment. To simplify the calculation, we often employ statistical tables, graphs, and formulas that provide guidelines for sample size selection. For each different form of experimental response, underlying treatment effect, desired level of power, and so forth, a different sample size table or formula is required. For further details on sample size tables, a number of useful sources may be recommended, including Casagrande et al. (31), Haseman (32), Kastenbaum et al. (33,34), or Neter et al. (18).

Allocation schemes can also be constructed with the goal of estimating a parameter of pharmaceutical relevance. For example, the area under the concentration–time curve (AUC) is a critical endpoint for evaluating the bioavailability of a compound (35), or for the bioequivalence of different drugs or different formulations of a single drug (36,37). For AUC estimation, the dose allocation question is formulated as two (related) questions: Which sampling times should be considered? and, for destructive samples: How many experimental units should be measured at each time? One criterion is to allocate experimental units to minimize the mean squared error associated with the AUC estimator. For destructive sampling studies with specified sampling times, Piegorsch and Bailer (38) showed that an optimal allocation should be inversely related to the response variance at each sampling time. Notice that this calculation requires preliminary estimates or other information on the expected pattern and variation of response. Other optimality criteria are also possible (5,7).

V. DOSE SELECTION

An important, yet oft-overlooked aspect of an experiment's design is the selection and specification of the actual treatment levels. When the experiment concerns the dose-related effects of some quantifiable stimulus, such as a toxin, it is important to select the dose levels with control and forethought. Here is an important, motivating example from regulatory toxicology.

Example 5. Observed-Effect Levels. The identification of the lowest or least potent concentration of a chemical at which toxicity is observed is an important issue when setting regulatory exposure standards for toxins. The lowest concentration at which a toxic effect is observed is called the *lowest-observed-effect concentration* (LOEC), or *lowest-observed-effect level* (LOEL); the LOEL is sometimes called the *least effective dose* (LED). Generally, this involves comparing each treatment group (nonzero concentration condition) with the control group. The LOEC is the lowest concentration group that does not differ from the control group. Lying below the LOEL or LOEC may be the highest concentration at which no toxicity is observed: the *no-observed-effect concentration* (NOEC), or *no-observed-effect level* (NOEL). (A NOEC may not exist if the responses in the lowest tested concentration exceed the responses in the zero concentration group.) These quantities, NOEC and LOEC, are determined statistically by comparing each concentration with the zero-concentration control group (39). The issues of sample size and power discussed in the foregoing are important for the determination of a LOEC or NOEC: a design that allocates too few experimental units to the exposure levels may overestimate or even fail to identify the LOEC or NOEC.

Also, an important concern raised when calculating a NOEC or LOEC is that they must, by definition, correspond to actual levels of the quantitative factor under study. Thus, the spacing of test doses are intimately tied to these summary values and, ultimately, to the resulting exposure standards based on them. Dose selection must be performed carefully, and include both a dense enough grid of dose levels and adequate resources at each level, to estimate LOEC or NOEC, or both, with sufficient sensitivity. The difficulties and excessive resource requirements for achieving this sensitivity have led to concern that observed-effect levels are poor summary statistics for dose–response data (40–42).

A. Nonlinear Dose Response

When selecting doses in a toxicity study, it is important to recognize that the experimental units may exhibit a dose–response that is nonlinear [i.e., that deviates from a simple, easily interpreted straight line (43)]. For instance, a *threshold model* occurs when doses below a threshold point fail to elicit any substantive toxic response (a form of NOEC). It is critical to include dose levels above the threshold; if not, no data will be produced that illustrate the toxic effect and the statistical analysis will be pointless.

If threshold levels exist in a particular experimental setting, they are usually unknown. Hence, the dose selection must proceed with some preliminary information on the nature of the dose–response. Previous experiments, or data on chemical disposition and pharmacokinetic effects may prove useful here (44,45).

In other settings, the dose–response may be extremely nonlinear, and even inflect and change direction. Here is a short example.

Example 6. Beneficial Effects Preceding Toxicity. Nonlinear responses are observed in many different toxicological studies and can include swings or even downturns in the dose–response. The influences underlying these effects are not always detrimental: some chemicals may be beneficial at low concentrations, enhancing growth, survival, or reproduction of organisms exposed at these concentrations. As concentrations increase beyond the nutritive levels, however, toxic response may take over. An upward trend in the concentration response, followed by a toxic downturn pattern, results naturally from the organisms' physiological processing of the chemical. The effect is known as *hormesis* (46). Careful dose selection is required here to be sure to identify the points near or at which the response changes.

B. Maximum-Tolerated Doses in Chronic Exposure Studies

In practice, doses at which downturns, thresholds, or other nonlinear phenomena occur are not known in advance. To select experimental dose levels to include these important points, investigators must employ some prior information on the dose–response. This can include prior results on a similar chemical or exposure regimen, concurrent laboratory results with similar strains or species, or as is common with chronic, long-term exposure studies, use of preliminary subchronic studies to determine the appropriate dose range for the chronic study. From these various sources, one attempts to estimate the maximum dose at which the experimental units tolerate exposure to a toxic stimulus, express their maximal response before a downturn, pass a threshold event, or achieve some other critical milestone.

For example, in long-term, chronic exposure studies of laboratory animal carcinogenicity, dose selection centers around estimation of the *maximum tolerated dose* (MTD). This is the highest dose of the carcinogen that animals can accept that, when applied throughout the chronic exposure period, is not expected to shorten their longevity by any non-carcinogenic toxic effects (13,47). Unfortunately, the MTD may be difficult to estimate from subchronic or preliminary exposure data, owing to differences in the animals' responses between short-term and long-term exposures, in vivo metabolic changes in the carcinogen over longer periods, or cellular damage thresholds that are reached after extended exposures. Modern quantitative methods aid in this estimation process, and some works have appeared that employ various parameters from the subchronic data to estimate the MTD and explore its interrelation with carcinogenesis (48–50).

When estimating MTD for chronic exposure carcinogenesis studies in rodents, it is common to employ prechronic studies: for example, a 14-day repeated dose study and a 90-day subchronic exposure study (51). Large decreases (over 10%) in body weight gain or survivorship of animals at high doses usually suggest extreme toxicity, and the MTD is often taken as the lowest dose below which these extreme effects are observed. We should warn, however, that this is an oversimplification of the effort and attention required to estimate an MTD. Indeed, multidisciplinary coordination is required in MTD selection based on prechronic data; the required input includes pathology on the existence and nature of any preneoplastic lesions observed at high doses, pharmacology and biochemistry of any metabolic or molecular changes the chemical undergoes after exposure or ingestion, toxicology of any chemical-related effects seen in similar species or with other endpoints such as mutagenesis, and, statistics to guide analysis and interpretation of the prechronic data. Indeed, modern toxicological testing requires interaction among all appropriate disciplines to design a useful long-term study. Dose selection is an important consequence of this interaction (52).

Once estimated, the MTD is employed as the highest dose in the chronic exposure study. Lower doses are usually taken at fractional values of the MTD (e.g., at one-half and one-fourth the MTD). Coupled with a zero-dose control, this would achieve a four-level dosage regimen. This sort of four-dose design is common in long-term, carcinogenesis studies (53). Sample sizes for such a study often involve balanced designs, with typically 50 animals randomly allocated to each of the four dose levels.

C. Sequential Dosing

If possible, it may be useful to employ a *sequential approach* to dose application. In a sequential experiment, dose selection is a concurrent effort: as a dose level is selected, it is employed and response data at that level are recorded. The study stops when sufficient data have accumulated for analysis. Sequential designs possess many resource-conserving attributes, including potentially lower numbers of doses and lower sample sizes (54). Conversely, the designs are often more complex to undertake than a fixed-term design, especially in long-term chronic exposure experiments, and they can, in some settings, require even greater resources for start-up and laboratory preparation.

VI. SUMMARY

In this chapter, basic concepts were given for the conduct and design of experiments. Control of extraneous variables, inclusion of control groups, identification of experimental units, sampling of observations, randomization of experimental units to treatment conditions, determining appropriate sample sizes, and spacing of quantitative factor levels were some of the basic issues addressed. The motivation for considering these issues before conducting a study can be stated simply: No amount of sophisticated statistical analyses can salvage a poorly designed or poorly conducted experiment.

It is worth reiterating that experimental designs can take on more complicated forms than those considered here. The nature of treatments or other factors can be much more complicated than, say, fixed factors with a potential blocking variable. Common variations encountered in pharmacological studies include factors nested within other factors, during which unique levels of one factor occur within levels of another factor, or repeated measures experiments (55) in which each experimental unit is measured repeatedly or over time. Readers interested in these advanced topics are encouraged to explore sources devoted specifically to the design and analysis of experiments, such as Hinkelmann and Kempthorne (2), or Kuehl (3).

REFERENCES

1. Moore DS, McCabe GP. Introduction to the Practice of Statistics. New York: WH Freeman & Co, 1993.
2. Hinkelmann K, Kempthorne O. Design and Analysis of Experiments. New York: Wiley, 1994.
3. Kuehl RO. Statistical Principles of Research Design and Analysis. Belmont, CA: Duxbury Press, 1994.
4. Cochran WG, Cox GM. Experimental Designs. New York: Wiley, 1957.
5. Al-Banna MK, Kelman AW, Whiting B. Experimental design and efficient parameter estimation in population pharmacokinetics. J Pharmacokinet Biopharm 18:347–360, 1990.

6.   Powers JD. Statistical considerations in pharmacokinetic study design. Clin Pharmacokinet 24:380–387, 1993.

7.   Ette EI, Howie CA, Kelman AW, Whiting B. Experimental design and efficient parameter estimation in preclinical pharmacokinetic studies. Pharm Res 12:729–737, 1995.

8.   Galloway SM, Bloom AD, Resnick M, Margolin BH, Nakamura F, Archer P, Zeiger E. Development of a standardized protocol for in vitro cytogenetic testing with Chinese hamster ovary cells. Comparisons of results for 22 compounds in two laboratories. Environ Mutagen 7:1–51, 1985.

9.   Margolin BH, Resnick MA, Rimpo JY, Archer P, Galloway SM, Bloom AD, Zeiger E. Statistical analyses for in vitro cytogenetic assays using Chinese hamster ovary cells. Environ Mutagen 8:183–204, 1986.

10. Portier CJ. Quantitative risk assessment. In: Ragsdale NN, Menzer RE, eds. Carcinogenicity and Pesticides. Principles, Issues, and Relationships. Washington, DC: American Chemical Society, 1989, pp 164–174.

11. Sheiner LB. Analysis of pharmacokinetic data using parametric models — 1: regression models. J Pharmacokinet Biopharm 12:93–117, 1984.

12. Haseman JK. Statistical issues in the design, analysis and interpretation of animal carcinogenicity studies. Environ Health Perspect 58:385–392, 1984.

13. Robens JF, Piegorsch WW, Schueler RL. Methods of testing for carcinogenicity. In: Hayes AW, ed. Principles and Methods of Toxicology (2nd ed.). New York: Raven Press, 1989, pp 251–274.

14. Haseman JK, Huff JE, Rao GN, Arnold JE, Boorman GA, McConnell EE. Neoplasms observed in untreated and corn oil gavage control groups of F344/N rats and (C57BL/6N × C3H/HeN)F₁ mice. J Natl Cancer Inst 75:975–984, 1985.

15. Haseman JK, Winbush JS, O'Donnell MW Jr. Use of dual control groups to estimate false positive rates in laboratory animal carcinogenicity studies. Fundam Appl Toxicol 7:573–584, 1986.

16. Margolin BH. The use of multiple control groups in designed experiments. Stat Sci 2:308–310, 1987.

17. Rosenbaum PR. The role of a second control group in an observational study (with discussion). Stat Sci 2:292–316, 1987.

18. Neter J, Kutner MH, Nachtsheim CJ, Wasserman W. Applied Linear Statistical Models. Chicago: RD Irwin, 1996.

19. Steinberg DM, Hunter WG. Experimental design: review and comment. Technometrics 26:71–130, 1984.

20. Samuels ML, Casella G, McCabe GP. Evaluating the efficiency of blocking without assuming compound symmetry. J Stat Plann Inf 38:237–248, 1994.

21. Federer WT. Sampling, blocking, and model considerations for the r-row by c-column experiment design. Biom Z. 18:595–607, 1976.

22. Schwetz BA, Harris MW. Developmental toxicology: status of the field and

contribution of the National Toxicology Program. Environ Health Perspect 100:269–282, 1993.

23. Haseman JK, Hogan MD. Selection of the experimental unit in teratology studies. Teratology 12:165–172, 1975.

24. Haseman JK, Piegorsch WW. Statistical analysis of developmental toxicity data. In: Kimmel C, Buelke-Sam J, eds. Developmental Toxicology. New York: Raven Press, 1994, pp 349–361.

25. Ames BN, McCann J, Yamasaki E. Methods for detecting carcinogens and mutagens with the *Salmonella*/mammalian microsome mutagenicity test. Mutat Res 31:347–364, 1975.

26. Zeiger E, Risko KJ, Margolin BH. Strategies to reduce the cost of mutagenicity screening with the *Salmonella* assay. Environ Mutagen 7:901–911, 1985.

27. Scheaffer RL, Mendenhall W, Ott L. Elementary Survey Sampling (5th ed.). Belmont, CA: Wadsworth, 1996.

28. Snedecor GW, Cochran WG. Statistical Methods. Ames, IO: Iowa State University Press, 1980.

29. Iman RL. A Data-Based Approach to Statistics. Belmont, CA: Duxbury Press, 1994.

30. Muller KE, Benignus VA. Increasing scientific power with statistical power. Neurotoxicol Teratol 14:211–219, 1992.

31. Casagrande JT, Pike MC, Smith PG. An improved approximate formula for calculating sample sizes for comparing two binomial proportions. Biometrics 34:483–486, 1978.

32. Haseman JK. Exact sample sizes for use with the Fisher–Irwin test for 2 × 2 tables. Biometrics 34:106–109, 1978.

33. Kastenbaum MA, Hoel DG, Bowman KO. Sample size requirements: one-way analysis of variance. Biometrika 57:421–430, 1970.

34. Kastenbaum MA, Hoel DG, Bowman KO. Sample size requirements: randomized block designs. Biometrika 57:573–577, 1970.

35. Rescigno A, Marzo A. Area under the curve, bioavailability, and clearance (with discussion). J Pharmacokinet Biopharm 19:473–482, 1991.

36. Westlake WJ. Bioavailability and bioequivalence of pharmaceutical formulations. In: Peace K, ed. Biopharmaceutical Statistics for Drug Development. New York: Marcel Dekker, 1988, pp 329–352.

37. Liu J-P, Chow S-C. On the assessment of variability in bioavailability/bioequivalence studies. Commun Statist Theory Methods 21:2591–2607, 1992.

38. Piegorsch WW, Bailer AJ. Optimal allocations for estimating area under curves for studies employing destructive sampling. J Pharmacokinet Biopharm 17:493–507, 1989.

39. Yanagawa T, Kikuchi Y, Brown KG. Statistical issues on the no-observed-adverse-effect level in categorical response. Environ Health Perspect 102(suppl 1):95–104, 1994.

40. Leisenring W, Ryan L. Statistical properties of the NOAEL. Regul Toxicol Pharmacol 15:161–171, 1992.
41. Suter GW. Abuse of hypothesis testing statistics in ecological risk assessment. Hum Ecol Risk Assess 2:331–347, 1996.
42. Chapman PM, Caldwell RS, Chapman PF. A warning: NOECs are inappropriate for regulatory use. Environ Toxicol Chem 15:77–79, 1996.
43. Bourne DWA. Mathematical Modeling of Pharmacokinetic Data. Lancaster, PA: Technomic Publishing, 1995.
44. Reitz RH, Ramsey JC, Andersen ME, Gehring PJ. Integration of pharmacokinetics and pathological data in dose selection for chronic bioassays. In: Grice HC, Ciminera JL, eds. Carcinogenicity: The Design, Analysis, and Interpretation of Long-Term Animal Studies. New York: Springer-Verlag, 1988, pp 56–64.
45. Hashimoto Y, Sheiner LB. Designs for population pharmacokinetics: value of pharmacokinetic data and population analysis. J Pharmacokinet Biopharm 19:333–353, 1991.
46. Stebbing ARD. Hormesis—the stimulation of growth by low levels of inhibitors. Sci Total Environ 22:213–234, 1982.
47. Gart JJ, Chu KC, Tarone RE. Statistical issues in interpretation of chronic bioassay tests for carcinogenicity. J Natl Cancer Inst 62:957–974, 1979.
48. Gombar VK, Enslein K, Hart JB, Blake BW, Borgstedt, HH. Estimation of maximum tolerated dose for long-term bioassays from acute lethal dose and structure by QSAR. Risk Anal 11:509–517, 1991.
49. Rosenkranz HS, Klopman G. Structural relationships between mutagenicity, maximum tolerated dose, and carcinogenicity in rodents. Environ Mol Mutagen 21:193–206, 1993.
50. Haseman JK, Lockhart A. The relationship between use of the maximum tolerated dose and study sensitivity for detecting rodent carcinogenicity. Fundam Appl Toxicol 22:382–391, 1994.
51. Huff JE, Haseman JK, McConnell EE, Moore JA. The National Toxicology Program toxicology data evaluation techniques and long-term carcinogenesis studies. In: Lloyd, WE, ed. Safety Evaluation of Drugs and Chemicals. Washington, DC: Hemisphere Publishing, 1986, pp 411–446.
52. Halperin-Walega E, Yacobi A, Batra VK. Toxicokinetic study design and integrated programs. In: Welling PG, de la Iglesia FA, eds. Drug Toxicokinetics. New York: Marcel Dekker, 1993, pp 85–104.
53. Portier CP, Hoel DG. Optimal design of the chronic animal bioassay. J Toxicol Environ Health 12:1–19, 1983.
54. Bergman SW, Turnbull BW. Efficient sequential designs for destructive life testing with application to animal serial sacrifice experiments. Biometrika 70:305–314, 1983.
55. Davidian M, Giltinan DM. Nonlinear Models for Repeated Measurement Data. New York: Chapman & Hall, 1995.

3

Interval Estimation with Small Samples for Median Lethal Dose or Median Effective Dose

KEITH A. SOPER

Merck Research Laboratories, West Point, Pennsylvania

I. INTRODUCTION

For many years there has been increasing interest in reducing the number of animals required for biomedical experiments. This is particularly true for experiments that screen for acute toxicity of a compound. When potential human risk requires such studies, we wish to expose as few animals as possible. Similarly, in early human studies of a novel drug, we need to estimate an effective dose while exposing as few patients as possible. Acute toxicity studies in recent years routinely have such small sample sizes that all statistical methods in common use today either fail to provide a confidence interval or give confidence intervals that may not have the nominal coverage probability.

We describe a new small-sample method that uses no large-sample approximations and always yields a confidence interval. Moreover, we show the new method guarantees the nominal coverage probability, given assumptions that can be calculated from the study design.

Consider the common situation for which our response parameter is dichotomous: success or failure of treatment, survival or death, occurrence or not of some event. The parameter is observed in every subject soon after dosing, so that time to event is not of interest. For each subject, we assume there is a minimum dose sufficient to elicit the response, called the *tolerance* for that subject. The frequency distribution of tolerance doses in a population is called the *tolerance distribution*. Often we are interested in estimating the median of the tolerance distribution, because that dose has 50% chance of producing a response in a randomly selected subject. When the event of interest is death soon after dosing, this is called the LD_{50}: LD for lethal dose. When the event is response to a novel drug, this is called the ED_{50}: ED for effective dose.

If we could somehow measure for each subject the precise dose necessary to elicit the response, then the LD_{50} could be estimated by the sample median, but this is not the usual situation. Instead, we know only whether or not the event occurred at a single dose. For example, in an acute toxicity study we might have 5 dose groups with 5 animals per group, or 25 animals in all. Given the number of responders in each dose group, we require an estimate of the population LD_{50} along with a 95% confidence interval.

The international Office of Economic Cooperation and Development (OECD) guidelines for acute toxicity testing reflect efforts to reduce sample size and animal suffering. The OECD Guideline 401 (1981) calls for at least three dose groups with ten animals per group, five of each sex. A "limit test" consisting of a single-dose group with ten animals is deemed sufficient when a compound causes no mortality at a dose of 5000 mg/kg; it yields a lower bound, but no point estimate for the LD_{50}. Statistical analysis including a point estimate and 95% confidence interval is required except for the limit test.

In the fixed-dose method (OECD Guideline 420, adopted in 1992), doses expected to be lethal are avoided. A preliminary sighting study with one animal per dose is used to estimate a minimum lethal dose. Then in the main study ten animals (five male and five female) are given the same dose of compound, at a dose deemed just under the minimum lethal dose. The dose is fixed at either 5, 50, 500, or 2000 mg/kg. If any die, ten animals are tested at the next lower fixed dose, whereas if there is no evident toxicity ten animals are tested at the next higher fixed dose. In the usual circumstance that the data consist of ten animals at a single dose, there is no way to directly estimate an LD_{50}, but interpretation of results includes a presumed range for the LD_{50}. For example, if all survive at 50 mg/kg, but there is evident toxicity, then the LD_{50} is presumed to fall somewhere between 200 and 2000 mg/kg. Van den Heuvel et al. (1990) present a validation study for the method, and Whitehead and Curnow (1992) discuss the mathematical basis for it. We will not consider LD_{50} estimation for the fixed-dose method.

The acute toxic class method has been the subject of a validation study (Schlede et al., 1992), biometric evaluation (Diener et al., 1994), and is in draft form to become a new OECD guideline. This method uses death as principal endpoint, but seeks to minimize the number of animals tested and the number of deaths. Broad categories for the LD_{50} are selected, rather than point estimates with confidence intervals. In Diener's (1994) paper, fixed doses of 5, 25, 200, 2000, or 5000 mg/kg are used. Three animals of one sex are tested at one of the doses, then, depending on the number of deaths, the study may terminate, or another three animals are tested. The next three animals tested may be of the other sex at the same dose, of the same sex at the next lower dose, or of the same sex at the next higher dose. A total of 3–18 animals may be needed to complete the study. Diener calculates an expected total of 4.4–14.3 animals per study, with an expected 0.9–5.5 deaths, depending on the true LD_{50}, slope of the dose–response curve, and categories used for the LD_{50}. Schlede et al. (1992) report that classification of compounds by the acute toxic class method agreed with LD_{50} tests for 86% of compounds, whereas in 5% the acute toxic class was lower, and in 9% it was higher. If additional refinement is desired, an additional three to six animals may be tested at 5, 50, or 500 mg/kg. One of the purposes for additional testing may be to enable estimation of the LD_{50} by maximum likelihood. Many computer programs require two dose groups, with death rates higher than 0%, but less than 100% (Diener, 1994). We believe that additional animals should not be added merely to satisfy assumptions convenient for statistical analysis. Instead, statistical methods are described in this chapter that always provide an LD_{50} estimate and confidence interval.

For simplicity this chapter is restricted to fixed, not sequential, study designs. Because the foregoing guidelines tend to have fixed doses, we cannot assume that the doses in a study span the range from nearly 0 to nearly 100% response, or even that the LD_{50} lies within the dose range. Despite this limitation, our goal is to describe point and interval estimates for the LD_{50} (ED_{50}) that

1. Always yield a confidence interval
2. Guarantee nominal coverage probability, even with small samples
3. For large samples, yields results similar to conventional parametric methods

Section II describes assumptions and notation. Section III describes a common nonparametric method, and Section IV the method of maximum likelihood. An exact parametric confidence interval is described in Section V, but restrictive assumptions are required. In Section VI we show how to combine maximum likelihood and the exact interval to obtain a small-sample confidence interval for the LD_{50} without restrictive assumptions. Actual coverage probabilities for the alternative methods are compared in Section VII, with discussion and conclusions in Section VIII.

II. NOTATION AND ASSUMPTIONS

Let $J \geq 1$ denote the number of dose groups. Each animal in group j gets dose $d_j > 0$ of a compound, and we observe whether or not each animal exhibits a response. Order the doses $d_1 < \cdots < d_J$. In each group j we denote the number of animals by n_j and the number of "responders" by $r_j, j = 1, \ldots, J$. We restrict attention to "fixed" study designs, so each n_j is fixed in advance of the study with $n_j \geq 1$. Take r_j to be a realization of a random variable R_j, with independence among all R_j. Each R_j is taken to follow a binomial distribution with parameters n_j and unknown P_j. To simplify the presentation we will consider the response to be death, so the problem is to find an interval estimate for the LD_{50}.

It will be useful to have notation describing the range of doses at which deaths are observed, or not observed. Let X_{eL} be a random variable denoting the lowest dose ($\log_{10}$ scale) with a death, and let X_{eH} denote the highest dose with a death. The subscript e stands for the event of interest. So $R_j = 0$ whenever $x_j < X_{eL}$ or $x_j > X_{eH}$. Similarly, let X_{nL} be a random variable denoting the lowest dose ($\log_{10}$ scale) with any survivors, and let X_{nH} denote the highest dose with any survivors. The subscript n stands for a nonevent. So $R_j = n_j$ whenever $x_j < X_{nL}$ or $x_j > X_{nH}$.

In most experiments of this type we can safely assume that the probability of response is progressive with dose. For convenience we shall assume that the logit of P_j is linearly related to log dose, in other words

$$Y(x) = \log\left(\frac{P(x)}{1 - P(x)}\right) = \alpha + \beta x$$

for all $\qquad -\infty < x < \infty, \qquad$ where $\qquad x = \log_{10}(d) \qquad (1)$

Base 10 logarithms are used for dose to conform with common practice. This β is called the *slope* of the dose–response function. In the usual case $\beta > 0$, this model implicitly assumes zero probability of death in control animals with zero dose.

$P(x)$ is related to $Y(x)$ and x by

$$P = \frac{\exp(Y)}{1 + \exp(Y)} \qquad \text{and}$$

$$\log(1 - P(x)) = -\log[1 + \exp(\alpha + \beta x)] \qquad (2)$$

When $0 < |\beta| < \infty$, these $Y(x)$ and $P(x)$ are continuous and strictly monotone in x, with a unique value μ such that $Y(\mu) = 0$ and $P(\mu) = 0.5$. Converting back to the original scale, 10^μ is called the LD_{50}. From Eq. (1) we have

$$\mu = -\frac{\alpha}{\beta} \qquad \text{and} \qquad Y(x) = \beta(x - \mu)$$

provided $\qquad 0 < |\beta| < \infty \qquad (3)$

Describe the model with the triplet $\theta = (\alpha, \mu, \beta)$, with $-\infty \le \alpha \le \infty$, $-\infty \le \beta \le \infty$, and μ satisfying Eq. (3); μ is indeterminate when $\beta = 0$. Step functions ($\beta = \pm\infty$) are included because they arise later in maximum-likelihood estimation.

In practice, we usually know whether the dose–response curve is rising or falling. For simplicity we assume in the following that we know $0 < \beta < \infty$.

Various issues in LD_{50} estimation are illustrated in the 12 data sets of Table 1, with three to five dose groups and a total of 10–200 observations. Doses are taken to be equally spaced in a log scale for simplicity. Data sets a, c, and g are actual results from acute toxicity experiments. Data set b shows results from a study of flasks "spiked" with a compound to find the lower limit of detection of an assay. Data sets d, e, and f are taken from Williams (1986). Data set h is a modification of study g. Data sets i, j, k, and l are hypothetical results from a study with

TABLE 1 Example Data Sets. List Responders/
Total (r_j/n_j) by Dose Group

	Log dose				
Study	−2	−1	0	1	2
a	—	0/3	0/3	3/3	1/1
b	—	0/15	0/15	11/15	15/15
c	0/3	1/3	2/3	1/1	1/1
d	2/40	12/40	18/40	23/40	31/40
e	1/5	3/5	2/5	4/5	5/5
f	3/5	2/5	3/5	4/5	5/5
g	—	1/4	0/4	2/4	—
h	0/4	1/4	0/4	2/4	—
i	—	0/3	1/3	2/3	3/3
j	—	0/3	0/3	0/3	0/3
k	—	1/3	3/3	0/3	2/3
l	—	0/3	3/3	3/3	3/3

four dose groups equally spaced on a logarithmic scale, three animals per dose.

III. SPEARMAN–KÄRBER METHOD

This nonparametric method (Spearman, 1908; Kärber, 1931) is widely used because it is simple and makes no assumptions about the shape of the underlying dose–response curve. First, the underlying distribution of doses necessary to elicit a response is discretized to $(J + 1)$ points in the log scale, $x_j^* = (x_j + x_{j+1})/2$ for $j = 0, \ldots, J$. This requires selecting log dose values x_0 and x_{j+1} outside the observed dose range, with the assumption that the probability of response at or below x_0 is zero, whereas the probability of response at or above x_{J+1} is 1. If a randomly selected individual is given dose x_j, the probability of a response is P_j, with $P_0 = 0$ and $P_{J+1} = 1$. This means the discrete probability associated with x_j^* is $P_{j+1} - P_j$. The mean μ_{sk} of the discretized distribution is defined to be the parameter of interest, that is

$$\mu_{sk} = \sum_{j=0}^{J} (P_{j+1} - P_j)x_j^* = \sum_{j=0}^{J} \frac{(P_{j+1} - P_j)(x_j + x_{j+1})}{2}$$

Note that $\mu_{sk} \neq \mu$ in general, although symmetry of the logistic function suggests they will be similar. In simplest form, a natural estimate for μ_{sk} is obtained by substituting the estimates $\tilde{P}_j = r_j/n_j$ for the unknown P_j to obtain

$$\hat{\mu}_{sk} = \sum_{j=0}^{J} \frac{(\tilde{P}_{j+1} - \tilde{P}_j)(x_j + x_{j+1})}{2} \tag{4}$$

with estimated variance

$$\widehat{\text{var}}(\hat{\mu}_{sk}) = \sum_{j=1}^{J} \frac{(x_{j+1} - x_{j-1})^2 \tilde{P}_j(1 - \tilde{P}_j)}{4(n_j - 1)} \tag{5}$$

If $n_j = 1$ so that $\tilde{P}_j$ is either 0 or 1, then the jth term in the variance estimate is set to zero. Note that $(n_j - 1)$ appears in the denominator, rather than n_j so that the variance estimate is unbiased (except when $n_j = 1$). Finney (1978; p 395) pointed out this is important when sample sizes are small. If samples are large enough that $\hat{\mu}_{sk}$ follows nearly a gaussian distribution, then a 95% confidence interval for μ_{sk} is given by $\hat{\mu}_{sk} \pm 1.96[\widehat{var(\hat{\mu}_{sk})}]^{1/2}$. For additional discussion of this and related nonparametric methods, see Finney (1978; p 394–403).

Particularly with equally spaced doses one might pick $x_0 = 2x_1 - x_2$ and $x_{J+1} = 2x_J - x_{J+1}$. When $\tilde{P}_1 = 0$ and $\tilde{P}_J = 1$, the limiting values x_0 and x_{J+1} need not be explicitly stated because they drop out of the formulas.

This estimate is most easily interpretable when $\tilde{P}_1$ is near 0, the $\tilde{P}_j$ are monotonically increasing, and $\tilde{P}_J$ is near 1. It is common to require an upper bound on $\tilde{P}_1$ and lower bound on $\tilde{P}_J$ to apply the method, because we assume $P_0 = 0$ and $P_{J+1} = 1$. In this chapter we arbitrarily require $\tilde{P}_1 \leq 0.25$ and $\tilde{P}_J \geq 0.75$; otherwise, the method is said to fail (e.g., in data sets f, g, h, j, and k). It also is considered to have failed if $\widehat{var}(\hat{\mu}_{sk}) = 0$, since this implies a confidence interval of zero width (data sets a and l). Hamilton et al. (1977, 1978) describe ways to force monotonicity on the $\tilde{P}_j$, and redefine a truncated mean as the parameter to be estimated when data indicate either $P_1 \gg 0$ or $P_J \ll 1$. Their method will always yield a point estimate and confidence interval provided the observed data show adequate dose–response and bracket the LD_{50}. Similar to the Spearman–Kärber method, their method relies on large-sample theory, and coverage probability with small samples remains a topic for investigation.

Bross (1950) presents calculations to support his contention that the Spearman–Kärber method is more accurate in small samples compared with maximum likelihood, even when the logistic model is correct. He considers two study designs, each with four equally spaced dose groups. One study has two animals per dose, the other five animals per dose. Laboring in the days before computers, he considers only nine models θ for the first design and two models for the second design. Moreover, in the first design he evaluates only 30 of the 81 possible outcomes, and in the second design he evaluates only 300 of the 1296 possible outcomes. Cornfield and Mantel (1951) object strongly to Bross' conclusions, arguing that his conclusions arise in part from the data sets he chose to include or ignore. Given modern computers, we present in this chapter calculations similar to those in Bross' paper, but do complete enumeration of all possible outcomes and evaluate over 50,000 models (dose–response curves) θ. Our conclusions in the following differ from Bross', but are consistent with those of Cornfield and Mantel (1951).

There is reason to be concerned that Eq. (5) may be a poor estimate of the variance when $\tilde{P}_j = 0$ or 1, because the estimated variance is then zero. Data set b is an extreme example where the Spearman–Kärber method assigns a variance of zero to every dose group except log dose 1. Data set c shows another extreme situation for which the method necessarily assigns a zero variance to log doses 1 and 2 because there is only one observation per dose. Also, because the confidence interval is accepted only when $\tilde{P}_1$ is near 0 and $\tilde{P}_J$ is near 1, the effective conditioning implies the variance estimate is not unbiased. We shall see in Section VI that confidence intervals generated by this method can indeed be too narrow for small samples, in the sense that they fail to provide the nominal 95% coverage.

IV. MAXIMUM LIKELIHOOD

Because each random variable R_j follows a binomial distribution and these J variables are independent, the likelihood function is a product of binomial distributions, namely

$$\prod_{j=1}^{J} \binom{n_j}{r_j} (P_j)^{r_j} (1 - P_j)^{n_j - r_j}$$

The log likelihood function is proportional to

$$L = \sum_{j=1}^{J} r_j \log(P_j) + \sum_{j=1}^{J} (n_j - r_j) \log(1 - P_j)$$

$$= \sum_{j=1}^{J} r_j Y_j + \sum_{j=1}^{J} n_j \log(1 - P_j)$$

$$= \sum_{j=1}^{J} r_j (\alpha + \beta x_j) - \sum_{j=1}^{J} n_j \log[1 + \exp(\alpha + \beta x_j)]. \tag{6}$$

Let $+$ in a subscript denote summation; so, for example, $n_+ = \sum_{j=1}^{J} n_j$ is the total number of animals in the experiment. We will use extensively the two summary statistics

$$A = \sum_{j=1}^{J} R_j = R_+ \quad \text{and} \quad B(u) = \sum_{j=1}^{J} R_j(x_j - u)$$

When $\beta > 0$ is known, this A is sufficient for μ because the n_j are fixed. Similarly, when μ is known, this $B(\mu)$ is sufficient for β. For any u the pair of statistics $[A, B(u)]$ are jointly sufficient for θ. The observed values of these random variables will be denoted by a and $b(u)$.

Many computer programs for maximum likelihood estimation require that there are at least two dose groups with response rate greater than 0%, but less than 100%, a stringent condition when there are only a few animals per dose group. This is not in fact required for maximum likelihood estimation, or for using Fieller's theorem to generate a confidence region. Fieller's theorem can be applied as long as the estimated slope $\hat{\beta}_{ml}$ is nonzero and finite, and this can occur even when there is only one animal per dose group. We describe now minimal requirements for maximum likelihood estimates and for use of Fieller's theorem.

Suppose there are at least two dose groups. Existence and uniqueness of a maximum likelihood estimate for θ depends on overlap of the dose range for deaths $[x_{eL}, x_{eH}]$ and that for survivors $[x_{nL}, x_{nH}]$. Silvapulle (1981) showed that there is a unique maximum likelihood estimate with finite slope (β) when the overlap is an interval of nonzero width, or is a single point in the interior of one interval (e.g., $x_{eL} < x_{nL} = x_{nH} < x_{eH}$). If the overlap is a single point on the boundary of one interval [e.g., data set b], the maximum likelihood solution is unique, but is a step function (has infinite slope β). If the intervals are disjoint, the maximum likelihood estimate can be any step function such that the "step" occurs in the gap between the intervals. To establish uniqueness in this case we arbitrarily set the step at the midpoint of the gap. For example, in data set a, maximum likelihood gives $\hat{\beta}_{ml} = \infty$ and the step can be anywhere between 0 and 1, set $\hat{\mu}_{ml} = 0.5$. If there are no deaths (data set j), or no survivors, then the maximum likelihood estimate can be any step function with step on one side the dose range, but we do not attempt to fit a parametric model in this case.

So the method of maximum likelihood uniquely defines a point estimate $(\hat{\alpha}_{ml}, \hat{\beta}_{ml})$. When $\hat{\beta}_{ml} = \pm \infty$, the corresponding estimated covariance matrix consists of all zeros because the model is degenerate. In data set b, for example, $\hat{\mu}_{ml} = 1$ and the corresponding confidence interval $[1, 1]$ has width zero. In data set a the confidence interval is $[0, 1]$. Otherwise, the estimated covariance matrix is

$$
\begin{pmatrix} \hat{v}_a & \hat{v}_{ab} \\ \hat{v}_{ab} & \hat{v}_b \end{pmatrix} = \begin{pmatrix} -\dfrac{\partial^2 L}{\partial \alpha^2} & -\dfrac{\partial^2 L}{\partial \alpha \partial \beta} \\ -\dfrac{\partial^2 L}{\partial \alpha \partial \beta} & -\dfrac{\partial^2 L}{\partial \beta^2} \end{pmatrix}^{-1}
$$

where the partial derivatives are evaluated at $(\hat{\alpha}_{ml}, \hat{\beta}_{ml})$. See Finney (1971) for details.

Assuming $0 < |\hat{\beta}_{ml}| < \infty$, an asymptotic confidence region for μ can be constructed using Fieller's theorem (see Finney, 1978; pp 80–82). Take the large-sample approximation that the point estimates follow a joint normal distribution with unknown expectation (α, β) and known positive definite covariance matrix. Under the null hypothesis $H_0: \mu = \mu_0$, note that $(\hat{\alpha}_{ml} + \mu_0 \hat{\beta}_{ml})$ follows a normal distribution with mean zero and variance $(v_a + 2\mu_0 v_{ab} + \mu_0^2 v_b)$, so we accept the hypothesis whenever

$$
\frac{(\hat{\alpha}_{ml} + \mu_0 \hat{\beta}_{ml})^2}{(v_a + 2\mu_0 v_{ab} + \mu_0^2 v_b)} \leq z_{\text{crit}}^2
$$

where z_{crit} is a critical value for the standard normal distribution. Set $g = z_{\text{crit}}^2 v_b / \hat{\beta}_{ml}^2$, so $g < 1$ implies that $\hat{\beta}_{ml}$ is significantly different from 0 at this level of significance. When $g < 1$, Fieller's theorem provides an interval with both lower and upper bounds finite, whereas if $g > 1$ the confidence region will have neither a lower nor an upper bound. To be specific, if $g < 1$, the confidence region for μ is the interval

$$
\left[\hat{\mu}_{ml} + \frac{g v_{ab}}{v_b} \pm \frac{z_{\text{crit}}}{\hat{\beta}_{ml}} \left\{ v_a + 2\hat{\mu}_{ml} v_{ab} + \hat{\mu}_{ml}^2 v_b - g \left(v_a - \frac{v_{ab}^2}{v_b} \right) \right\}^{1/2} \right] / (1 - g) \tag{7}
$$

The limits in Eq. (7) are guaranteed to exist when $g < 1$. If $g > 1$ then the confidence region is the complement of the interval Eq. (7). When $g > 1$ the limits in Eq. (7) may not exist, and in that case Fieller's theorem gives the unbounded confidence interval $(-\infty, \infty)$. If $g = 1$ and $\hat{\mu}_{ml} \neq -v_{ab}/v_b$, then the confidence region consists of all μ such that

$$2\left(\hat{\mu}_{ml} + \frac{v_{ab}}{v_b}\right)\mu \geq \left(\hat{\mu}_{ml}^2 - \frac{v_a}{v_b}\right)$$

yielding a confidence region with one finite bound. Finally, if $g = 1$ and $\hat{\mu}_{ml} = -v_{ab}/v_b$, the confidence region is $(-\infty, \infty)$.

Given our assumption $\beta > 0$, we shall say the data do not support a bounded confidence interval when $\hat{\beta}_{ml} \leq 0$, and the Fieller's method fails to give a confidence interval. We shall also say the method fails when $\hat{\beta}_{ml} = \infty$. Fieller's method always yields a confidence region provided $0 < \hat{\beta}_{ml} < \infty$. The confidence region does not place any finite bound on μ, however, unless the slope estimate $\hat{\beta}_{ml}$ is statistically significantly greater than 0 (equivalently, when $g \leq 1$).

Williams (1986) proposed a confidence interval for μ based on an asymptotic likelihood ratio test rather than Fieller's theorem. The resulting confidence interval always exists, even when $\hat{\beta}_{ml} = \infty$ or $\hat{\beta}_{ml} \leq 0$. Moreover, Williams reports simulations showing his interval is virtually always shorter than the interval Eq. (7) for samples of 20–30 spread over four to six groups. Coverage probability in his simulations tended to be less than the nominal 95%, but rarely, below 93%. Failure to cover the true μ most often occurred when $\hat{\beta}_{ml} = \infty$. Williams suggested imposing an arbitrary upper bound $\hat{\beta}_{ml}(x_{j+1} - x_j) \leq 4$ to correct the problem. Our principal concern with Williams' method is that it relies on an asymptotic test procedure that may not be accurate with very small samples.

We turn now to a modified maximum likelihood procedure that does not use any large-sample approximations, and refer to it in this chapter as the *small-sample* method. To set the stage, point and interval estimates for three data sets appear in Table 2. Four statistical methods are compared: Spearman–Kärber, maximum likelihood with Fieller's theorem, Williams' method, and the small-sample method proposed in the following. The data sets and results for Williams' method are taken from Table 1 of Williams (1986). (In data set f, we obtained a different maximum likelihood point estimate for μ than did Williams 1986. We verified directly that our estimate had greater likelihood than could be obtained for any β with Williams' estimate for μ, and that the partial derivatives were zero at our estimate. Our results agreed with Williams for data set e.) All parametric methods including the small-sample method yield similar results for data set d, an experiment with 40 observations per group and doses that appear to well bracket the LD_{50}. They also

TABLE 2 Alternative Methods for Three Data Sets: Estimated μ
(95% Confidence Interval), Log Scale

Method	Data set d	Data set e	Data set f
Spearman–Kärber	0.35	−0.50	Failed
	[0.05, 0.65]	[−1.38, 0.38]	
Maximum likelihood	0.45	−0.61	−1.45
Fieller's theorem	[0.06, 0.89]	[−3.36, 0.75]	[−∞, 0.18] +
			[6.12, ∞]
Maximum likelihood	0.45	−0.61	−1.45
Williams' method	[0.06, 0.88]	[−2.63, 0.49]	[−∞, 0.01] +
			[24.8, ∞]
Proposed small-sample	0.45	−0.62	−1.47
method	[0.05, 0.85]	[−1.82, 0.53]	[−∞, 0.16]

agree well for data set e. The Spearman–Kärber interval is substantially narrower compared with maximum likelihood for data sets d and e, whereas the method fails for data set f because the bottom of the dose range has greater than 25% mortality. For data set f both Williams' method and Fieller's theorem yield two intervals for the confidence region, although the upper interval might be excluded as not plausible. The small-sample method yields a single interval similar to the lower interval for Fieller's theorem. In fact, our method is constructed so it always yields a single interval.

V. MOTIVATING CASE: KNOWN SLOPE

Consider temporarily the problem of constructing an exact 95% confidence interval when $0 < \beta < \infty$ is known. This simpler problem illustrates that β is the principal complication in our estimation problem, and yields insights we use to construct a small-sample confidence interval when β is unknown.

For this section the experiment can be as small as $J = 1$ group with $n_1 = 1$ observation. Equation (3) tells us that estimation of μ and α are equivalent for known $\beta > 0$, so we consider α. The log-likelihood function has derivative

$$\frac{\partial L}{\partial \alpha} = a - \sum_{j=1}^{J} n_j P_j = a - E[A] \tag{8}$$

The maximum likelihood estimate $\hat{\alpha}_{ml}$ satisfies $a = E[A]$, with $\hat{\alpha}_{ml} = -\infty$ when $a = 0$ and $\hat{\alpha}_{ml} = \infty$ when $a = n_+$. Since A is a complete sufficient statistic for α when β is fixed (Lehman, 1983; p 46), a confidence interval for α (or μ) can be based on A alone.

Fix any $\theta_0 = (\alpha_0, \mu_0, \beta)$. To test the null hypothesis $H_0:\theta = \theta_0$ against the two-sided alternative $H_1:\theta \neq \theta_0$ at the 0.05 level, we accept H_0 provided

$$Pr[A \leq a; \theta_0] > 0.025 \qquad \text{and} \qquad Pr[A \geq a; \theta_0] > 0.025.$$

Because A is discrete, this test has level *less than or equal to* 0.05. The set of all α_0 for which the null hypothesis is accepted defines a 95% confidence region. It is always an interval, say $[\tilde{\alpha}_L(\beta), \tilde{\alpha}_H(\beta)]$. We write it as a function of β to emphasize that the interval depends on the slope. The corresponding confidence interval for μ is

$$\tilde{\mu}_L(\beta) = \frac{-\tilde{\alpha}_H(\beta)}{\beta} \qquad \text{and} \qquad \tilde{\mu}_H(\beta) = \frac{-\tilde{\alpha}_L(\beta)}{\beta}. \tag{9}$$

We compute $\tilde{\alpha}_L(\beta)$ as the unique solution to the strictly increasing function

$$Pr[A \geq a; (\tilde{\alpha}_L(\beta), \tilde{\mu}_H(\beta), \beta)] = 0.025$$

$$\text{if } a \geq 1; \quad \text{or} \quad \tilde{\alpha}_L(\beta) = -\infty \quad \text{if } a = 0. \tag{10}$$

Similarly, $\tilde{\alpha}_H(\beta)$ is the unique solution to the strictly decreasing function

$$Pr[A \leq a; (\tilde{\alpha}_H(\beta), \tilde{\mu}_L(\beta), \beta)] = 0.025$$

$$\text{if } a \leq n_+ - 1; \text{ or } \tilde{\alpha}_H(\beta) = \infty \text{ if } a = n_+. \tag{11}$$

According to these equations the confidence interval does not include its endpoints, but we will always include finite endpoints in the confidence interval to acknowledge that calculations are done with finite precision, and for consistency with confidence intervals defined in the following.

The confidence interval makes no use of "large-sample" approximations. It always exists and, if the data include at least one death and one survivor, has finite width. Because the interval is based on a complete sufficient statistic, it uses all the information in the data. It bounds the risk of error on either side of the interval, guaranteeing $Pr[\mu < \tilde{\mu}_L(\beta)] \leq 0.025$ and $Pr[\mu > \tilde{\mu}_H(\beta)] \leq 0.025$. Depending on μ the actual coverage probability may be greater than 95% owing to the discreteness of A.

It is instructive to examine how the interval changes as a function of β. Figure 1 shows 95% interval estimates for μ given data set a. A horizontal line drawn from any $0.5 \le \beta \le 8$ intersects the curves at the corresponding 95% interval. For example, in the display, a line is drawn at $\beta = 4.22$, yielding the 95% confidence interval $[-0.21, 1.22]$ for μ. The steeper the slope of the dose–response curve, the more we know about μ from each observed rate r_j/n_j and the narrower the confidence interval becomes. In this example the confidence interval at any β_0 encloses the confidence interval for all $\beta > \beta_0$, as will usually be true when the data bracket the LD_{50}. If one were given a priori a lower bound $\beta_0 > 0$, then a conservative confidence interval can be defined using the method of this section with $\beta = \beta_0$. Unfortunately, a lower bound on β is not usually available.

Figure 1 suggests that a good small-sample LD_{50} interval might be obtained using the foregoing interval, substituting an estimated $\hat{\beta}$ for the unknown β. This idea is developed in the next section.

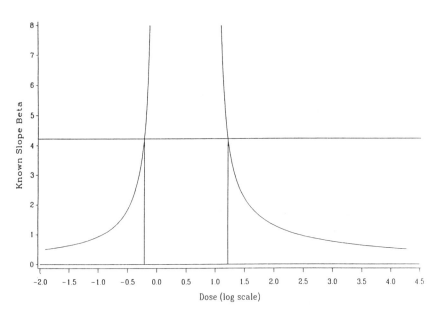

FIGURE 1   The 95% confidence intervals for μ (log LD_{50}) as a function of β, assumed known. Data example a.

VI. A METHOD FOR SMALL SAMPLES

We prefer a parametric confidence interval based on sufficient statistics, as best summarizing all information available from data. When data do not support parametric estimation, we resort to a nonparametric bound so our method always gives a confidence interval. Criteria for abandoning parametric estimation are given explicitly later. We dare not use large-sample approximations for acute toxicity designs in use today, and need the interval to be reliable even if μ falls outside the dose range. To summarize, our goal for this section is to define an estimate for μ with a confidence interval that

Always exists
Uses no large-sample approximations
Covers the true μ with 95% confidence, even if μ is outside the dose range
Is based on sufficient statistics

Several special cases are discussed in the following definitions. Although the idea of the method is simple, special cases are inevitable, given our goal to define an interval for all possible results from any study design.

Our strategy is to begin with the maximum likelihood estimate $\hat{\theta}_{ml} = (\hat{\alpha}_{ml}, \hat{\mu}_{ml}, \hat{\beta}_{ml})$. We then modify the estimates to avoid implausible estimates, such as $\hat{\beta}_{ml} = \infty$, and so that they are median unbiased in a certain sense, yielding say $\hat{\theta}^* = (\hat{\alpha}^*, \hat{\mu}^*, \hat{\beta}^*)$. The confidence interval from the previous section with $\beta = \hat{\beta}^*$ then defines the interval.

What if the data do not support use of a parametric model? We consider the data to be insufficient for parametric estimation if any of the following conditions are found:

1. There is only one dose group ($J = 1$).
2. There are no survivors ($r_+ = n_+$), or no deaths ($r_+ = 0$).
3. $\hat{\beta}_{ml} \leq 0$.
4. $\hat{\beta}^* \leq 0$.
5. $\hat{\mu} < x_1$, or $\hat{\mu}^* > x_J$.

In cases 1 and 2 there is no way to estimate a slope β for the dose-response curve (data set j). In cases 3 and 4 (data set k), the data do not support a point estimate for β because we are assuming the true $\beta > 0$. Case 5 (data set g) requires extrapolation that relies heavily on the assumed shape of the dose–response curve, an assumption untestable with small data sets. In any of these cases we abandon parametric modeling, but we still attempt to bound the LD_{50} with a nonparametric confidence interval as described later.

The first task is to define our point estimate $\hat{\theta}$. We start with the maximum likelihood estimate $\hat{\theta}_{ml}$. Because $\hat{\beta}_{ml}$ can be infinite, as for example, in data sets a and b, we take one step away from maximum likelihood by defining $\hat{\beta}*$ to be median unbiased in a certain sense with $\mu = \hat{\mu}_{ml}$ fixed. Let $b_{min}(\mu)$ and $b_{max}(\mu)$ be the minimum and maximum possible values for the statistic $B(\mu)$. To guarantee the estimate is unique and finite we define $\hat{\beta}*$ to be the solution to

$$Pr[B(\hat{\mu}_{ml}) \leq b(\hat{\mu}_{ml}); \theta_1] = Pr[B(\hat{\mu}_{ml}) \geq b(\hat{\mu}_{ml}); \theta_1]$$

$$\text{if } b_{min}(\hat{\mu}_{ml}) < b(\hat{\mu}_{ml}) < b_{max}(\hat{\mu}_{ml})$$

$$Pr[B(\hat{\mu}_{ml}) = b_{min}(\hat{\mu}_{ml}); \theta_1] = 0.5, \text{ if } b(\hat{\mu}_{ml}) = b_{min}(\hat{\mu}_{ml})$$

$$Pr[B(\hat{\mu}_{ml}) = b_{max}(\hat{\mu}_{ml}); \theta_1] = 0.5, \text{ if } b(\hat{\mu}_{ml}) = b_{max}(\hat{\mu}_{ml}) \qquad (11)$$

where θ_1 is defined by $\mu_1 = \hat{\mu}_{ml}$, $\beta_1 = \hat{\beta}*$, and $\alpha_1 = -\mu_1\beta_1$.

Next, to ensure that our point estimate always lies inside any confidence interval, we take a second step away from maximum likelihood and define $\hat{\mu}*$ to be median unbiased in a certain sense given β fixed at $\hat{\beta}*$. Specifically, $\hat{\mu}*$ is the unique solution to

$$Pr[A \leq a; \hat{\theta}*] = Pr[A \geq a; \hat{\theta}*], \text{ if } 1 \leq a \leq n_+ - 1$$

$$Pr[A = 0; \hat{\theta}*] = 0.5, \text{ if } a = 0$$

$$Pr[A = n_+; \hat{\theta}*] = 0.5, \text{ if } a = n_+ \qquad (12)$$

where $\hat{\theta}* = (\hat{\alpha}*, \hat{\mu}*, \hat{\beta}*)$. Here $\hat{\beta}*$ is fixed from Eq. (11) and $\hat{\alpha} = -\hat{\mu}*\hat{\beta}*$.

These two steps uniquely define the point estimate $\hat{\theta}*$. A preliminary confidence interval $[\hat{\mu}_L, \hat{\mu}_H]$ for μ is now constructed as defined in Section V with $\beta = \hat{\beta}*$ considered fixed. Mathematically, the confidence interval is "exact" when $\beta = \hat{\beta}*$ and the dose–response curve holds exactly. We note two special cases for which the confidence interval should be widened to reflect that neither assumption is exact. To avoid extrapolation, when the lower bound $\hat{\mu}_L$ is strictly greater any dose with a survivor ($\hat{\mu}_L^* > X_{nH}$), we decrease the lower bound to the top dose with a survivor. When the lower bound $\hat{\mu}_L$ is strictly less than the lowest dose x_1, we do not set any lower bound, since the data cannot refute with 95% confidence the hypothesis that every dose studied is above the LD_{50}. Setting a lower bound in this situation requires an accurate estimate of the dose–response slope β, an unsafe assumption given the small sample sizes available. In symbols, we define our final parametric lower bound to be

$$\hat{\mu}_L^* = \begin{cases} -\infty, & \text{if } \hat{\mu}_L < x_1 \\ \hat{\mu}_L, & \text{if } x_1 \leq \hat{\mu}_L \leq x_{nH} \\ x_{nH}, & \text{if } \hat{\mu}_L > x_{nH} \end{cases}$$

Recalling that x_{eL} is the lowest dose group with an event (death) and x_J is the top dose group, we define similar limits for the parametric upper bound:

$$\hat{\mu}_H^* = \begin{cases} x_{eL}, & \text{if } \hat{\mu}_H < x_{eL} \\ \hat{\mu}_H, & \text{if } x_{eL} \leq \hat{\mu}_H \leq x_J \\ \infty, & \text{if } \hat{\mu}_H > x_J \end{cases}$$

As an example of the first special case, suppose the results for data set b were 0/15, 0/15, 15/15, 15/15. The parametric 95% confidence interval with β fixed at $\hat{\beta}^*$ lies strictly inside the interval (0, 1) but we expand the limits to [0, 1]. With smaller sample sizes such as example a the parametric interval encloses [0, 1] so no change is needed.

Consider data set 1 as a second example. Even though there are no deaths at the bottom log dose of -1, the sample size is only 3 so we cannot say with confidence that μ is within the dose range even though $\hat{\mu}^* = -0.5$. Moreover, we do not know much about the slope of the dose–response curve given only these data. So the foregoing definitions result in $\hat{\mu}_L^* = -\infty$ to indicate that the data are not sufficient to place a lower bound on the LD_{50} at the desired level of confidence.

It remains to describe the nonparametric bound we use when the parametric model is abandoned for any of the five conditions listed earlier. The bound is designed only to determine whether the doses are well below or above the LD_{50}. This is enough because it is used only when the doses are so narrowly spaced that a dose–response cannot be established, when all doses appear to lie on one side of the LD_{50}, or for limit studies with a single dose group.

First pool the dose groups and compare $A = \sum_{j=1}^{J} R_j$ with a binomial random variable with parameters n_+ and $P = 0.5$. If $Pr[A \leq a] \leq 0.025$, then we reject $H_0:P = 0.5$ and bound μ below by the bottom dose x_1: our interval for μ is $[x_1, \infty)$. If $Pr[A \geq a] \leq 0.025$, then we reject $H_0:P = 0.5$ and bound μ above by the highest dose x_J: our interval for μ is $(-\infty, x_J]$. Otherwise the interval is $(-\infty, \infty)$. We interpret an unbounded confidence interval as warning that the data are insufficient to draw any conclusion about μ with 95% confidence.

Next, attempt to tighten the nonparametric bounds in a stepwise fashion, as long as two conditions are met. Suppose we have already accepted the lower bound $\mu \in [x_{j'}, \infty]$. Let $r' = \Sigma_{j>j'} r_j$ and $n' = \Sigma_{j>j'} n_j$ describe the average response above dose j'. To tighten the lower bound to the next higher dose, the first condition requires monotonicity above $x_{j'}$ in the sense that $r_{j'}/n_{j'} \le r'/n'$. The second condition is $Pr[R' \le r'] \le 0.025$ when R' is considered to follow a binomial distribution with parameters n' and $P = 0.5$. If both conditions are met, then we tighten the lower bound to $[x_{j'+1}, \infty]$. This procedure continues until we fail either condition. Note the stepwise nature of the procedure, the bound $[x_3, \infty]$ cannot be attempted until both $[x_1, \infty]$ and $[x_2, \infty]$ are shown to satisfy the conditions. Stepwise construction is necessary to protect the final coverage probability. The tightest possible lower bound is $[x_J, \infty]$. The procedure for establishing and tightening an upper bound for μ is similar.

For example, consider data set j with no deaths at any dose. These data do not provide information to estimate the slope of the dose–response curve, but we can use the nonparametric method to bound the LD_{50}. In step 1, we start with 0/12 deaths; since $Pr[R_+ \le 0] = 0.0002$ assuming a binomial distribution with $P = 0.5$, we accept the confidence interval $[-1, \infty)$. In step 2 the monotonicity bound is satisfied, so drop the bottom dose; with 0/9 deaths we have $Pr[R' \le 0] = 0.002$, so tighten the interval to $[0, \infty)$. In step 3, with 0/6 deaths we have $Pr[R'' \le 0] = 0.016$, so tighten the interval to $[1, \infty)$. In step 4 we have 0/3 deaths with probability of 0.125, so the process stops. The final confidence interval is $[1, \infty)$.

Table 3 shows estimated LD_{50} and 95% confidence intervals for each of the 12 example data sets in Table 1. The small sample method is designed to yield a confidence interval in all cases, whereas the Spearman–Kärber and Fieller methods fail for several data sets. Data set c is included as a real example for which conventional requirements for both Spearman–Kärber and Fieller's method are satisfied, but sample sizes are so small that use of large-sample approximations is suspect. For all these data sets, the small-sample confidence interval encloses the Spearman–Kärber interval if it exists. If the Fieller method yields a single interval, it nearly always encloses the small-sample interval. The Fieller method can yield a peculiar confidence region consisting of the union of two half-open intervals (data sets f and h), but this cannot happen with the small-

TABLE 3 Results for 12 Data Sets: Estimated/Slope $\hat{\beta}$, LD_{50} ($\hat{\mu}$) and 95% Confidence Interval for $\hat{\mu}$, Log Scale

Data set	Method	$\hat{\beta}$	$\hat{\mu}$	Confidence region for $\hat{\mu}$
a	Spearman–Kärber	—	0.50	Failed
	Fieller's method	∞	0.50	Failed
	Small-sample	4.22	0.50	[−0.21, 1.22]
b	Spearman–Kärber	—	0.77	[0.54, 1.00]
	Fieller's method	∞	1.00	Failed
	Small-sample	3.77	0.79	[0.49, 1.07]
c	Spearman–Kärber	—	−0.50	[−1.42, 0.42]
	Fieller's method	2.15	−0.47	[−∞, ∞]
	Small-sample	1.90	−0.47	[−1.48, 0.60]
d	Spearman–Kärber	—	0.35	[0.05, 0.65]
	Fieller's method	0.84	0.45	[0.06, 0.89]
	Small-sample	0.83	0.45	[0.05, 0.85]
e	Spearman–Kärber	—	−0.50	[−1.38, 0.38]
	Fieller's method	0.92	−0.61	[−3.36, 0.75]
	Small-sample	0.89	−0.62	[−1.82, 0.53]
f	Spearman–Kärber	—	—	Failed
	Fieller's method	0.61	−1.45	[−∞, 0.18] + [6.12, ∞]
	Small-sample	0.59	−1.47	[−∞, 0.16]
g	Spearman–Kärber	—	—	Failed
	Fieller's method	0.70	1.68	[−∞, ∞]
	Small-sample	—	—	[−∞, ∞]
h	Spearman–Kärber	—	—	Failed
	Fieller's method	0.98	1.36	[−∞, −1.50] + [−0.07, ∞]
	Small-sample	—	—	[−2.00, ∞]
i	Spearman–Kärber	—	0.50	[−0.42, 1.42]
	Fieller's method	2.30	0.50	[−∞, ∞]
	Small-sample	2.05	0.50	[−0.45, 1.45]
j	Spearman–Kärber	—	—	Failed
	Fieller's method	—	—	Failed
	Small-sample	—	—	[1.00, ∞]
k	Spearman–Kärber	—	—	Failed
	Fieller's method	—	—	Failed
	Small-sample	—	—	[−∞, ∞]
l	Spearman–Kärber	—	−0.50	Failed
	Fieller's method	∞	−0.50	Failed
	Small-sample	4.22	−0.50	[−∞, 0.21]

sample method. In data sets f and g the small-sample method gives a lower confidence limit of $-\infty$ to warn that all doses studied may be above the LD_{50}. Results in data set g are close enough that inclusion of one more low-dose group with zero deaths (data set h) is sufficient to bound the LD_{50} with 95% confidence by the small-sample method, although not by Fieller's method. Data set i satisfies the requirements for all three statistical methods, but Fieller's method gives an unbounded confidence interval. Data set j, with zero deaths, permits a lower bound, but not a point estimate for the LD_{50}. Data set k gives no information about the LD_{50} because the data were insufficient to demonstrate an increasing response with dose. For data set l a parametric model could be fit, but the parametric lower bound for the LD_{50} was below the lowest-dose group and so was extended to $-\infty$.

Now that we have seen how the proposed small-sample method handles a variety of data sets with small and large samples, we evaluate its small-sample behavior in comparison with Fieller's theorem and Spearman–Kärber's method.

VII. SMALL-SAMPLE COVERAGE

The small-sample method, similar to all methods discussed in this chapter, cannot guarantee 95% coverage for any study design and any dose-response curve $\theta = (\alpha, \mu, \beta)$ unless β is known. For the small-sample 95% confidence interval, we can show there exists a $\beta_0 < \infty$, such that the actual coverage probability is at least 0.95 for any $-\infty < \mu < \infty$ provided $\beta > \beta_0$. The value of β_0 depends on the study design and sample size (e.g., given four groups at equally spaced log doses and three animals per group, $\beta_0 = 1.1[x_j - x_{j-1}]$). A more practical question is to study the small sample behavior of alternative methods for a wide range of dose–response curves. In this section we compare the proposed small-sample method with maximum likelihood followed by Fieller's theorem, and with the Spearman–Kärber method.

Rather than study a wide variety of designs and a few choices for θ, we chose to fix a single-study design, three choices for sample size, and a wide range of θ. Our study design for this section is four dose groups (log doses -1, 0, 1, 2). Our sample sizes are 3 per group, 5 per group, or 10 per group, corresponding to a total of 12, 20, or 40 animals in the experiment. Sample sizes of 3 per group have been used in recent years for acute toxicity studies (e.g., in the acute toxic class protocol; Schlede et al., 1992). The earlier OECD Guideline 401 (1981) calls for five animals per group per sex, resulting in ten animals per group if sexes can be pooled.

We consider an interval defined for the Spearman–Kärber method only if the observed response rate at the bottom dose is 0.25 or less, and the rate at the top dose is 0.75 or greater; otherwise, the method is said to fail. Limits of this sort are routinely used for the Spearman–Kärber method because it assumes 0% risk of death below the bottom dose and 100% risk of death above the top dose. Similarly, the method fails if the estimated standard error is 0 because the confidence interval has width 0. For maximum likelihood followed by Fieller's theorem, the method is considered to have failed if the data set contains no survivors, no deaths, if $\hat{\beta}_{ml} \leq 0$, or $\hat{\beta}_{ml} = \infty$. Calculated coverage probabilities in this section are conditional on obtaining a valid confidence region, by which we mean the method yields a confidence region, and it has non-0 width. Conditional coverage probabilities are not provided in these displays when the probability of obtaining a valid confidence region drops below 0.0005. For the small-sample method, on the other hand, coverage probabilities are unconditional because the method is guaranteed to yield a confidence interval of width greater than 0.

Nominal coverage probability in all cases is 95%. Actual exact coverage probabilities and other statistics are computed by direct calculation. Direct calculation is feasible because the number of different possible outcomes is not huge (there are 256 outcomes when $n_j = 3$, 1,296 outcomes when $n_j = 5$, and 14,641 outcomes when $n_j = 10$). We carried out calculations for 56 choices of β from 0.005 to 25.0, and for all μ from -4.00 to 5.00 in steps of 0.01, a total of 50,456 dose–response curves θ.

We start by examining exact coverage probability (conditional on obtaining a valid confidence region) when the true unknown $\beta = 2.0$. Figures 2–4 show coverage probability for each method as a function of the true unknown μ given sample sizes of three, five, and ten per group, respectively. Coverage probability for each method follows a jagged curve, as is inevitable for small studies, because each possible confidence region has a discrete probability mass, so the curve "steps" up or down as μ crosses the boundary of a confidence region. Horizontal lines are plotted at the nominal 0.950 coverage level, at 0.975, and at the maximal level 1.000. Vertical lines show the dose range for the experiment.

In Fig. 2 the Fieller method is most conservative, with coverage probability of 0.996 or greater for any μ. This is because when $n_j = 3$ the Fieller method always yields a confidence region of infinite width,

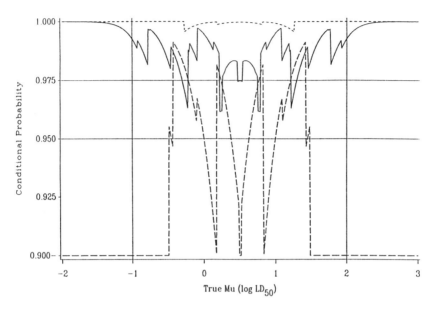

FIGURE 2 Exact coverage probability for μ (log LD$_{50}$) given 12 animals, 3 per dose group. True dose–response slope is $\beta = 2.0$; study with log doses -1, 0, 1, 2. (Line is dashed for Spearman–Kärber, solid for small-sample, dotted for Fieller.)

either the whole real line or a union of two intervals with one finite endpoint. The small-sample method has uniformly lower coverage probability compared with the Fieller method, but always greater than the nominal 0.95 level. Even if β were known exactly, the resulting exact confidence interval guarantees only at least 95% coverage owing to discreteness. Coverage probability for the Spearman–Kärber method is often lower than the nominal 0.95 level, even for values of μ well inside the dose range. Poor performance of the Spearman–Kärber interval arises in part because the interval is defined only when there is clear a dose-response from nearly 0% to nearly 100% mortality over the observed dose range. See Table 5 for a summary of the risk each method fails to yield a confidence interval when the true $\beta = 2$.

Figure 3, with five animals per group, has results similar to those for Fig. 2. The Fieller confidence regions are generally the most conservative, although not quite uniformly so compared with the small-sample method. The Spearman–Kärber intervals do not usually attain true 95%

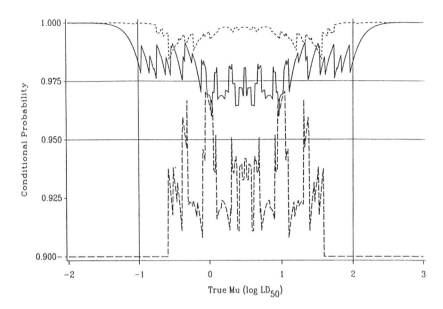

FIGURE 3 Exact coverage probability for μ (log LD_{50}) given 20 animals, 5 per dose group. True dose–response slope is $\beta = 2.0$; study with log doses -1, 0, 1, 2. (Line is dashed for Spearman–Kärber, solid for small sample, dotted for Fieller.)

coverage. The small-sample method guarantees 95% coverage probability when $\beta = 2$. In fact, coverage probability is at or above 97.5% when μ is not near the center of the dose range. This is because the confidence intervals are designed to have 2.5% risk of falling above (below) the true μ. When μ is near the bottom of the dose range there is no way for the confidence interval to lie entirely below μ, given samples of five animals per group, so the only risk is that the confidence interval lies above μ. See Table 6 for a summary of the risk each method fails to yield a confidence interval when the true $\beta = 2$.

Even with ten animals per group the Fieller method is conservative (Fig. 4). The small-sample method is less conservative than the Fieller method when μ is near the center of the dose range, but still has coverage probability at least equal to the nominal 0.950 level. The methods have similar coverage probability for μ in the outer thirds of the dose range, and the small-sample method is more conservative for μ outside the dose range. The Spearman–Kärber intervals never attain the nominal 0.95

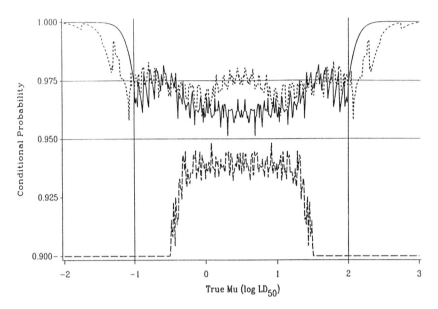

FIGURE 4 Exact coverage probability for μ (log LD_{50}) given 40 animals, 10 per dose group. True dose–response slope is $\beta = 2.0$; study with log doses -1, 0, 1, 2. (Line is dashed for Spearman–Kärber, solid for small-sample, dotted for Fieller.)

coverage probability, regardless of μ. See Table 7 for a summary of the risk each method fails to yield a confidence interval when the true $\beta = 2$. Even with ten animals per group, a substantial dose–response curve $\beta = 2$, and μ near the center the dose range there is nonneglible risk that the Fieller or Spearman–Kärber method will fail to yield a valid confidence region.

Space does not permit providing graphs of coverage probability for all 55 remaining values of β studied. To summarize our findings, we present results for the six values of β in Table 4. Because a value of β conveys little by itself, Table 4 also shows for each β the maximum possible rise in probability of a response between two adjacent dose groups. Tables 5–10 give summary information for these six values of β and sample sizes of three, five, or ten per group. Exact probabilities were calculated for all μ from -4.00 to 5.00 in steps of 0.01, but we summarize results by averaging over intervals of μ in these tables. The intervals for μ are the inner third of the dose range (0.00–1.00), the outer thirds of

TABLE 4   Maximum Possible Rise in
$P(x)$ for a Change of Δ_x in Log Dose, for
Various Slopes β

Dose effect $\beta(\Delta_x)$	Maximum Rise in $P(x)$
0.1	0.49–0.51
0.5	0.44–0.56
1.0	0.38–0.62
2.0	0.27–0.73
4.0	0.12–0.88
10.0	0.01–0.99

the dose range (-1.00 to -0.01 and 1.01–2.00), one dose step outside the dose range (-2.00 to -1.01 and 2.01–3.00), and values of μ "far out" of the dose range (-4.00 to -2.01 and 3.01 to 5.00). Results for values of μ still farther out than -4.00 or 5.00 are evident given the results for -2.01 to -4.00 or 3.01–5.00.

Tables 5–7 show the risk that each method will fail to yield a valid confidence region. When β is small and μ is near the center of the dose range, Spearman–Kärber or Fieller is likely to fail because the data are insufficient to establish a dose–response. In these cases the small-sample method yields the infinite interval ($-\infty$, ∞), indicating data were insufficient to make any statement about μ with 95% confidence. We feel this can be important information to provide the investigator. When β is large, Spearman–Kärber or Fieller are likely to fail because three or four dose groups have the extreme response of 0% or 100% deaths. This type of outcome is becoming increasingly common because many acute toxicity studies employ a wide dose-spacing. These tables show that the Spearman–Kärber and Fieller methods have a substantial risk of failing to yield a confidence interval unless doses are chosen so that $\beta(x_j - x_{j-1})$ is near 1 and sample sizes are at least five. The small-sample method by construction always yields a confidence region summarizing the information in the data.

We turn next to an examination of coverage probability for each of the three methods. Table 8 shows coverage probability averaged over selected ranges of μ, and Table 6 shows the minimum coverage probability for any μ in the range. In both displays coverage is conditional on obtaining a valid confidence region, and is omitted if the probability of obtaining a valid confidence region drops below 0.0005.

TABLE 5   Study with Three Animals per Group at Log Doses
$-1, 0, 1, 2$: Average Probability Each Method Fails to Provide
a Confidence Region for μ, the Log LD_{50}

True slope		μ Within dose range[b]		μ Outside dose range[c]	
$\beta(x_j - x_{j-1})$	Method[a]	Inner third	Outer thirds	Adjacent	Far out
0.1	SKB	0.977	0.978	0.978	0.980
	FLR	0.484	0.485	0.486	0.491
	SS	0.000	0.000	0.000	0.000
0.5	SKB	0.910	0.925	0.957	0.989
	FLR	0.241	0.265	0.341	0.537
	SS	0.000	0.000	0.000	0.000
1.0	SKB	0.739	0.842	0.968	0.999
	FLR	0.179	0.255	0.502	0.837
	SS	0.000	0.000	0.000	0.000
2.0	SKB	0.405	0.738	0.992	1.000
	FLR	0.481	0.559	0.844	0.987
	SS	0.000	0.000	0.000	0.000
4.0	SKB	0.370	0.716	0.999	1.000
	FLR	0.897	0.909	0.987	1.000
	SS	0.000	0.000	0.000	0.000
10.0	SKB	0.696	0.854	1.000	1.000
	FLR	1.000	1.000	1.000	1.000
	SS	0.000	0.000	0.000	0.000

[a]SKB, Spearman–Kärber; FLR, Fieller's theorem; SS, small-sample.
[b]Log dose 0.00–1.00 (inner third); -1.00 to -0.01 or 1.01–2.00 (outer thirds).
[c]Log dose -2.00 to -1.01 or 2.01–3.00 (adjacent); -4.00 to -2.01 or 3.01–5.00
(far out).

For the Spearman-Kärber method, average coverage probability in
Table 8 almost always falls below the nominal 95% level, the only exception occuring when the true μ falls in the inner third of the dose range
and the slope is quite steep $\beta \geq 4$. These conditions are necessary to
satisfy the assumption made by the method that the dose range encloses
nearly the entire span of mortality form 0% to 100%. It may be argued
that sample sizes of three are too small for the method, but even with
sample sizes of five (Table 9) or ten (Table 10), coverage probabilities
remain below the nominal 0.95 level unless μ falls near the center of the
dose range and β is large enough that a clear dose–response can be

TABLE 6 Study with Five Animals per Group at Log Doses $-1, 0, 1, 2$: Average Probability Each Method Fails to Provide a Confidence Region for μ, the Log LD_{50}

True slope $\beta(x_j - x_{j-1})$	Method[a]	μ Within dose range[b]		μ Outside dose range[c]	
		Inner third	Outer thirds	Adjacent	Far out
0.1	SKB	0.944	0.944	0.946	0.951
	FLR	0.439	0.440	0.440	0.442
	SS	0.000	0.000	0.000	0.000
0.5	SKB	0.768	0.813	0.899	0.976
	FLR	0.129	0.140	0.182	0.351
	SS	0.000	0.000	0.000	0.000
1.0	SKB	0.429	0.647	0.921	0.997
	FLR	0.036	0.071	0.281	0.737
	SS	0.000	0.000	0.000	0.000
2.0	SKB	0.086	0.458	0.960	1.000
	FLR	0.249	0.323	0.744	0.978
	SS	0.000	0.000	0.000	0.000
4.0	SKB	0.161	0.396	0.981	1.000
	FLR	0.799	0.817	0.978	1.000
	SS	0.000	0.000	0.000	0.000
10.0	SKB	0.579	0.679	0.993	1.000
	FLR	0.999	0.999	1.000	1.000
	SS	0.000	0.000	0.000	0.000

[a]SKB, Spearman–Kärber; FLR, Fieller's theorem; SS, small-sample.
[b]Log dose 0.00–1.00 (inner third); -1.00 to -0.01 or 1.01–2.00 (outer thirds).
[c]Log dose -2.00 to -1.01 or 2.01–3.00 (adjacent); -4.00 to -2.01 or 3.01–5.00 (far out).

established, but not so large that most dose groups have 0% or 100% mortality.

Confidence regions generated by Fieller's theorem, on the other hand, always have average coverage probability above the nominal 95% level, often far above 95% (see Tables 8–10). The principal drawback of Fieller's method is that risk of failure to yield a confidence region is substantial given the sample sizes considered in this chapter (see Tables 5–7).

The small-sample method has average coverage probabilities ranging from 0.948 to 1.000 for μ within the dose range and sample sizes of three, five, or ten per group (see Tables 8, 9, or 10, respectively).

TABLE 7 Study with Ten Animals per Group at Log Doses
−1, 0, 1, 2: Average Probability Each Method Fails to Provide a
Confidence Region for μ, the Log LD_{50}

True slope $\beta(x_j - x_{j-1})$	Method[a]	μ Within dose range[b] Inner third	Outer thirds	μ Outside dose range[c] Adjacent	Far out
0.1	SKB	0.993	0.993	0.993	0.994
	FLR	0.388	0.388	0.389	0.390
	SS	0.000	0.000	0.000	0.000
0.5	SKB	0.896	0.931	0.980	0.998
	FLR	0.046	0.052	0.070	0.150
	SS	0.000	0.000	0.000	0.000
1.0	SKB	0.507	0.789	0.986	1.000
	FLR	0.001	0.004	0.071	0.535
	SS	0.000	0.000	0.000	0.000
2.0	SKB	0.047	0.535	0.993	1.000
	FLR	0.048	0.086	0.559	0.955
	SS	0.000	0.000	0.000	0.000
4.0	SKB	0.031	0.314	0.997	1.000
	FLR	0.582	0.610	0.957	1.000
	SS	0.000	0.000	0.000	0.000
10.0	SKB	0.433	0.552	0.999	1.000
	FLR	0.997	0.997	1.000	1.000
	SS	0.000	0.000	0.000	0.000

[a]SKB, Spearman–Kärber; FLR, Fieller's theorem; SS, small-sample.
[b]Log dose 0.00–1.00 (inner third); −1.00 to −0.01 or 1.01–2.00 (outer thirds).
[c]Log dose −2.00 to −1.01 or 2.01–3.00 (adjacent); −4.00 to −2.01 or 3.01–5.00
(far out).

Nominal coverage probability is achieved on average for μ outside the dose range, provided the slope $\beta \geq 0.5$. This corresponds (see Table 4) to a maximum rise in mortality rate of only 0.44–0.56 between adjacent dose groups, a quite shallow dose–response curve for the widely spaced doses commonly used in acute toxicity studies.

VIII. DISCUSSION

The Spearman–Kärber method, as defined here, gives confidence intervals that have far less than the nominal 95% coverage probability; therefore, they should not be used with small sample sizes. Just as seriously,

TABLE 8   Study with Three Animals per Group at Log Doses −1, 0, 1, 2: Average Probability a Nominal 95% Region Covers μ, Conditional on Obtaining a Valid Region[d]

True slope $\beta(x_j - x_{j-1})$	Method[a]	μ Within dose range[b] Inner third	Outer thirds	μ Outside dose range[c] Adjacent	Far out
0.1	SKB	0.868	0.410	0.000	0.000
	FLR	0.990	0.999	1.000	1.000
	SS	0.991	0.957	0.914	0.937
0.5	SKB	0.890	0.519	0.000	0.000
	FLR	0.993	0.999	1.000	1.000
	SS	0.984	0.955	0.955	0.994
1.0	SKB	0.911	0.627	0.000	0.000
	FLR	0.996	0.999	1.000	1.000
	SS	0.979	0.968	0.986	1.000
2.0	SKB	0.943	0.733	0.000	—
	FLR	0.999	0.999	1.000	1.000
	SS	0.984	0.987	0.999	1.000
4.0	SKB	0.981	0.795	0.000	—
	FLR	1.000	1.000	1.000	—
	SS	0.995	0.997	1.000	1.000
10.0	SKB	0.999	0.819	—	—
	FLR	—	—	—	—
	SS	1.000	1.000	1.000	1.000

[a]SKB, Spearman–Kärber; FLR, Fieller's theorem; SS, small-sample.
[b]Log dose 0.00–1.00 (inner third); −1.00 to −0.01 or 1.01–2.00 (outer thirds).
[c]Log dose −2.00 to −1.01 or 2.01–3.00 (adjacent); −4.00 to −2.01 or 3.01–5.00 (far out).
[d]A confidence region is valid if it exists and has nonzero width.

the method requires estimation of the entire dose–response curve because the parameter μ_{sk} is a mean, not a median, so doses causing up to risk of 100% mortality must be administered to substantial numbers of animals. This alone makes the Spearman-Kärber method inappropriate for modern acute toxicity studies.

Sitter and Wu (1993) concluded that confidence intervals, based on Fieller's theorem, are generally superior to those based on an alternative asymptotic method. However, the smallest sample size considered in their simulation is ten animals per dose group. They remark (p 1024) that Fieller intervals do not have good coverage when the sample size is small

TABLE 9 Study with Five Animals per Group at Log Doses
−1, 0, 1, 2: Average Probability a Nominal 95% Region Covers μ,
Conditional on Obtaining a Valid Region[d]

True slope $\beta(x_j - x_{j-1})$	Method[a]	μ Within dose range[b] Inner third	Outer thirds	μ Outside dose range[c] Adjacent	Far out
0.1	SKB	0.917	0.372	0.000	0.000
	FLR	0.962	0.976	0.971	0.968
	SS	0.994	0.956	0.921	0.946
0.5	SKB	0.929	0.535	0.003	0.000
	FLR	0.969	0.983	0.986	0.989
	SS	0.983	0.952	0.958	0.996
1.0	SKB	0.934	0.723	0.018	0.000
	FLR	0.980	0.986	0.996	0.998
	SS	0.970	0.963	0.987	1.000
2.0	SKB	0.932	0.884	0.059	—
	FLR	0.997	0.995	1.000	1.000
	SS	0.971	0.983	0.998	1.000
4.0	SKB	0.956	0.957	0.086	—
	FLR	1.000	1.000	1.000	—
	SS	0.993	0.997	1.000	1.000
10.0	SKB	0.996	0.997	0.148	—
	FLR	1.000	1.000	—	—
	SS	0.999	0.999	1.000	1.000

[a]SKB, Spearman–Kärber; FLR, Fieller's theorem; SS, small-sample.
[b]Log dose 0.00–1.00 (inner third); −1.00 to −0.01 or 1.01–2.00 (outer thirds).
[c]Log dose −2.00 to −1.01 or 2.01–3.00 (adjacent); −4.00 to −2.01 or 3.01–5.00 (far out).
[d]A confidence region is valid if it exists and has nonzero width.

or the design is highly asymmetric. As found in this paper and noted also in Milliken (1982), Fieller intervals are conservative. Moreover, for the sample sizes and dose spacing commonly used in acute toxicity testing, a more serious problem frequently arises. The maximum likelihood estimate for the slope β can be infinite, for which the Fieller interval does not exist.

Williams (1986) and Aitkin (1986) independently suggested that confidence intervals for acute toxicity testing should be based on the profile likelihood function. Confidence intervals are guaranteed to exist.

TABLE 10 Study with 10 Animals per Group at Log Doses −1, 0, 1, 2: Average Probability a Nominal 95% Region Covers μ, Conditional on Obtaining a Valid Region[d]

True slope $\beta(x_j - x_{j-1})$	Method[a]	μ Within dose range[b]		μ Outside dose range[c]	
		Inner third	Outer thirds	Adjacent	Far out
0.1	SKB	0.875	0.148	0.000	0.000
	FLR	0.955	0.966	0.963	0.962
	SS	0.993	0.953	0.921	0.954
0.5	SKB	0.913	0.275	0.000	0.000
	FLR	0.956	0.968	0.974	0.980
	SS	0.978	0.948	0.964	0.998
1.0	SKB	0.938	0.494	0.000	—
	FLR	0.959	0.961	0.976	0.997
	SS	0.965	0.960	0.985	1.000
2.0	SKB	0.939	0.765	0.000	—
	FLR	0.973	0.973	0.990	1.000
	SS	0.962	0.970	0.998	1.000
4.0	SKB	0.931	0.852	0.000	—
	FLR	0.993	0.993	0.995	—
	SS	0.986	0.990	1.000	1.000
10.0	SKB	0.892	0.828	0.000	—
	FLR	0.994	0.995	—	—
	SS	0.999	1.000	1.000	1.000

[a]SKB: Spearman-Kärber; FLR: Fieller's theorem; SS: small-sample.
[b]Log dose 0.00–1.00 (inner third); −1.00 or −0.01 or 1.01–2.00 (outer thirds).
[c]Log dose −2.00 to −1.01 or 2.01–3.00 (adjacent); −4.00 to −2.01 or 3.01–5.00 (far out).
[d]A confidence region is valid if it exists and has nonzero width.

If $\tilde{\beta}(\mu)$ is the maximum likelihood estimate for β given fixed μ, then the profile log likelihood function is defined to be

$$L(\mu) = \sum_{j=1}^{J} r_j(\alpha + \tilde{\beta}(\mu)x_j) - \sum_{j=1}^{J} n_j \log\{1 + \exp[\alpha + \tilde{\beta}(\mu)x_j]\}$$

An asymptotic confidence interval for μ can be defined by accepting all μ such that $2[L(\hat{\mu}_{ml}) - L(\mu)] \leq c$, where c is the appropriate critical value for a χ^2 distribution with one degree of freedom. Williams (1986) did not feel his method is satisfactory when $\hat{\beta}_{ml} = \pm \infty$ is a strong possibility. He recommended placing an upper bound $\hat{\beta} \leq 4/(x_j - x_{j-1})$. His upper bound is based on the observation that investigators design their studies with doses spaced such that the true β can be expected to satisfy the bound. In this way "prior knowledge" of β is built into the test.

Grieve (1996) noted that the profile likelihood takes no account of the uncertainty in the estimated nuisance parameter β. He proposed Bayesian methods to solve the problem; see also Racine et al. (1986). Bayesian methods formally build prior knowledge into the statistical procedure.

Storer (1993) considered the problem of small-sample confidence intervals for μ, primarily for sequential designs used in phase I clinical trials. Just as in our paper, he started with a small-sample test for the null hypothesis $H_0{:}\mu = \mu_0$ with discrete distribution calculated exactly for given β. To handle uncertainty in the nuisance parameter β, he considered including μ_0 in the confidence interval if the test of $H_0{:}\mu = \mu_0$ was accepted *for any* $\beta > 0$. This yields a confidence interval that guarantees nominal coverage. Unfortunately, for the study designs used for acute toxicity testing today, this approach is too conservative, often resulting in the uninformative interval $(-\infty, \infty)$. Perhaps for this reason, as well as for computational simplicity, Storer (1993) proposed using the estimate $\tilde{\beta}(\mu_0)$ for β when testing $H_0{:}\mu = \mu_0$. By using a likelihood ratio test, Storer's (1993) method thus returns to the profile likelihood function, although he uses the exact discrete distribution rather than a χ^2 approximation.

Recent acute toxicity test designs claim to yield results comparable with those with classic LD_{50} designs, but with far fewer animals and deaths. For example, in one international validation study of the acute toxic class method, Schlede et al. (1995) report their method required an average sample size of 14.3 animals with 4.1 deaths, and yet yielded results quite comparable with more traditional LD_{50} experiments employing 20–30 animals and aiming for an overall death rate near 50%. The acute toxic class method uses only three or six animals per dose. We believe experiments with such small samples can succeed only because they rely, either implicitly or explicitly, on prior belief about the slope β of the dose–response curve. These designs yield information meaningful to the toxicologist, because he or she believes the doses are "widely spaced," in other words that $\beta(x_j - x_{j-1})$ is large. Fieller intervals are useless for the design studied in Section VII with three animals per group because whenever they exist they always have infinite width. The Fieller method fails because it requires the data to show $\beta > 0$ to a high level of confidence. We believe that useful confidence intervals for these very small designs must also in some way use the prior belief that doses are widely spaced, that $\beta(x_j - x_{j-1})$ is large.

Our small-sample confidence intervals are useful to the toxicologist in at least three ways. First, when they have finite width they help describe the variability in the information; second, when they are infinite they warn that the observed dose range was insufficient to place a bound on μ with the desired confidence; and third, the vague assumption that doses are widely spaced is made precise in the sense that nominal coverage is not guaranteed unless $\beta(x_j - x_{j-1})$ is above a threshold that can be calculated for any selected study design.

It is not immediately obvious how to build the assumption that doses are widely spaced into a statistical method, because most investigators, in our experience, are unwilling to place a precise lower bound on the dose–response slope β, let alone come up with a complete prior distribution. We resolve the dilemma by fixing β at our best estimate $\hat{\beta}^*$. Some of the uncertainty in our estimate is addressed by using a median unbiased criterion. This does more than ensure the estimate is finite. Because the confidence intervals for μ enclose all preceding intervals as β decreases toward zero (see Fig. 1), we can hope the confidence interval, based on a median unbiased criterion, will have about the right width to guarantee nominal coverage. We can verify our hope for any given β by direct calculation. In addition, we give explicit rules to limit our reliance on the point estimate $\hat{\beta}^*$, either by prohibiting extrapolation beyond the observed dose range or by dropping parametric modeling altogether.

Our small-sample method can be used with unequal numbers of animals per dose and unequal dose spacing. There can be any number of dose groups and any sample size including $n_j = 1$. It is, however, computationally intensive. This is not an impediment for small studies. By the time sample sizes are so large that a desktop computer takes more than a few minutes to complete the computations, we are quite willing to make the large-sample approximations inherent in Fieller's theorem or Williams' method. Our small-sample method is admittedly somewhat ad hoc in that we cannot offer mathematical arguments showing all our choices are "optimal." Mathematical optimality is seldom attainable, however, except with extremely restrictive mathematical assumptions or large-sample theory.

In very small studies our small-sample confidence method is likely to give $(-\infty, \infty)$. For example given two dose groups, with two animals per dose, our small-sample method gives an infinite 95% confidence interval regardless of the outcome. In such circumstances the only way to provide a finite confidence interval appears to be to use external information to place a lower bound β_0 on the slope, and then calculate a confidence interval at β_0 by the "exact" method of Section V. When the doses are spaced closely together, unbounded intervals $(-\infty, \infty)$ in the log scale contribute substantially to achieving the nominal coverage rate. Experiments should be designed to avoid this unhappy outcome, a quantitative statement that the data fail to provide any information about the LD_{50} at the desired level of confidence. Doses should be spaced far enough apart that the risk of a completely uninformative confidence interval is small.

The toxicology literature does not seem to have reached consensus on what constitutes wide spacing between doses. This depends on the slope β of the dose–response curve. Williams (1986) said studies should be designed such that $1 \leq \beta(x_j - x_{j-1}) \leq 2$. Diener (1994) in evaluating the acute toxic class method assumed that $2.1 \leq \beta(x_j - x_{j-1}) \leq 13.8$. The acute toxic class method uses eight- to tenfold steps between doses. For the small-sample design in this chapter using three animals per group, $\beta(x_j - x_{j-1}) \geq 1.1$ is sufficient to guarantee 95% coverage for any μ. Although the small-sample method may not guarantee 95% coverage for small β, it does guarantee 95% coverage, regardless of how large β may be. Given widely spaced doses it is common to observe no deaths up to one dose and 100% deaths at all higher doses, so it is practical to have a method that can handle such cases.

Investigators routinely use confidence intervals based on asymptotic theory, intervals that achieve only the nominal 95% confidence level on average, not for arbitrary μ. But if one chooses to calculate a lower bound $\beta_0(x_j - x_{j-1})$ to guarantee 95% coverage for any μ, what if the bound on β is unacceptably high? One can always lower the bound by sufficiently increasing the sample size, but there are at least four alternatives to using more animals.

1. Make the doses more widely spaced.
2. Use a sequential design that ensures the final data set will show a good dose–response.
3. Replace the median unbiased criterion for $\hat{\beta}^*$ with a more severe requirement, say the lower bound of a one-sided $100\rho\%$ confidence interval, with $\rho > 0.5$.
4. Tukey noted that if the jagged nature of the coverage probability function (Figs. 2–4) is smoothed out, then the desired cover-

age probability can more easily be obtained. Smoothing can be obtained by choosing a small random shift in the dose levels, before the experiment. The shift would be taken from a uniform distribution on $[-0.5\delta, 0.5\delta]$ where δ is the average distance between adjacent doses in a log scale. Coverage probabilities as a function of μ would then be averaged into a smooth curve. Because acute toxicity studies are performed before much is known about the shape or location of the dose–response curve, such a random shift is not a severe imposition on the study design.

We undertook this project largely because conventional statistical methods often fail to yield a confidence interval with small-sample sizes in common use today for acute toxicity studies. The size of an experiment should never be increased simply to satisfy the assumptions of conventional statistical methods designed during a time when large studies were routine. The small-sample method described in this chapter provides a method of generating a confidence interval that never fails to provide a confidence interval, that uses no large-sample approximations, and that maintains 95% coverage with small samples, provided the doses are not spaced closely together. It can provide a bound on μ even for limit studies with a single dose group. Consequently, it is well suited to acute toxicity testing as practiced today.

REFERENCES

Aitkin M. Statistical modelling: the likelihood approach. Statistician 35:102–113, 1986.

Bross I. Estimates of the LD_{50}, a critique. Biometrics 6:413–423, 1950.

Cornfield J, Mantel N. Some comments on "estimates of the LD_{50}: a critique." Biometrics 7:295–298, 1951.

Diener W, Siccha L, Mischke U, Kayser D, Schlede E. The biometric evaluation of the acute toxic-class method (oral). Arch Toxicol 68:599–610, 1994.

Finney DJ. Probit analysis, 3rd ed. London: Cambridge University Press, 1971, pp 52–57.

Finney DJ. Statistical method in biological assay, 3rd ed. New York: Macmillan Publishing, 1978, pp 80–82.

Grieve AP. On likelihood and Bayesian methods for interval estimation of the LD_{50}, In: Morgan BJT, ed, Statistics in Toxicology. Royal Statistical Society Lecture Note Series 3, Oxford: Clarendon Press, 1996, pp 87–100.

Hamilton MA, Russo RC, Thurston RV. Trimmed Spearman–Kärber method for estimating median lethal concentrations in toxicity bioassays. Environ Sci Technol 11:714–719, 1977.

Hamilton MA, Russo RC, Thurston RV. Correction to "trimmed Spearman-Kärber method for estimating median lethal concentrations in toxicity bioassays. Environ Sci Technol 12:417, 1978.

Karber G. Beitrag zur kollektiven Behandlung pharmakologischer Reihenversuche. Arch Exp Pathol Pharmakol 162:480–487, 1931.

Lehman EL. Theory of point estimation. New York: John Wiley & Sons, 1983, pp 46–47.

Milliken GA. On a confidence interval about a parameter estimated by a ratio of normal random variables. Commun Stat Theory Methods 11:1985–1995, 1982.

OECD. Guideline for testing of chemicals No. 401: acute oral toxicity. Paris: Office of Economic Cooperation and Development, 1981.

OECD. Guideline for testing of chemicals No. 420: acute oral toxicity – fixed dose method. Paris: Office of Economic Cooperation and Development, 1992.

Racine A, Grieve AP, Fluhler H, Smith AFM. Bayesian methods in practice: experiences in the pharmaceutical industry. Appl Stat 35:93–150, 1986.

Schlede E, Mischke U, Roll R, Kayser D. A national validation study of the acute-toxic-class method – an alternative to the LD_{50} test. Arch Toxicol 66: 455–470, 1992.

Schlede E, Mischke U, Diener W, Kayser D. The international validation study of the acute toxic class method (oral). Arch Toxicol 69:659–670, 1995.

Silvapulle MJ. On the existence of maximum likelihood estimators for the binomial response model. J R Stat Soc Ser B 43:310–313, 1981.

Sitter RR, Wu CFJ. On the accuracy of Fieller intervals for binary response data. J Am Stat Assoc 88:1021–1025, 1993.

Spearman C. The method of "right and wrong" cases ('constant stimuli') without Gauss's formulae. Br J Psychol 2:227–242, 1908.

Storer BE. Small-sample confidence sets for the MTD in a phase I clinical trial. Biometrics 49:1117–1125, 1993.

Van den Heuvel MJ, Clark DG, Fielder RJ, Koundakjian PP, Oliver GJA, Pelling D, Tomlison NJ, Walker AP. The international validation study of a fixed-dose procedure as an alternative to the classical LD_{50} test. Food Chem Toxicol 28:469–482, 1990.

Whitehead A, Curnow RN. Statistical evaluation of the fixed-dose procedure. Food Chem Toxicol 30:313–324, 1992.

Williams DA. Interval estimation of the median lethal dose. Biometrics 42:641–645, 1986.

4

Principles in Statistical Testing in Randomized Toxicological Studies

Ludwig A. Hothorn
University of Hannover, Hannover, Germany

Dieter Hauschke
Byk Gulden Pharmaceuticals, Konstanz, Germany

I. BRIEF DESCRIPTION OF PURPOSE AND DESIGN OF RANDOMIZED TOXICOLOGICAL STUDIES

The purpose of randomized toxicological studies is the safety assessment of a new drug or a chemical substance under investigation. According to the guidelines, several types of studies in the so-called regulatory toxicology can be distinguished: repeated toxicity, mutagenicity, reprotoxicity, and carcinogenicity studies. The objective of these studies is to determine global toxic, mutagenic, teratogenic, and carcinogenic effects. In vivo (e.g., long-term carcinogenicity studies on rats) as well as in vitro (e.g., Ames assay using a special strain of *Salmonella typhimurium* bacteria) studies are used. In animal studies the duration varies from 1 week to 2 years. The route of administration (e.g., per os) depends on the type of intended clinical administration. Normally, two species, selected from rodents and nonrodents, are used and toxicological studies are performed as a battery of tests (e.g., Ames assay, 4-week study on rats, reprotoxicological study, 6-month study on dogs, and a carcinogenicity study on rats). From a statistical perspective, each study is analyzed independently. Decision making based on all studies together is very important, but adequate biostatistical methods are still missing.

All these studies rest on the following many-to-one design: C^-, D_1, . . . , D_k, with D_i denoting different doses. Extensions of this design are the two-way layout, including the factor sex; the two-way layout, including the factor time (repeated measures of selected endpoints, e.g., body mass); and the hierarchical design (e.g., for pregnant females in repro-toxicological studies [dose* pregnant female > litter > sex; where * denotes cross-classification and > hierarchical classification, respectively]. However, the statistical analysis is carried out only for the one-way layout; and lower bounds for the required sample sizes are recommended by the corresponding guidelines.

II. PRINCIPLES AND CLASSIFICATION CRITERIA

With the exception of acute toxicity studies, the many-to-one design *treatments versus negative control* (i.e., $k + 1$ experimental groups) is applied in all toxicological studies. From a statistical point of view, the following types can be distinguished:

1. Dose–response design: C^-, D_1, . . . , $\mathbf{D}_k$, with D_i denoting different doses; $C^- = 0 < D_1 < \ldots < D_k$ (k not to large, i.e.; $\in$ [2, 3, or 4]).
2. Unrestricted design: C^-, $\mathbf{T}_1$, . . . , $\mathbf{T}_k$, with T_i denoting different treatments (e.g., different substances, application forms, or combinations of substances).
3. Extended design including a positive control: C^-, $\mathbf{D}_1$, . . . , $\mathbf{D}_k$, C^+.
4. Complex design: C^-, $\mathbf{C}^0$, substance A $(\mathbf{D}_1, \ldots, \mathbf{D}_k)$, substance B $(\mathbf{D}_1, \ldots, \mathbf{D}_k)$, C^+.

where C^- denotes the negative control administrated with the vehicle, $\mathbf{C}^0$ the empty control, and C^+ the positive control, using a known toxic substance.

The formulation of the hypotheses and the corresponding statistical analyses will be presented in detail for the first two designs, and the other two designs will be discussed only briefly. Usually, these one-way designs are included in a factorial layout with factors, such as sex and time. Assuming in advance an interaction between and within these factors, an independent analysis is performed separately for a dose effect by sex and time. Therefore, only methods for the one-way design are described here. Some of the designs are univariate, with only one endpoint (e.g., number of revertants in the Ames assay). However, the major part of the studies are multivariate with numerous endpoints (e.g., different tumor sites in a carcinogenicity study). The univariate approach will be discussed predominantly and some remarks are given for the multivariate situation.

This chapter describes primarily parametric and nonparametric methods and corresponding methods for dichotomous endpoints. Mortality-adjusted comparisons of tumor rates, per-litter–defined tests (overdispersed binomial data), and special dose–response problems for mutagenicity data are only briefly mentioned. For details, see Chapters 8, 10, and 12.

The question of whether the analysis of toxicological studies is of confirmatory or exploratory nature is not simple to answer. From the point of decision making, confirmatory testing should dominate. However, in toxicological practice the sample sizes are defined by guidelines and not designed for a specific experimental question. Furthermore, owing to the large number of multiple endpoints, a mixture of both strategies seems to be reasonable, as proposed in a recent recommendation for design and analysis of repeated toxicity studies (Hothorn et al., 1997). Nevertheless, this chapter is directed at only the confirmatory analysis.

A. Test on Difference Versus Test on Equivalence

In Chapter 6, the principle of adequate hypotheses formulation is addressed in detail for safety studies. The basic idea is that, in these studies, the primarily consumer risk should be controlled. Consequently, instead of applying procedures for testing differences while controlling only the producer risk, equivalence procedures should be used according to Hauschke (1995, 1997) and Neuhäuser and Hothorn (1995, 1997a). However, until now only conventional procedures for testing differences represent the state of art for numerous scenarios in multiple testing. Moreover, in toxicological studies serious problems may consist in the a priori definition of a tolerance level δ, essentially in studies with multiple endpoints (e.g., repeated toxicity and carcinogenicity studies). Some of these studies represent screening studies without a decision in the sense of balancing false-negative and false-positive error rates. Gad and Weil (1986) described this scenario as: "Most toxicity studies . . . are of a shot gun nature. They are designed to detect and identify any and all effect." Therefore, the following methods are based on traditional hypotheses for differences. However, the discussion of these methods is focused on the problem of achieving maximum power, which is equivalent to minimizing the false-negative error rate (i.e., the consumer risk).

B. Global Test Versus Multiple Comparison Procedure

The difference between a global test and a multiple comparison procedure (MCP) consists of the single versus multiple decision for the $(k + 1)$-sample problem. Global tests can be performed by tests on homogeneity (i.e., F-test of ANOVA [or by the Kruskal–Wallis, 1952 test, the nonparametric analogon]) with the decision that the treatment effects are homogeneous or not. The application of homogeneity tests might not be of relevance in all toxicological studies, although they can be used as pretests (see Sec. II). Another type of a global test is the trend test with the decision that the treatment effects are ordered in a monotonic fashion (see Sec. II.K). The decision against the null hypothesis is global in the sense that there is no information that groups are heterogeneous or from which dose there is a monotonic increase in the effects. (Trend tests and MCPs are defined here in a one-sided sense. From a statistical point of view a two-sided version is possible.) It is obvious that in many cases this information is not sufficient because the primary question is which dose groups are different from the control. On the other hand, the failure to reject the global null hypothesis is a probable outcome in toxicological studies. Therefore, a global test is frequently the starting point in multiple decision procedures (see Sec. II).

For some assays, the global decision (e.g., heterogeneity or trend) is sufficient (e.g., for the Ames mutagenicity assay). Only the decision of positive (effect) or negative (no effect) is needed because the dose levels are arbitrary and, therefore, no further test for determining the no-observed-adverse-effect level (NOAEL; for definition, see Chap. 6) will be performed. A bridge between global test and MCP is the closure principle according to Marcus et al. (1976). Based on any specific test — also based on a global test — multiple decision procedures can be constructed (for details, see Sec. IV.A).

C. MCPs: Many-to-One Comparisons, All-Pair Comparisons or Any-Pair Comparisons or A Priori-Ordered Comparisons

In the $(k + 1)$-sample situation the following types of comparison procedures can be distinguished:

1. Many-to-one comparisons: comparisons with C^- only
2. All-pair comparisons: comparisons with each other
3. Any-pair comparisons: predefined comparisons
4. A priori-ordered comparisons: comparisons based on an a priori-defined order of importance
5. All-or-none comparisons: comparisons based on the intersection union test

The choice among these procedures depends on the design, the restriction of the alternative, the experimental question, and the objective to reduce type II error. The usual way for analyzing a design including C^- is done by a many-to-one MCP; this represents the typical situation in toxicological studies. In some special cases, the comparisons between all treatment groups (all-pair comparisons) or predefined selected ones (any-pair comparisons; e.g., comparisons of C^- versus C^0 and C^- versus all-dose groups, but not the comparisons of C^0 versus the dose groups in the complex design; see foregoing) might be of importance and this should be clearly pointed out in advance. This choice is not a statistical problem and depends on only the toxicological questions to be answered by the study. Many-to-one MCPs are described in detail in Section IV. Several versions of all-pair MCPs exist; the most popular one is Tukey's studentized range test (1953; available in SAS GLM or PROBMC; Anonymous, 1995). Any-pair comparisons can be constructed by α-adjustment methods when the number of the relevant comparisons can be specified in advance. A priori-ordered comparisons can be illustrated by the extended design, including a positive control $\{C^- D_1, \ldots, D_k, C^+\}$. According to Hothorn (1995), the hypotheses are ordered starting with the test on sensitivity by the comparison C^- versus C^+ followed by tests on substance effects C^- versus D_i. All tests can be performed at level α, but if the hypothesis on sensitivity is not rejected, the procedures stops and no further test on substance effect is allowed. A detailed description of a priori-ordered procedures, including multiple treatments, or multiple endpoints, multiple time points, is given in Vollmar (1995). An extreme form of multiple comparison is based on the intersection union test (Berger, 1982; Casella and Berger, 1990): H_0 is rejected if and only if *all* individual comparisons are rejected at level α. In toxicology this scenario is hard to understand, but in some clinical trials such problems exist (e.g., a fixed dose combination should be more efficient than the monotherapies).

However, for most procedures, the type II error increases by the

TABLE 1   Power Comparison Between All-Pair and Many-to-One MCP

	All-pair procedure	Many-to-one procedure
	6 comparisons	3 comparisons
Type II error β	0.17	0.11

number of comparisons. In Table 1 the corresponding power is given for
a ($k = 3 + 1$) design with $\alpha = 0.05$, $n_i = 24$, $\sigma/d = 1$, one-sided, σ^2
denoting the variance and d the toxicologically important difference.
Hence, many-to-one MCPs should be generally preferred in toxicology
and the lowest number of treatment (dose) groups should be selected at
the design stage.

The ($k + 1$)-sample problem can be tested by a MCP or by independent two-sample tests, each at level α and for each of the three
aforementioned types. The choice between the experiment-wise error rate
(α_{exp}) and the comparison-wise error (α_{comp}) represents the problem of
balancing between false-positive error and false-negative error rates.
MCPs control the experiment-wise error rate α_{exp}, resulting in a larger
false-negative rate β. Independent two-sample tests exceed α_{exp}, but reveal the smallest false-negative rate β.

D. Testing Procedures Versus Simultaneous
Confidence Intervals

Several outcomes of the multiple decisions in MCPs can be used: (adjusted) p-values, yes or no decisions for the null hypotheses at a predefined level α (usually $\alpha = 0.05$, 0.01, or 0.001 corresponding to the
symbols *, **, ***) or simultaneous confidence intervals (CI) for the
differences to control. Several advantages make the CIs the method of
choice: they are scale variant (endpoint-specific region, easy for interpretation), containing quantitative information about the variance, the sample size, the dimension k, the actual α-level and about derivation from
the null hypotheses. Furthermore, simultaneous confidence intervals can
be used in the safety approach with an a posteriori-defined minimally
relevant safety difference δ (for definition, see Chap. 6). However, CIs
are up to now mostly available for single-step procedure only (Hsu,
1996) but stepwise procedures guarantee higher power. Moreover, CIs
are not yet available for all MCPs.

E. Simultaneous Procedures Versus α-Adjustment Methods

The MCPs controlling the experiment-wise error rate can be constructed by

1. Using multivariate distributions (e.g., the multivariate t-distribution taking the correlation between the comparisons into account)
2. α-Adjustment methods
3. Resampling approaches (e.g., Westfall and Young, 1993; Troendle, 1995)

If the ANOVA assumptions are fulfilled, then for all values of k, α, and n_i the following relation holds true: $\pi_{\text{simultaneous}} \geq \pi_{\alpha\text{-adjustment}}$, with $\pi = 1 - \beta$ denoting the power. However, for small dimension of k (up to about five for many-to-one comparisons, which is typical in toxicology) the difference is small from a practical point of view. Therefore, under certain conditions, the use of α-adjustments makes sense if multivariate distributions are not available in the computer software, if for the specific endpoint a simultaneous MCP does not exist, if the variances are heterogeneous, if discrete endpoints should be analyzed, or if the same procedure should be used for all endpoints. From the point of maximizing the power, the choice seems to be simple. However, single-step simultaneous MCPs have the advantage that simultaneous confidence intervals for the differences with the control are available.

F. Single-Step Versus Stepwise MCPs

Simultaneous procedures and α-adjustment methods can be performed either as single-step or stepwise procedures (Table 2). Again, considering the power, stepwise procedures should be used because of $\pi_{\text{stepwise}} \geq$

TABLE 2 Stepwise Parametric MCPs

Approach	Simultaneous procedures	α-Adjustment procedures
Step-down	Marcus et al., 1976	Holm, 1976
Step-up	Dunnett and Tamhane, 1992	Hommel, 1988; Hochberg, 1988
Step-up and down	Tamhane and Dunnett, 1996	

$\pi_{\text{single-step}}$. However, simultaneous confidence intervals are not yet available for all stepwise procedures. Stepwise procedures can be performed in step-up or step-down manner and are presented in the following as α-adjustment procedures.

1. Step-down: starting with the smallest p-value and conditional testing with α/k, $\alpha/(k - 1)$, . . . , α
2. Step-up: starting with the largest p-value and conditional testing with α, $\alpha/2$, . . . , α/k

G. The Concept of Adjusted p-Values

In multiple testing problems, elementary (unadjusted) p-values can be used and compared with adjusted levels (e.g., with Bonferroni-bounds). However, more intuitively is the use of adjusted p-values; all multiple adjustments include this value; therefore, they can be directly compared with the nominal α-level. In the case of a single-step simultaneous MCP, the adjusted p-values can be computed as the smallest possible α-levels of the multivariate t-distribution. In the case of the α-adjustment approach the adjusted p-values p_i^{adj}, based on the two-sample p-values p_i according to Wright (1992), Tamhane (1996), and Westfall and Young (1993), are computed as follows (based on the ordered p-values $p_{(1)} \leq p_{(2)} \leq \ldots \leq p_{(k)}$):

Bonferroni: $p_i^{\text{adj}} = \min\{1, kp_i\}$

Holm: $p_{(i)}^{\text{adj}} = \min[1, \min\{kp_{(k)}, (k - 1)p_{(k-1)}, \ldots, ip_{(i)}\}]$
            $(1 \leq i \leq k)$

Hochberg: $p_{(i)}^{\text{adj}} = \min[1, \max\{p_{(1)}, 2p_{(2)}, \ldots, ip_{(i)}\}]$ $(1 \leq i \leq k)$

It is easy to show, that Hochberg's procedure is at least as powerful as that of Holm and Holm's procedure is at least as powerful as that of Bonferroni, depending on the structure of the p_i values. Hochberg's procedure is based on the Simes (1986) procedure and assumes that the p_i values are independent; the adjusted p-values of Hochberg's procedures cannot be larger than the largest unadjusted p-value.

H. One-Sided Versus Two-Sided Hypotheses Formulation

In the literature for randomized clinical trials a controversy exists between one- and two-sided testing. In principle the decision is simple: if there is any doubt about the direction of the effect, then two-sided testing is indicated. If there is no doubt about the direction *and* if the decision in the noninteresting direction has the same predictive value as H_0, then one-sided testing for increase or decrease should be performed. Two examples from toxicological studies are the endpoints body mass (two-sided) and the number of revertants in the Ames assay (one-sided). The advantage of one-sided testing is important under the aspect of power consideration; the two-sample t-test with $\alpha = 0.05$, $\sigma/d = 1$, and $n_i = 15$, yields a power of $\pi_{\text{one-sided}} = 0.848$, but only $\pi_{\text{two-sided}} = 0.753$. Therefore, one-sided testing should be preferred in toxicology wherever possible. In long-term carcinogenicity studies an increase or decrease of tumor rates may be observed; hence, one could argue for two-sided testing. However, in relation to the objective of the carcinogenicity study (reveals any neoplastic risk of the substance?), one-sided testing should be performed because of the dramatic loss in power for two-sided testing: two-sample χ^2-test with $\alpha = 0.05$, a spontaneous rate in the control of 1%, a tumor rate during treatment of 5%, $n_i = 50$ results in $\pi_{\text{one-sided}} = 0.143$, but $\pi_{\text{two-sided}} = 0.083$. Sometimes in the literature only the possibility for the decision of no difference or a difference is described, postulating that a further decision about the direction (increase or decrease) is not possible. However, using the closure principle Hauschke and Steinjians (1996) demonstrated that a directional decision is possible without an α-adjustment.

I. Testing Hierarchies

In some text books (e.g., Gad and Weil, 1986; Salsburg, 1986) and publications (e.g., Little, 1990), testing hierarchies for adapting suitable tests on the actual data conditions are described (so-called decision trees). The idea is to characterize the condition of the data and to select a suitable test procedure. For instance, starting with a test on gaussian distribution and variance homogeneity, a nonparametric test is selected if the hypotheses are rejected. In the next step a test on homogeneity of the means is performed and for a significant test result an MCP is selected. There are two arguments against this kind of decision-tree approach. The validity tests (pretests) have to be formulated as statistical tests on equivalence (e.g., rejecting H_0 to demonstrate gaussian distribution). However, these equivalence tests are either not yet available or their power is very low relative to the power of the main test. Even if the pretest for gaussian distribution would be used in the traditional manner, the power for usual sample sizes per treatment group (e.g., 20, 10, or even 3 animals in primate studies) is very low. Solutions that "mimic" the equivalence character by using higher α-levels for the pretests are still controversial.

  Therefore, the "data-driven" decision approach seems not to be useful. The decision between parametric and nonparametric methods should be based in advance on historical data (e.g., negative controls). In the two-sample parametric case, a decision between variance homogeneity and heterogeneity is not necessary if the Welch t-test will be used in general, because in the homogeneous case, it represents the standard pairwise t-test. Moreover, the combination of a global test (e.g., F- or Kruskal–Wallis test) and MCPs is popular within such decision trees. But this approach is not a procedure controlling the α-level. Recently, Hsu (1996, p. 178) concluded that "To consider MCP as to be performed only if the F-test for homogeneity rejects is a mistake." However, a correct approach for combing global and local decisions is simply available by the closure principle (see Sec. IV.A.1.c). For that reason, global tests should be avoided in the sense of a pretest before executing an MCP.

J. Point Zero Versus Shifted Null Hypotheses

Assuming a one-sided two-sample problem, the hypotheses for difference are usually formulated as follows, with μ_i describing the expected value of group i:

$$H_0:\mu_{C_-} - \mu_{D_i} = 0$$
$$H_1:\mu_{C_-} - \mu_{D_i} < 0$$

  That means that for very small variances or large sample sizes a rejection of the null hypothesis may occur. This phenomenon arises in some mutagenicity assays if in a group nearly the same counts will be observed. The point zero hypothesis will be rejected even if the increase in the means is biologically irrelevantly low. The situation is described in the literature as the difference between statistical significance and biological importance. Hence, the point zero null hypothesis is not appropriate for biological experiments and toxicological studies. Therefore, the so called relevance-shifted null hypothesis should be used:

$$H_0:\mu_{C_-} - \mu_{D_i} = \varepsilon$$
$$H_1:\mu_{C_-} - \mu_{D_i} < \varepsilon$$

The relevance shift parameter ε has to be defined a priori. Modifications can be simply performed in the two-sample situation [t-test and Wilcoxon (1945)–Mann/Whitney (1947) u-test]. Dunnett and Tamhane (1991) published related versions for many-to-one comparisons and Meng et al. (1993) for the Bartholomew trend test, respectively. However, in comparison with a point zero null hypothesis test, there can be situations for which a shifted test needs a larger sample size. This problem is directly related to one-sided tests for equivalence (see Chap. 6).

K. Restriction of the Alternative Hypothesis for the Dose–Response Design

The restriction of the alternative hypothesis is an important concept to increase the power, thereby, reducing the type II error rate. A simple justification is Paracelsius law that the dose makes the poison. The most effective restriction, one-sided instead of two-sided, has already been described. The alternative of the many-to-one dose–response design can be restricted to

1. Totally order: $H_i{:}\mu_{C^-} \leq \mu_{D_1} \leq \mu_{D_2} \leq \ldots \leq \mu_{D_k}$ with at least $\mu_{C^-} < \mu_{D_k}$
2. Simple tree order: $H_1{:}\mu_{C^-} < [\mu_{D_1}, \ldots, \mu_{D_k}]$
3. Partial order: $H_1{:}\mu_{C^-} < \mu_{D_i} \ni i \in (1, \ldots, k) \mid \mu_{C^-} \leq \mu_{D_1} \leq \mu_{D_2} \leq \ldots \leq \mu_{D_k}$
4. Simple loop order: $H_1{:}\mu_{C^-} < [\mu_{D_1}, \ldots, \mu_{D_j}] \leq \ldots \leq \mu_{D_k}]$
5. Umbrella order: $H_1{:}\mu_{C^-} \leq \mu_{D_1} \leq \ldots \leq \mu_u \geq \ldots \geq \mu_{D_k}$

The question arises whether the restriction of the alternative yields a substantial increase in power in comparison with that for the unrestricted alternative. If the dose–response is monotonic—with any kind of shape—the answer is yes. However, possible downturns at higher doses has to be taken into account in toxicological studies. Some publications described the application of umbrella tests in this situation, but the experimental question is not to detect an umbrella shape. The primary question is to detect one-sided increasing effect, frequently monotonic, but with the possibility of a downturn at higher doses; therefore, order-restricted approaches protecting against downturns should be used. Between both extremes of unrestricted and total order, the partial order (Shaffer, 1986) and the simple tree order exist as a compromise. If the real data are ordered, the power is only slightly smaller than the power for the optimal order procedure, but if the means are ordered in a non-monotonic way, the decision is correct. To restrict or not to restrict the alternative a priori is finally a question of balancing between robustness and optimal power. The restriction of the alternative to total order guarantees a high power if the dose–response is monotonic, but a serious power loss occurs if downturns at high doses appear. Without an a priori restriction the power is relatively low, but this procedure is robust against any pattern of mean values.

L. Hypotheses Formulation for Mean Values, Stochastic Order, Distribution Functions, and Location Scale

Hypotheses for tests and MCPs should be primarily endpoint-specific (e.g., for parametric, nonparametric, dichotomous, or Poisson-distributed endpoints). For continuous endpoints, the question arises of whether the hypothesis restricted on the mean (expected value) μ_i is the best way. The distributions of the two populations can be compared using the Kolmogorov–Smirnov test. However, the sample size needed for an acceptable α/β ratio is much higher than practicable in toxicological studies. Therefore, under the assumption of the gaussian distribution and homogeneous variances (which implies equal skewness and kurtosis), the comparison of the populations can be replaced by comparison of the mean values. Many endpoints do not fulfill these conditions; hence, a nonparametric test is indicated. However, the nonparametric alternative is called stochastic ordering, which means that the high dose is stochastic larger than the control. From the practical point of view, the biological interpretation of this alternative is difficult. Moreover, nonparametric tests also assume variance homogeneity, but in the form of homomorphy for the distribution functions (the cumulative distribution functions should not cross) (Horn and Vollandt, 1995). The situation with variance heterogeneity can be solved by the Welch or Satterthwaite approach in the parametric setup. Another approach considers changes in location and scale as substance effects. This is called informative variance heterogeneity and some location–scale trend tests are available (Brandt and Hothorn, 1995). One model assumes a mixing distribution of responder (substance effect) and nonresponder (control effect) under the alternative; a biological reasoning for such an approach was given by Hothorn (1994) for the micronucleus assay.

M. Outliers

The adequate treatment of outliers in toxicological studies is a difficult task. One objective is to identify extreme individual measures in the sense of pathological values. On the other hand, extreme values could be outliers without any relation to substance effects. In contrast to statistical methods for detecting outliers, such a formal approach should be avoided in toxicology. Declaring an extreme value as an outlier should be based on only technical or biological reasons. Nevertheless, as a first step of data analysis exploratory methods for detection of outliers (e.g., groupwise box-plots) can be helpful to identify such single, extreme values from the huge amount of data.

III. TREND TESTS

A. Principles

1. Including Dose Levels into Statistics Versus Qualitative Consideration of the Dose Levels

Trend tests can be characterized whether the dose levels are incorporated into the test statistic in a direct or in only a qualitative manner. It could be assumed that the qualitative consideration yields an information loss and, consequently, a reduction in power. However, in general, this is not true; the dose levels may be not optimal and scores should be used in a better way (Tukey et al., 1985). On the other side, dose levels are often selected in expectation of a linear dose–response relation for either linear or logarithmic dose scale. For an unknown profile of the dose–response relation, model-based trend tests reveal a low power if the preselected model and the experimental data differ. Moreover, in the parametric context, all trend tests can be identified as contrast tests. Barlow et al. (1972) demonstrated that the likelihood ratio test is a contrast test with infinite contrasts. Robertson et al. (1988) revealed that the MLE test (Williams, 1971, 1972) is a special multiple contrast test (consisting of a pairwise and several reverse Helmert contrasts). Mehta et al. (1984) has shown that the regression approach according to Tukey et al. (1985) is equivalent to multiple contrast tests.

2. Asymptotic Versus Permutative Test Statistics

Only for large-sample sizes some test statistics (e.g., the Cochran (1954)–Armitage (1955) trend test] are asymptotically gaussian distributed. Under the ANOVA assumptions of gaussian distribution and variance homogeneity, other test statistics are distributed according to a suitable distribution (e.g., the Helmert contrast test is univariate t-distributed). Nonparametric tests [e.g., the Jonckheere (1954) trend test] are asymptotically gaussian distributed under the assumption of continuously distributed random variables. In practice, however, ties occur frequently, and the distribution is no longer valid [Weller and Ryan (1996) provided an approximation for a ties correction of the variance estimator]. Permutation tests require no assumption about ANOVA conditions, sample size, ties, or other. The principle of these test procedures consists in defining "any suitable" test statistics, computing the empirical test value for the underlying data set, and then performing all permutations under the null hypothesis. Under the validity of H_0 the probability for the membership of an experimental unit to any treatment group is the same (Good, 1994); therefore, the p-value can be estimated by a simple counting process. Several computational procedures have been developed to realize all permutations [e.g., the network algorithm (Mehta and Patel, 1983), the shift algorithm (Streitberg and Röhmel, 1987), or the so-called simulation-based algorithm (Berry, 1995)]. In the meantime, high-speed PCs and workstations are available, and permutation tests represent an alternative to the traditional distribution-based tests, but permutative tests can become rather conservative owing to their discrete nature. For dichotomous endpoints the use of unconditional versions can reduce this conservativeness (Storer and Kim, 1990). The simple mid-p-value approach (Lancaster, 1961) can be used, but it does not guarantee a correct α-level test. For censored data (e.g., for analyzing mortality-adjusted small tumor rates) the equality of censoring patterns is an additional condition for applying permutative tests (Fairweather et al., 1997).

3.   Influence of the Dose–Response Profile on Power

One of the problems in the application of trend tests consists in their sensitivity to the unknown shape of the dose–response profile. With use of Pitman's concept of asymptotic relative efficacy, several contrasts were compared for selected dose–response profiles (Neuhäueser, 1996); the results for $k = 3$ are presented in Table 3. The Pitman efficacy is roughly the ratio of the slopes of the power functions of two tests near α, assuming infinite sample sizes.

Table 3 shows that the loss in power for nonoptimal contrast tests is large for unknown profiles and occurs over a broad region of the noncentrality parameter. The power of the Helmert contrast (dotted line) and reverse Helmert contrast (line) (Fligner and Wolfe, 1982) can be

TABLE 3   Ratio of Pitman Efficiencies Relative to the Shape-Optimal
Contrast (for the Definition of the Contrasts, see Table 4)

Contrast	Linear profile	Convex profile	Concave profile
Helmert contrast	0.60	Optimal contrast	0.11
Reverse Helmert contrast	0.60	0.11	Optimal contrast
Maximin contrast	0.97	0.65	0.65
Linear contrast	Optimal contrast	0.60	0.60
Jonckheere–Analogon contrast	0.84	0.93	0.28
Pairwise contrast	0.90	0.67	0.67

simply computed by using the noncentral t-distribution and are given in
Fig. 1 for convex and concave shapes, $k = 4$, $n_i = 10$, $\alpha = 0.05$.

It is easy to see that for convex profiles, the Helmert contrast is
much more powerful than the reverse Helmert contrast, for concave
profiles it is just the other way around. Even for small shifts the differences in power are dramatic. Clearly, in principle, the shape of the dose–

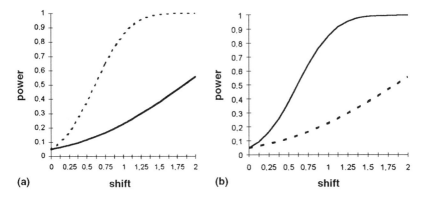

FIGURE 1   Power functions for (a) convex and (b) concave shapes.

response relation is a priori unknown. Several concepts can be used now to solve this problem:

1. Ignoring this important fact is a common practice, but cannot be accepted in safety studies.
2. Looking at the data, characterizing a profile type and selection of the best suitable trend test represents one kind of hunting for significance.
3. The LRT test, according to Bartholomew (1959, 1961), can be chosen, but the test is limited to some ideal conditions.
4. Applying the adjustive approach (Neuhäuser, 1996).

B. Parametric Trend Tests

1. Contrast Tests

Contrast tests are defined by simply linear combination of the mean values and univariate distributed:

$$ t_C^{\text{parametric}} = \frac{\sum_{i=0}^{k} c_i \overline{X}_i}{\sqrt{MSE \sum_{i=0}^{k} c_i^2/n_i}} \propto t_{v,1-\alpha} $$

with $\sum_{i=0}^{k} c_i = 0$ ($i = 0$ represent C^-), where $v = \sum_{i=0}^{k} n_i - (k + 1)$ denotes the degree of freedom, $MSE = \sum_{i=0}^{k} \sum_{j=1}^{n_i} (X_{ij} - \overline{X}_{i.})^2/(N - (k + 1))$ the mean square error and $t_{v,1-\alpha}$ the central univariate t-distribution with v the degree of freedom. The choice of the contrasts coefficients c_i is "free," and several versions were described in the literature (see Table 4).

In the situation of variance homogeneity the correlation between two contrasts is

$$ \rho_{a,b} = \frac{\sum_{i=0}^{k} a_i b_i/n_i}{\sqrt{\left(\sum_{i=0}^{k} a_i^2/n_i\right)\left(\sum_{i=0}^{k} b_i^2/n_i\right)}} $$

(Bechhofer and Dunnett, 1982); if $\sum_{i=0}^{k} a_i b_i = 0$ the contrasts are orthogonal and uncorrelated.

A series of articles exist for the power comparison of several contrast tests (including comparisons with other trend tests). The statements

TABLE 4 Contrast Tests

Contrast type	Ref	Coefficients
Helmert contrast	Ruberg, 1989	$c_i = -1, i = 0, \ldots, k-1$ $c_k = k$
Reverse Helmert contrast	Fligner and Wolfe, 1982	$c_0 = -k$ $c_i = 1, i = 1, 2, \ldots, k$
Maximin contrast	Abelson and Tukey, 1963	$c_i = \sqrt{i\left(1 - \dfrac{i}{k+1}\right)}$ $- \sqrt{(i+1)\left(1 - \dfrac{i+1}{k+1}\right)}$
Pairwise contrast	Hothorn and Lehmacher, 1991	$c_0 = -1$ $c_i = 0, i = 1, 2, \ldots, k-1$ $c_k = 1$
Linear contrast	Rom et al., 1994	$c_0 = -k$ $c_i = c_{i-1} + 2, i = 1, 2, \ldots, k$
Jonkheere–Analogon contrast	Neuhäuser, 1996	$c_0 = -1$ $c_i = \left(\displaystyle\sum_{j=k-i+1}^{k} 1/j\right) - 1, i = 1, 2, \ldots, k-1$ $c_k = \displaystyle\sum_{j=1}^{k} 1/j$

concerning the advantage of a selected contrast test are not correct owing to ignorance of the a priori unknown shape. It is obvious that if the contrast fits the empirical shape, then the test must be optimal in power (e.g., linear shape $\Rightarrow$ linear contrast; convex shape $\Rightarrow$ Helmert contrast). An approach to stabilize the power relative to shape has been published by McDermott and Mudholkar (1993). This procedure is based on the nested decompensation method (decompensation of a global trend test in $k, k-1, \ldots,$ 2-dimensional Helmert contrasts with zero correlation) and using Fisher's Liptak's, or Tippett's criterion for combining the $(k-1)$ p values. McDermott and Mudholkar demonstrated superior power in comparison with the LRT. However, their method is based on several shape-specific combination criteria; therefore, the conclusion of superiority is not correct (Hothorn et al., 1996).

A further approach for stabilizing the power is the so-called multiple contrast test $T_{\text{mult}} = \max(T_m), m \in \{1, \ldots, k\}$ (Mukerjee et al.,

1986). The distribution of T_{mult} depends on the correlation coefficients between the k contrasts tests and may be complex. One mentioned approach is based on Bonferroni's adjustment and the other on the k-dimensional t-distribution with zero correlation between the orthogonal contrasts. Neuhäuser (1996) generalized this approach for

1. Two or more tests
2. Adjustment by either Bonferronization, using multivariate distributions (parametric), or permutations techniques (nonparametric, dichotomous)
3. Selection from standardized statistics, not only from different contrasts, but also from different dose scores, different p-value combinations (modification of the McDermott approach) and tests sensitive for a special pattern of time-to-event data (Tarone, 1981)
4. Selection of statistics with low correlation and a high sensitivity for an extreme behavior [e.g., optimal in power for convex and concave profiles, according to the principle of maximum efficiency robustness (Gastwirth, 1970, 1985)].

2. The Likelihood Ratio Test

The likelihood ratio test for a total monotonic order in the case of unknown, homogeneous variances was derived by Bartholomew (1959, 1961):

$$E_k^2 = \sum_{i=0}^{k} n_i (\hat{\mu}_i - \overline{X}..)^2 / \sum_{i=0}^{k} \sum_{j=1}^{n_i} (X_{ij} - \hat{\mu}_i)^2 \text{ with } \hat{\mu}_i$$

$$\mu_i = \max_{0 \le u \le i} \min_{i \le v \le k} \sum_{q=u}^{v} \overline{X}_q / (v - u + 1) \ i \in \{0, \ldots, k\}$$

being the maximum likelihood estimator under order restriction. This test statistics is distributed according to a weighted sums of β-variables (see Barlow et al., 1972; Robertson et al., 1988). In the general case, quantiles or p-values are numerically difficult to determine, and for balanced total ordering, quantiles were tabulated by Nelson (1977). Several algorithms for calculating the maximum likelihood estimator $\hat{\mu}_i$ were published by Robertson et al. (1988, p. 56), and Chase (1974) extended the method for an increased precision in one group.

3. Maximum Likelihood Trend Test

Williams (1971, 1972) published a MCP for the order-restricted many-to-one design. The first test in this step-down procedure is the comparison of the kth dose group with the control; therefore, it represents a global test for the totally ordered hypothesis:

$$tw_k = \frac{\hat{\mu}_k - \overline{X}_0}{\sqrt{\text{MSE}(1/n_k + 1/n_0)}} \propto \overline{t}_{k,\nu,\rho_{il},\text{one-sided},1-\alpha}$$

where $\hat{\mu}_k$ denotes the maximum likelihood estimator under order restriction excluding $\overline{X}_0$. Tabulated quantiles for the $\overline{t}$-distribution are available in the original publications; approximations are provided by Hothorn (1994b), and software is accessible (SAS-PROBMC "williams" instead of "dunnett"; however, this is not documented in Anonymous 1995). The maximum likelihood estimators $\hat{\mu}_i$ corresponds to that one in Bartholomew's test, but without considering $\overline{X}_0$.

4. Linear Regression Tests

Model-based tests can also be used as trend tests. However, the correct model selection for an a priori unknown shape is an open question. The difficulties with using a pretest were discussed in Section II. Tukey et al. (1985) proposed the use of the three-dose transformations arithmetic, ordinal and arithmetic-logarithmic without any α correction. Capizzi et al. (1992) improved approach using a trivariate t-distribution. Mehta et al. (1984) proved the equivalence of the regression approach with multiple contrasts, and Neuhäuser (1996) demonstrated that Capizzi's test is an adjustive contrast test, with high correlations between the scores. Especially for nonlinear shapes, the power of the adjustive contrast test based on Helmert contrast is much higher owing to the lower correlation. Antonello et al. (1993) described the application of Tukey et al. (1985) test in the field of reproductive toxicity studies.

Example 1. In a repeated toxicity study on Wistar rats the body weight was measured after 2 weeks. The summary data for the body weights are presented in Table 5, the raw data in the Appendix.

TABLE 5 Summary Data

Group	Mean	SD	n_i
C^-	291.45	11.75	15
D_{low}	280.83	16.12	15
D_{med}	276.71	17.27	15
D_{high}	260.43	16.62	15

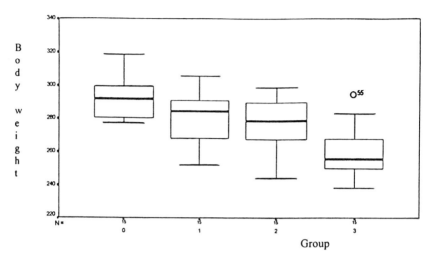

FIGURE 2   Box-plots.

The variable is a continuous endpoint and the assumption of an approximate gaussian distribution is fulfilled, as seen from the Box-plots presented in Fig. 2.

Moreover, approximate homogeneity of the variances can also be assumed. The MSE = 243.07 and $v = 60 - 4 = 56$. With the following SAS program the several contrasts for the global test ($k = 3 + 1$) can be calculated (with the class variable dose and the endpoint body w):

```
proc glm;
class dose;
model bodyw=dose;
contrast 'Helmert contrast' dose -1 -1 -1 3;
contrast 'Reverse Helmert c.' dose -3 1 1 1;
contrast 'Maximin contrast' dose -0.866025 -0.133975 0.133975 0.866025;
contrast 'Linear contrast' dose -3 -1 1 3;
contrast 'Pairwise contrast' dose -1 0 0 1;
contrast 'Jonckheere-anal.c.' dose -1 -0.66666667 -0.16666666 1.8333333;
```

The output is as follows:

Contrast	DF	Contrast SS	Mean Square	F Value	Pr > F
Helmert contrast	1	5726.85605556	5726.85605556	23.56	0.0001
Reverse Helmert c.	1	3971.50138889	3971.50138889	16.34	0.0002
Maximin contrast	1	7338.12251342	7338.12251342	30.19	0.0001
Linear contrast	1	7081.02083333	7081.02083333	29.13	0.0001
Pairwise contrast	1	7213.70133333	7213.70133333	29.68	0.0001
Jonckheere-anal.c.	1	6950.81858103	6950.81858103	28.60	0.0001

It can be seen that all contrast tests reject the null hypothesis, but the maximin contrast is the most sensitive one having the maximum test value. These p-values are defined two-sided. The mean values are monotonically ordered; hence, the MLE equals the mean values: $\hat{\mu}_i = \overline{X}_i$. Therefore, the test statistics $\overline{E}^2_{k=4} = 0.548$. Based on the approximate 0.95 quantile for this test (see in Barlow et al., 1972; Table A4) with a value of 0.071, the null hypothesis can also be rejected. Williams' trend test can be simply calculated by $tw_k = (\hat{\mu}_k - \overline{X}_0)/\sqrt{\text{MSE} (1/n_k + 1/n_0} = (260.43 - 291.44)/\sqrt{243.07 \cdot 2/15} = -5.45$ and the corresponding quantile can be estimated in SAS by: $\bar{t} = \text{PROBMC('Williams', . , 0.95, 56, 3)}$; with $\bar{t} = 1.78355$. Again, the null hypothesis is rejected, the p-value is 0.00000055893. The function PROBMC can be used in SAS (Anonymous, 1992) to calculate quantiles or p-values for Tukey's ("range"), Dunnett's ("dunnett1"/"dunnett2", one-sided/two-sided) and Williams' ("williams") procedure using: value = PROBMC("test," quantile, $(1 - p)$-value, v, k, < correlation coefficients >).

C. Nonparametric Trend Tests

1. Contrast Tests

In applied articles, Jonckheere's (1954) trend test is usually performed as a nonparametric contrast test. However, it belongs to a general class of nonparametric contrast tests and several kinds of ranking can be used.

    a. k-*Ranking Nonparametric Contrast Tests.* In analogy with the parametric contrast tests (see Sec. III.B) the sample means $\overline{X}_i$ are replaced by the means of the k-rankings $\overline{R}_i$ (ranking over all individuals in all groups)

$$t^{\text{nonparametric}}_{C,k-\text{ranking}} = \frac{\sum_{i=0}^{k} c_i a_N (\overline{R}_i)}{\sqrt{\text{var}(a_N) \sum_{i=0}^{k} c_i^2/n_i}} \underset{\text{asympt.}}{\propto} z_{1-\alpha} \text{ with } \sum_{i=0}^{k} c_i = 0;$$

$$\text{var}(a_N) = \frac{1}{N-1} \sum_{i=0}^{k} (a_N(i) - \bar{a}_N)^2 \text{ and}$$

$$a_N(\overline{R}_i) = \frac{1}{n_i} \sum_{j=1}^{n_i} a_N(R_{ij})$$

The coefficients c_i can be chosen according to Table 4. Several well-known nonparametric scores a_N can be used (e.g., Wilcoxon scores for location tests, or Conover and Salsburg (1988) scores for responder-nonresponder distributions); Brandt and Hothorn (1995) described scores for location-scale alternatives.

    b. Pairwise-Ranking Nonparametric Contrast Tests. According to several publications (e.g., Fairley and Fligner, 1986), pairwise-ranking (ranking only over each individuals in group i and group q) is more appropriate, especially for small-sample sizes. In analogy to parametric contrasts, they can be derived as a sum of two-sample tests: $\sum_{i=0}^{k} c_i \bar{X}_i = \sum_{i=0}^{k-1} \sum_{q=i+1}^{k} e_{qi}(\bar{X}_q - \bar{X}_i)$. The coefficients e_{qi} can be chosen according to the desired contrast (e.g., for the linear contrast all coefficients are equal to 1, whereas for Helmert contrast $e_{k0} = 1$ (or else 0). However, a more popular but analogously representation of such pairwise contrasts is the use of Mann–Whitney counts U_{iq} (e.g., Jonckheere's, 1954, trend test [asymptotic version]):

$$T_J = \frac{\left| \sum_{i=0}^{k-1} \sum_{q=i+1}^{k} U_{iq} - \left| \left(N^2 - \sum_{i=0}^{k} n_i^2 \right)/4 \right| \right|}{\sqrt{\left| N^2(2N + 3) - \sum_{i=0}^{k} n_i^2(2n_i + 3) \right|/72}} \propto z_{1-\alpha}$$

or Fligner and Wolfe's (1982) trend test, which equals the reverse Helmert contrast in the asymptotic version:

$$T_{JFW} = \frac{\left| \sum_{i=0}^{k-1} U_{0i} - (n_0/2) \sum_{i=1}^{k} n_i \right|}{\sqrt{\left| n_0 \left(\sum_{i=1}^{k} n_i \right) \left(\sum_{i=0}^{k} n_i + 1 \right) \right|/12}} \propto z_{1-\alpha}$$

2. The Likelihood Ratio Test

The likelihood ratio test can also be performed with k-rankings, but only as an asymptotic version. The first version was proposed by Chacko (1963), which was extended by Shorack (1967) for the unbalanced case. However, in a small-sample situation this modification loses the advantage of power (Robertson, 1988; Magel and Magel, 1986; Mahrer and Magel, 1995). In the nonparametric case this rather complicated test is without relevance compared with the simple contrast tests.

3. Maximum Likelihood Trend Test

The test statistics of Shirley (1977) for the kth dose group versus control represents a global test for the totally ordered hypothesis based on k-ranking ML-estimators:

$$ts_k = \frac{\hat{R}_k - \overline{R}_0}{\sqrt{N(N + 1)(1/n_k + 1/n_0)/12}} \propto \overline{t}_{k,df = \infty, p_{f0}, \text{one-sided}, 1 - \alpha}$$

with $\overline{R}_k$ denoting the ML-estimators under the ordered alternative of the k-rankings:

$$\hat{R}_i = \max_{1 \le u \le i} \min_{i \le v \le k} \frac{\sum\limits_{q=u}^{v} \overline{R}_q}{v - u + 1} \quad i \in (1, \ldots, k) \text{ (excluding } \overline{R}_0)$$

4. Linear Regression Tests

In analogy with parametric linear regression, Park (1989) published a k-ranking nonparametric regression test. This test is equivalent to a linear nonparametric contrast.

Example 2. In a repeated toxicity study with Wistar rats the liver enzyme aspartate aminotransferase (ASAT) was measured. The summary statistics are presented in Table 6 and the raw data in the Appendix, respectively. From historical data, it is known that this endpoint is right-skewed distributed; therefore, a nonparametric test will be used.

The pairwise and k-ranking trend test will be demonstrated using the Jonckheere's and Shirley's trend test. The Mann–Whitney counts are $U_{01} = 59$, $U_{02} = 77$, $U_{03} = 77.5$, $U_{12} = 74$, $U_{13} = 76$, $U_{23} = 62.5$. The asymptotic version of Jonckheere's test is:

$$T_J = \frac{\sum\limits_{i=0}^{k-1} \sum\limits_{q=i+1}^{k} U_{iq} - \left| N^2 - \sum\limits_{i=0}^{k} n_i^2 \right|/4}{\sqrt{\left| N^2(2N + 3) - \sum\limits_{i=0}^{k} n_i^2(2n_i + 3) \right|/72}} \propto z_{1-\alpha}$$

Given $N = 40$, $n_i = 10$, and $k = 3$, the test is $T_J = 3.04$ with a p-value of 0.0012. The k-ranking mean values are: $\overline{R}_0 = 14.15$; $\overline{R}_1 = 16.40$; $\overline{R}_2$

TABLE 6 Summary Data

Dose	n_i	Mean	SD
C^-	10	1.893	0.361
D_1	10	1.980	0.227
D_2	10	2.418	0.534
D_3	10	2.696	0.887

$= 24.35$; $\overline{R}_3 = 27.10$. Because $\overline{R}_1 < \overline{R}_2 < \overline{R}_3$ (excluding $\overline{R}_0$) the MLEs are the same values and Shirley's test is $ts_k = (27.10 - 14.15)/\sqrt{[40 \cdot 41(1/10 + 1/10)]/12} = 2.45$. Using PROBMC ($v \Rightarrow \infty$) a p value of 0.0081 results.

D. Trend Tests for Dichotomous Endpoints

For dichotomous endpoints in the $(k + 1)$-sample problem, the following contingency table will be used (see Table 7).

For dichotomous endpoints the Cochran (1954)–Armitage (1955) trend test (C-A-test) is the most popular favored by several authors (Gad and Weil, 1988; Litt et al., 1990) and even by *Federal Register* for analyzing tumorigenicity studies (Anonymous, 1985). The test statistic is asymptotic optimal for all monotonic alternatives (Tarone and Gart, 1980) and asymptotic gaussian distributed (Portier and Hoel, 1984; one-sided version):

$$T_{CA} = \sqrt{N/(N - r.)r.} \cdot \frac{\sum\limits_{i=0}^{k} (r_i - \frac{n_i}{N}r.)D_i}{\sqrt{\sum\limits_{i=0}^{k} \frac{n_j}{N} D_i^2 - \left(\sum\limits_{i=0}^{k} \frac{n_j}{N} D_i\right)^2}} \propto z_{1-\alpha}$$

with $r_i \sim \text{bin}(n_i, p_i)$ describing the number of successes in group i, where $N = \Sigma n_i$ is the total sample size, $r. = \Sigma r_i$ denotes the number of all successes and $p_i = r_i/n_i$ is the probability of an effect in group i. The power of the test depends strongly on the choice of the dose scores D_i. From a closed power formula by Nam (1986), the corresponding values are presented for three profiles and several dose scores (Table 8).

For a priori unknown shapes, Armitage (1955) and Graubard and Korn (1987) recommended equidistant scores. According to the adjustive approach (Neuhäuser and Hothorn, 1997), this problem can be solved in a more powerful manner.

In toxicology the sample sizes n_i are small, usually between 50

TABLE 7   Principle of a Contingency Table

	C^-	D_1	D_2	$\ldots$	D_k	Σ
Number with an effect	r_0	r_1	r_2		r_k	$r.$
Number at risk	n_0	n_1	n_2		n_k	N

TABLE 8   Shape Dependence of Power for Several
Dose Scores in the C-A-Trend Test

Dose scores	Linear	Convex	Concave
Equidistant	0.49	0.51	0.37
0, 2, 4, 8	0.48	0.59	0.31
0, 2, 10, 30	0.45	0.64	0.22
1, 10, 100, 1000	0.39	0.67	0.17
1, 1.1, 1.2, 4	0.38	0.67	0.17
1, 3.8, 3.9, 4	0.34	0.17	0.56

Source: Neuhäuser, 1996 ($n_i = 10$, $\alpha = 0.05$)

(carcinogenicity studies with rats) and 5 (repeated toxicity study on dogs). Williams (1988) and Koch (1996) demonstrated for *max{pairwise contrasts}* that the behavior (size and power) of the normal approximation is poor resulting in the requirement of an an exact version. On the other hand, conditional 2 by k table tests assume an a priori known and fixed total number of responders (marginal sum). In real data problems this seems to be unrealistic and an unconditional version is more appropriate. Because of the controversial discussion concerning the conditional and unconditional approach (e.g., Mehta and Hilton, 1990, 1993) both approaches will be mentioned here. Neuhäuser (1996) developed for the C-A-test an exact conditional version (based on Williams' procedure, 1988) and an asymptotic exact unconditional version (based on the method of Storer and Kim, 1990). Moreover, Neuhäuser and Hothorn (1997) presented an adjustive modification (permutation approach) for optimal dose scores selection; corresponding SAS programs are available (Neuhäuser, 1996). Both testing principles decrease the conservativeness of the asymptotic C-A-test, especially for small success rates, and the power is higher in comparison with the asymptotic version, particularly for small control rates $p_0 > 0.1$, which are relevant in toxicological studies.

1. Contrast Tests

For dichotomous data, contrast tests can be defined in the same way as the parametric and nonparametric versions. According to Barlow et al. (1972) and Robertson et al. (1988) the asymptotic test statistic is

$$t_C^{\text{dichotomous}} = \frac{\sum\limits_{i=0}^{k} c_i r_i / n_i}{\sqrt{p.(1 - p.)\sum\limits_{i=0}^{k} (c_i^2/n_i)}} \propto z_{1-\alpha} \text{ with } p. = \frac{r.}{N}$$

However, according to the foregoing arguments asymptotic tests should be avoided. Neuhäuser (1996) described exact conditional and unconditional contrast tests including the corresponding adjustive modification. Furthermore, the author presented a powerful modification of the Jonckheere contrast.

2. Likelihood Ratio Test

An isotonic regression test was given by Collins et al. (1981), and a likelihood ratio test was published by Robertson et al. (1988) and Oluyede (1994). However, these tests are only asymptotically valid and, therefore, they will be omitted here.

Example 3. In a repeated toxicity study, the design $\{C^-, D_1, D_2\}$, with more than 50 endpoints, was investigated. Table 9 gives the histopathological findings of the kidneys and should by analyzed statistically for an increase, assuming a monotonic dose–response relation (i.e., one-sided). The stepwise conditional testing using the asymptotic version of the C-A-test starts with the highest dose (based on the dose scores 0, 1, 2):

$$ta_{(k=2+1)} = \sqrt{75/(75 - 15) \cdot 15}$$

$$\frac{\left(1 - \frac{25}{75}15\right) \cdot 0 + \left(3 - \frac{25}{75}15\right) \cdot 1 + \left(11 - \frac{25}{75}15\right) \cdot 2}{\sqrt{\frac{25}{75}(0 + 1 + 4) - \left(\frac{25}{75} \cdot 3\right)^2}}$$

$ta_{(k=2+1)} = 3.53 > 1.644$, and the null hypothesis can be rejected and the trend test for C^- versus D_1 can be performed; $ta_{(k=1+1)} = 1.03$ the

TABLE 9   Number of Histopathological Findings

	C^-	D_1	D_2	Σ
With finding	1	3	11	15
n_i	25	25	25	75

null hypothesis cannot be rejected. Because the small sample sizes, the permutative version is more appropriate and SAS PROC MULTTEST is used (with 0 denoting no finding and 1 finding, respectively):

SAS-program

```
proc multtest data=vb_12 permutation;
  nsample=10000 pvals ;
  test ca(bef nobef / lowertailed);
  class dose;
  contrast 'CA linear trend' 0 1 2;
run;
```

SAS-output

```
                         MULTTEST PROCEDURE
Test for discrete variables:          Cochran-Armitage trend
Z-score approximation used:           Everywhere
Continuity correction:                0
Tails for discrete tests:             Lower-tailed
Strata adjustment?                    No
P-value adjustments:                  Permutation
Number of resamples:                  10000
Seed:                                 42449

                      MULTTEST COEFFICIENTS
                                Class
          Test                0      1        2
          CA linear trend     0      1        2
                CA linear trend     0.0002      0.0005
          BEF       Count           1.00        3.00        11.00
                    N               25.00       25.00       25.00
                    Percent         4.00        12.00       44.00
                    Test            Raw_p       Adj_p
                    CA linear trend 0.0002      0.00050
```

E. Trend Tests for Other Endpoints

1. Trend Test for Count Data

Count data frequently occurs in toxicological studies (e.g., number of micronuclei or the number of multiple tumors). Nonparametric trend tests can be applied if the variance estimator is corrected for ties; for the Jonckheere trend test a correction formula was given by Lehmann (1975). Another possibility is the permutative version of nonparametric trend tests (e.g., Jonckheere's trend test within the software package StatXact (Mehta and Patel, 1995).

Special asymptotic tests can be defined for count data, and Breslow (1990) published the following test:

$$
T_B = \frac{\sum\limits_{i=1}^{k} \overline{X}_{i.} n_i \, (D_i - \overline{D})}{k \sum\limits_{i=1}^{k} \sum\limits_{j=1}^{n_j} (X_{ij} - \overline{X}..)^2 (D_i - \overline{D})^2} \propto z_{1-\alpha}
$$

Weller and Ryan (1997) modified this test, incorporating an unadjusted variance estimator, and Lee (1985) gave an asymptotic contrast tests for Poisson endpoints

$$T_L = \frac{\left(\sum\limits_{i=1}^{k} i\overline{X}_{i.} - N\sum\limits_{i=1}^{k} in_i \right)/N}{\sqrt{N\left[\sum\limits_{i=1}^{k} i^2 n_i/N - \left(\sum\limits_{i=1}^{k} in_i/N \right)^2 \right]}} \propto z_{1-\alpha}$$

as well as an asymptotic C-A-test analogue by replacing i by D_i. The further inclusion of negative control data into this test statistics was solved by Tarone (1982).

2. Mortality-Adjusted Trend Tests for Dichotomous Endpoints

Frequently, censored trend tests are used for comparing tumor rates under competing risk of mortality. Three major types can be classified: the log-rank trend test (Tarone, 1975), the trend version of the statistic according to Hoel and Walburg (1972), and a combined test of fatal and incidental tumors (Petro et al., 1980). More recently, Graves (1994) compared the power of these trend tests under several conditions of competing risks. A simple alternative without considering the cause of death is the modified C-A-test according to Bailer and Portier (1988). Assuming Weibull hazards to tumor onset, the number of animals at risk n_i will be modified into $n_i^* = \Sigma_j (t_{ij}/T)^3$ (and $n_i^* \leq n_i$) if the animal j in group i died at time t_{ij} before the terminal time T, $t_{ij} < T$. This test was modified by Bieler and Williams (1993) using the delta method for variance estimation.

Because of the small number of animals and tumors in carcinogenicity studies, permutative versions were developed. However, in unequal censoring patterns, serious problems can occur. A possible solution consists in applying a statistic without involving the information concerning the cause of death (Bolderbuck et al., 1997).

3. Stratified Trend Tests for Dichotomous Data

In tumorigenicity studies, stratified trend tests play an important role in the analysis of dichotomous data. Possible strata are the following:

1. Time intervals for incidental tumors (e.g., ad hoc time strata; Peto et al., 1980) and fixed time intervals given by the National Toxicology Program (Lin and Ali, 1994)
2. Time intervals for fatal tumors

3. Combined analysis of fatal and incidental tumors
4. Combined analysis of several tumor origins or combining several tumor sites

In practice, small-sample sizes are allocated to the different strata; hence, permutative trend test should be used. Under the permutation argument, a stratified trend test is the sum of all single trend tests for each strata (Mehta et al., 1992). The problem of selecting the correct and suitable trend test becomes a serious problem because different shapes are probable. Graves and Pazdan (1995) suggested stratified C-A-test and stated that "the choice of (dose) scores should be very seriously considered." Therefore, Hothorn and Neuhäuser (1997) proposed adjustive permutative versions of the C-A-tests and a corresponding contrast test.

4. Trend Tests in the Presence of Extrabinomial Variation

Because of litter effects in reproductive and some mutagenicity studies, discrete endpoints have an extrabinomial variation. Many procedures have been developed and published (e.g., permutation and bootstrap methods, general estimation equation based test, and maximum quasi-likelihood estimation; Williams, 1987; Lockhart et al., 1992; Boos, 1993; Piegorsch, 1993).

IV. MANY-TO-ONE MCP

In the following, only many-to-one procedures for the one-way design are described; the corresponding simultaneous confidence intervals are discussed in Chapter 6. All-pair comparisons or multiple comparison with the best (Hochberg and Tamhane, 1987; Hsu, 1996) are not relevant for toxicological studies and will not be discussed here.

A. Many-to-One MCPs Without Order Restriction

1. Parametric MCP

a. Simultaneous MCPs: Dunnett's (1955) MCP. The $k + 1$ random variables X_{ij} are independent distributed according to $N(\mu_i, \sigma^2)$ ($i = 0, 1, \ldots, k$). For all $i = 1, 2, \ldots, k$ the null hypothesis $H_0^i: \mu_i = \mu_0$ is tested against the alternative:

1. $H_1^i: \mu_i > \mu_0$ (one-sided for an increase)
2. $H_1^i: \mu_i < \mu_0$ (one-sided for a decrease)
3. $H_1^i: \mu_i \neq \mu_0$ (two-sided for a difference)

From the pooled mean square estimator (MSE), the degrees of free-
dom $v = N - k - 1$ and the correlation coefficients $\rho_{i0} = \sqrt{n_i/(n_0 + n_i)}$,
the k test statistics:

$$td_i = \frac{\overline{X}_i - \overline{X}_o}{\sqrt{MSE(1/n_i + 1/n_0)}} \quad \forall\ i \in (1, \ldots, k)$$

will be compared with the quantile of the multivariate t-distribution
$d_{k,v,\text{one/two-sided},\rho_{i0},1-\alpha}$, which is the solution of the equation

$$\int_0^\infty \int_{-\infty}^\infty \prod_{i=1}^{k-1} [\Phi((\rho_{i0}x + dy)/((1 - \rho_{i0}^2)^{1/2})]d\Phi(x)\Theta(y)dy = 1 - \alpha$$

with Θ denoting the density of $\hat{\sigma}/\sigma$.
H_0^i will be rejected if

$td_i > d_{k,v,\text{one-sided},\rho_{i0},1-\alpha}$ (In case 1)
$td_i < d_{k,v,\text{one-sided},\rho_{i0},1-\alpha}$ (In case 2)
$|td_i| > d_{k,v,\text{two-sided},\rho_{i0},1-\alpha}$ (In case 3)

The quantiles $d_{k,v,\text{one/two-sided},\rho_{i0},1-\alpha}$ (or the related adjusted p values)
can be computed with the function PROBMC in SAS (Table 10) (Anony-
mous, 1995). In the absence of a computer program, the following simple approximation can be used (Hothorn, 1992)

$$d_{k,v,\text{one-sided},\rho=0.7071,1-\alpha=0.95} \approx (1.2708 + 0.52561w - 0.32498z$$
$$+ 0.23913w^5 + 0.034092z^3)t_{v,1-\alpha}$$

with $w = (k - 1)/(k + 1)$ and $z = (v - 1)(v + 1)$.
The dependence of the quantile on the correlation coefficient is
presented in Table 11 for an unbalanced design ($v = 30$, $k = 2$, $1 - \alpha$
$= 0.95$, one-sided).
In a series of articles many-to-one comparisons were published for
different designs: the two-way layout (Cheung and Holland, 1994), the
block design (e.g., Jacroux, 1989), the crossover design (Pigeon and
Raghavarao, 1987), and repeated measurements design (Majumdar,
1988); a Bayesian procedure was given by Brant et al. (1992).
A step-down procedure for the unbalanced case and a step-up procedure was published by Dunnett and Tamhane (1991, 1992). Only for
the step-up procedure in the unbalanced design was a valid proof provided; hence, this method will be described: the statistics td_i are ordered
in a decreasing manner (i.e., $td_{(k)} \geq td_{(k-1)} \geq \ldots \geq td_{(1)}$.

TABLE 10 Selected Quantiles of the Multivariate *t*- and Gaussian Distribution for Correlation Coefficient $\rho = 0.7071$, $n = $ const, and $1 - \alpha = 0.90/0.95/0.99$: a/b/c)

	One-sided			Two-sided		
ν	$k = 2$	$k = 3$	$k = 4$	$k = 2$	$k = 3$	$k = 4$
5	1.87[a]	2.09	2.25	2.43	2.67	2.83
	2.44[b]	2.68	2.85	3.03	3.29	3.48
	3.90[c]	4.21	4.43	4.63	4.98	5.22
10	1.71	1.90	2.02	2.15	2.34	2.47
	2.15	2.34	2.47	2.57	2.76	2.89
	3.11	3.31	3.45	3.53	3.74	3.88
15	1.67	1.84	1.96	2.05	2.23	2.34
	2.07	2.24	2.36	2.44	2.61	2.73
	2.91	2.08	3.20	3.25	3.43	3.55
20	1.64	1.81	1.93	2.05	2.22	2.33
	2.03	2.19	2.30	2.38	2.54	2.65
	2.81	2.97	3.08	3.13	3.29	3.40
30	1.62	1.79	1.90	1.99	2.14	2.25
	1.99	2.15	2.25	2.32	2.47	2.58
	2.72	2.87	2.97	3.01	3.15	3.25
60	1.60	1.76	1.87	1.95	2.10	2.20
	1.95	2.10	2.21	2.27	2.41	2.51
	2.64	2.78	2.87	2.90	3.03	3.12
120	1.59	1.75	1.85	1.93	2.08	2.18
	1.93	2.08	2.18	2.24	2.38	2.47
	2.60	2.73	2.82	2.85	2.97	3.06
∞	1.58	1.73	1.84	1.92	2.07	2.16
	1.92	2.09	2.16	2.21	2.35	2.44
	2.56	2.68	2.77	2.79	2.92	3.00

Step 1. If $td_{(k)} < d_{k,\nu,\text{one-sided},\rho_{i0},1-\alpha}$ then no null hypotheses can be rejected and the procedure stops. For a significant test result, reject the corresponding hypothesis and go to step 2.

Step 2. If $td_{(k-1)} < d_{k-1,\nu,\text{one-sided},\rho_{i0},1-\alpha}$ then no null hypotheses $j < k$ can be rejected, and the procedure stops. With a significant test result, reject the corresponding hypothesis and proceed to the next step.

This stepwise procedure is repeated until the failure to reject a null hypothesis stops the process.

TABLE 11   Quantiles from the Multivariate t-Distributions
for Different Correlations (Calculated with SAS PROBMC
Function; one-sided, $1 - \alpha = 0.95$)

n_i	ρ_{i0}	$d_{k,\nu,\delta_{i0},1-\alpha}$
11, 11, 11	0.7071, 0.7071	1.98907
13, 10, 10	0.6594, 0.6594	1.99880
15, 9, 9	0.6124, 0.6124	2.00639
17, 8, 8	0.5657, 0.5657	2.01241
19, 9, 5	0.5670, 0.4564	2.01816

Source: Anonymous, 1995.

b. α-Adjustment Methods. The α-adjustment represents an alternative approach to simultaneous MCPs that are based on the multivariate t-distribution. Single-step or step-down and step-up can be used. In the single-step case each of the k p-values from the pairwise parametric tests will be compared with α/k (Bonferroni inequality) or with $1 - (1 - \alpha)^{1/k}$ (Slepian–Sidak inequality). For the stepwise procedures these p-values have to ordered by their magnitude [i.e., $p_{(1)} \leq p_{(2)} \leq \ldots \leq p_{(k)}$]. The step-down approach (Holm, 1979) starts with the smallest p-value $p_{(1)}$ with conditional testing at level α/k, $\alpha/(k - 1)$, ..., α, whereas the step-up approach, according to Hochberg (1988), starts with the largest p-value $p_{(k)}$ with conditional testing at α, $\alpha/2$, ..., α/k. A more powerful approach was published by Hommel (1988) and a general approach by Liu (1996). In the parametric case, an α-adjustment seems senseless, because there exists more powerful simultaneous procedures. On the other hand, stepwise procedures based on Welch t-tests seem appropriate for the frequently occurring case of variance heterogeneity, in which simultaneous MCPs are not robust (Rudolph, 1988; Ortseifen and Hothorn, 1995). Only for small-sample sizes a markedly power loss occurs owing to the reduction in the degrees of freedom ($\nu_{0i} = n_i + n_0 - 1$ instead of ν). A SAS-macro was recently published by Ortseifen (1996) and is available via e-mail : hothorm@ifgb.uni-hannover.de.

Example 4. The data from Example 1 will be used here. The adjusted p-values for the one-sided Dunnett procedure for decrease and the 0.95 confidence intervals can be calculated by the simple SAS program:

TABLE 12 Adjusted p Values

Method	Adjusted p values		
	$p_{C\text{-}D\text{max}}$	$p_{C\text{-}D\text{med}}$	$p_{C\text{-}D\text{low}}$
Bonferroni	0.0003	0.0183	0.1014
Holm	0.0001	0.0122	0.1014
Hochberg	0.0001	0.0122	0.1014

```
proc glm;
class dose;
model bodyw=dose;
lsmeans dose/ pdiff=controll ('0') cl;
run;
```

The p-values are $p_{C\text{-}D\text{max}} = 0.0001$, $p_{C\text{-}D\text{med}} = 0.0164$, $p_{C\text{-}D\text{low}} = 0.0821$. For the step-down procedure the related p-values are $p_{C\text{-}D\text{max}} = 0.0001$, $p_{C\text{-}D\text{med}}$ eq 0.0118, $p_{C\text{-}D\text{low}} = 0.0338$. The one-sided confidence intervals are (SAS output):

```
General Linear Models Procedure

                         Least Squares Means
            Adjustment for multiple comparisons: Dunnett
               Least Squares Means for effect DOSE
            95% Confidence Limits for LSMEAN(i)-LSMEAN(j)

                    Simultaneous                       Simultaneous
                       Lower          Difference          Upper
                     Confidence        Between          Confidence
          i     j      Limit            Means             Limit
          2     1        .            -10.613333        1.381417
          3     1        .            -14.740000       -2.745249
          4     1        .            -31.013333      -19.018583
```

It is obvious that the decrease for the high and medium dose is significant but not for the low dose. An advantage of a confidence interval is that it is scale variant (e.g., 95% of a future population will show a maximum decrease of 19 g body weight in the high dose). The following one-sided unadjusted p-values for the many-to-one design are given for the t-tests based on MSE: $p_{C\text{-}D\text{max}} = 0.0001$, $p_{C\text{-}D\text{med}} = 0.0061$, $p_{C\text{-}D\text{low}} = 0.0338$. In this sequence the p-values are ordered, and the adjusted p-values can be simply estimated. The adjusted p-values for Bonferroni, Holm, and Hochberg α-adjustment procedures are given in Table 12.

c.   Closure Principle.   The closure principle, according to Marcus et al. (1976), represents an excellent way to combine global and local decisions without an additional α-effort. The construction principle is simple: define all elementary hypotheses to be tested and form all intersection hypotheses up to the global hypothesis. The testing hierarchy is simply starting with the test of the global hypothesis. If the null hypothesis cannot be rejected the procedure stops; a rejection permits the tests of all intersection hypotheses at the next stage. If a null hypothesis of the intersection hypotheses cannot be rejected, the corresponding implication cannot be tested. Each test can be performed at level α, and the choice of test is free. The partition hypotheses (e.g., $\{1, 2\} \cap \{3, 4\}$) can be tested by Fisher's product criterion or by Bonferroni's inequality. In Fig. 3 an example of a closure system is given for the all-pair comparison problem in the case of four groups (indicated by the numbers 1, 2, 3, and 4).

In Fig. 4, the scheme is restricted to the many-to-one design (one control and three treatments groups: C, 1, 2, 3) without order restriction.

The choice of the tests is free and, therefore, t-tests can be used for the elementary null hypotheses and F-tests for all other hypotheses (see

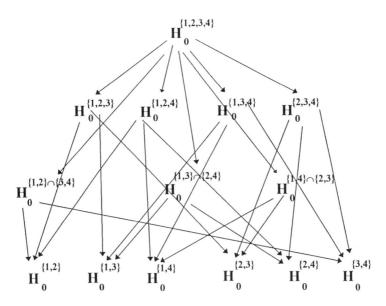

FIGURE 3   Closure system for all-pair comparisons.

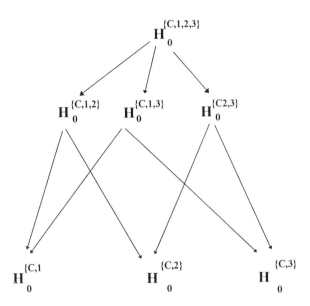

FIGURE 4   Closure system for unrestricted many-to-one comparisons.

foregoing testing hierarchies). More relevant to the many-to-one design is the application of Dunnett's test for each hypothesis:

$$td = \max_{i} \frac{\overline{X}_i - \overline{X}_0}{\sqrt{\text{MSE} \ (1/n_i + 1/n_0)}}$$

But a combination of F-test (global hypothesis) and pairwise contrasts $\{D_i$ vs. $C^-\}$ (all other hypotheses) can be used as well.

2. Nonparametric MCP

a. Simultaneous MCPs. According to the different ranking methods, the nonparametric many-to-one MCPs can be classified into pairwise ranking (Steel, 1959) and k-ranking procedures (Nemenyi, 1963). Several articles (e.g., Koziol and Reid, 1977) demonstrated the superiority of pairwise ranking for the finite situation. The pairwise-ranking procedure is based on the sum of ranks $R_{i.}$ in group i, ranking over the groups 0 and i.

*Exact Version for Small-Sample Sizes (*assuming $n_i = \text{const} = n$). H_0^i will be rejected if $R_{i.} > r_{k,n_0,n,\text{one-sided},1-\alpha}$,   (In case 1)

where $r_{k,n_0,n,\text{one/two-sided},1-\alpha}$ is the $(1 - \alpha)$ quantile of the distribution of $\max(R_{i.})$, and

if $n(n_0 + n + 1) - R_{i.} > r_{k,n_0,n,\text{one-sided},1-\alpha}$ (In case 2)

if $\max(R_{i.}, n(n_0 + n + 1) - R_{i.}) > r_{k,n_0,n,\text{two-sided},1-\alpha}$ (In case 3)

Selected quantiles $r_{k,n_0,n,\text{one/two-sided},1-\alpha}$ are published in Steel (1959) and an approximation formula is given by Hsu (1996).

Asymptotic Version for Larger-Sample Sizes.

1. $ds_i = \dfrac{R_{i.} - [n(n_0 + n + 1)/2] - 1/2}{\sqrt{nn_0(n_0 + n + 1)/12}}$

2. $ds_i = \dfrac{n(n_0 + n + 1) - R_{i.} - [n(n_0 + n + 1)/2] - 1/2}{\sqrt{nn_0(n_0 + n + 1)/12}}$

    $\forall\, i \in (1, \ldots, k)$

3. $ds_i = \dfrac{\max\{R_{i.}, n(n_0 + n + 1) - R_{i.}\} - [n(n_0 + n + 1)/2] - 1/2}{\sqrt{nn_0(n_0 + n + 1)/12}}$

    $\forall\, i \in (1, \ldots, k)$

H_0^i will be rejected

if $ds_i > d_{k,\infty,\text{one-sided},\rho_{i0},1-\alpha}$, (In case 1) with $d_{k,v=\infty,\text{one/two-sided},\rho_{i0},1-\alpha}$ denoting the $(1 - \alpha)$ quantile of the multivariate gaussian distribution with correlation coefficients $\rho_{i0} = \sqrt{n_i/(n_0 + n_i)}$,
if $ds_i < d_{k,\infty,\text{one-sided},\rho_{i0},1-\alpha}$, (In case 2)
if $|ds_i| > d_{k,\infty,\text{two-sided},\rho_{i0},1-\alpha}$ (In case 3)

For ties, the variance estimator can be adjusted according to Brandt (1996). Further nonparametric many-to-one procedures were published by Slivka (1970) (percentiles), Chakraborti and Gibbons (1991) (medians), and Steel (1959a) Rhyne and Steel (1965) (signs). A stepwise approach was given by Campbell and Skillings (1985).

b.   α-Adjustment Methods.   In analogy with the parametric case, single-step or stepwise approaches can be applied for nonparametric two-sample tests (e.g. *u*-test) or related permutative versions.

Example 5.   The data from Example 2 will be used here. The rank sums $R_{i.}$ are $R_{1.} = 114$, $R_{2.} = 132$, $R_{3.} = 132.5$ (which can be calculated from the Mann–Whitney counts U_{0i} using the relationship $R_{i.} = n_i(n_i + 1)/2 + U_{0i}$. Because of the relative large sample sizes $n_i = 10$, the asymptotic version will be used here for the one-sided problem testing for an increase:

$$ds_i = \frac{R_{i.} - [n(n_0 + n + 1)/2] - 1/2}{\sqrt{nn_0(n_0 + n + 1)/12}} \quad \forall\, i \in (1, \ldots, k)$$

The values of the test statistics are $ds_1 = 0.72$, $ds_2 = 2.08$, and $ds_3 = 2.12$. Using the multivariate normal distribution with equal correlation coefficients [based on SAS PROBMC("Dunnett1," 2.12, ... , ∞, 3)] the p-values are $p_1 = 0.44$, $p_2 = 0.048$, $p_3 = 0.044$. Alternatively, permutative u-tests can be used resulting in $p_1 = 0.258$, $p_2 = 0.0205$, and $p_3 = 0.0186$. The adjusted p-values for the many-to-one design based on Holm's procedure are $p_1 = 0.774$, $p_2 = 0.041$, and $p_3 = 0.0186$.

c.   Closure Principle.   The condition of the closure principle is any level-α test; therefore, this principle can be also used in the nonparametric situation. The Kruskal–Wallis test can be used in analogy with the F-test scenario, or Max–Steel test can be used in analogy with Dunnett's test scenario, or a combination of Kruskal–Wallis test (global hypothesis) and pairwise u-tests can be applied.

3.   MCPs for Dichotomous Endpoints

a.   Simultaneous MCPs.   Dichotomous data are discrete and the question arises for which sample size the test statistic fits approximately the asymptotic distribution. This is valid only for the case of large-sample sizes; therefore, exact versions will be discussed now. In analogy with 2×2 tables, the conditional Fisher's exact test assumes a priori known marginal sums. Nevertheless, the marginal sum has to be assumed as random and Suissa and Shuster (1985) published an exact version. Storer and Kim (1990) described an asymptotic exact unconditional distribution that has computational advantages.

Asymptotic Single-Step Simultaneous MCP.   Passing (1984) published the following MCP:

$$tc_i = \frac{(p_i - p_0)}{\sqrt{p.(1 - p.)(1/n_i + 1/n_0)}} \propto t_{k,\infty,\rho_{ij},1-\alpha} \quad \text{with}$$

$$\rho_{ij} = \sqrt{\frac{n_i}{n_i + n_0}}\sqrt{\frac{n_j}{n_j + n_0}}$$

Instead of the total pooled variance estimator, Bristol (1993) proposed an alternative with pairwise pooled variance:

$$tc_i^{\text{pairwise}} = \frac{(p_i - p_0)}{\sqrt{p_{0i}(1 - p_{0i})(1/n_i + 1/n_0)}} \propto t_{k,\infty,\rho_{ij},1-\alpha}$$

where

$$\rho_{ij} = \sqrt{\frac{n_i}{n_i + n_0}} \sqrt{\frac{n_j}{n_j + n_0}} \quad \text{and} \quad p_{0i} = \frac{(r_0 + r_i)}{(n_0 + n_i)}.$$

Koch (1996) demonstrated that this asymptotic version is valid only for very large sample sizes (e.g., > 200).

Exact Conditional MCP for Global Pooled Variance Estimator. An exact conditional many-to-one MCP was recently published by Koch (1996) (Table 13):

$$tc_i = \frac{(p_i - p_0)}{\sqrt{p.(1 - p.)(1/n_i + 1/n_0)}} \propto c_{k,n_i,1-\alpha}$$

Algorithms for computation of quantiles, p-values for any conditions, and an unconditional exact version (not assuming fixed and a priori known marginal sum of success rates) were derived by Koch (1996).

TABLE 13   Selected One-sided Quantiles of $c_{k,n,0.95}$

$n_0 = n_i = $ n.	$k = 2$	$k = 3$	$k = 4$	$k = 5$
10	1.96	2.25	2.35	2.35
15	2.00	2.20	2.24	2.24
20	1.94	2.09	2.22	2.29
25	1.99	2.13	2.27	2.32
30	2.02	2.11	2.20	2.33
40	2.02	2.10	2.24	2.27
50	2.01	2.09	2.22	2.26
60	1.95	2.09	2.21	2.26
80	1.94	2.11	2.22	2.26
100	1.98	2.13	2.18	2.28
200	1.94	2.12	2.21	2.28
∞	1.92	2.06	2.16	2.23

b. *α-Adjustment Methods.* In analogy with the parametric case, single-step or stepwise approaches can be applied for asymptotic two-sample tests (e.g., χ^2-tests; Fisher's exact test; tests according to Suissa and Shuster, 1985; or Storer and Kim, 1990). This approach can be further improved using the conservativeness of permutative tests (Tarone, 1990; Piegorsch, 1993). In the single-step approach a reduction in dimension is possible for all comparisons with $p_{i,\min} < \alpha/k$. This improvement is notable for small-sample sizes or high dimension of k. Recently, Roth (1996) discussed a powerful step-up modification.

Example 6. The data from Example 3 will be used here. A possible downturn at dose 2 should be considered a priori. Therefore, an unrestricted many-to-one MCP for proportions using the unconditional version based on the quantiles $c_{k,n,0.95}$ is applied.
Test statistics:

$$tc_i = \frac{(p_i - p_0)}{\sqrt{p.(1 - p.)(1/n_i + 1/n_0)}} \propto c_{k,n_j,1-\alpha}$$

With the proportions $p_0 = 1/25$, $p_{B1} = 3/25$, $p_{B2} = 11/25$ and $p. = 15/75$ the test statistics are:

$$tc_1 = (0.12 - 0.04)/\sqrt{(0.2(1 - 0.2)(1/25 + 1/25)} = 0.71$$

$$tc_2 = (0.44 - 0.04)/\sqrt{(0.2(1 - 0.2)(1/25 + 1/25)} = 3.54$$

Because $tc_1 = 0.71 < c_{k=3,n\text{-}25,0.95} = 2.13$ and $tc_2 = 3.54 > 2.13$ the null hypothesis is rejected only for the comparison C versus D_2 at level $\alpha = 0.05$.

4. MCPs for Multivariate Endpoints

Although the use of multivariate endpoints in toxicological studies is controversially discussed, a many-to-one modification of Hotelling's T^2-test (Higazi and Dayton, 1984), a many-to-one version of O'Brien's (1984) parametric summary statistics (Kropf et al., 1997), and α-adjustment methods can be performed.

5. Construction Principle for Other Endpoints

In toxicology, many more variables than continuous exist (e.g., Poisson distributed [number of tumors], censored variables [survival distribution], extrabinomial distributed [discrete findings within a teratogenicity study], or stratified test problems for combining fatal and incidental tumors). For these scenarios many-to-one MCPs are not yet available.

However, for small-dimension $k = 2, 3,$ or 4, simply the α-adjustment approach should be used.

B. Many-to-One MCPs with Order Restriction: Total Order

1. Parametric MCP

a. Simultaneous MCPs: Williams' (1971) MCP. Based on the pooled mean square error MSE, the degree of freedom $v = N - k - 1$, the correlation coefficients: $\rho_{i0} = \sqrt{n_i/(n_0 + n_i)}$, and the maximum likelihood estimators of the expected means under the totally ordered alternative $\hat{\mu}_i = \max_{1 \le u \le i} \min_{i \le v \le k} \sum_{q=u}^{v} \overline{X}_q/(v - u + 1)$ $i \in (1, \ldots, k)$ (excluding $\overline{X}_0$), the k test statistics will be computed as follows:

$$tw_i = \frac{\hat{\mu}_i - \overline{X}_0}{\sqrt{\mathrm{MSE}(1/n_i + 1/n_0)}} \quad \forall \; i \in (1, \ldots, k)$$

and H_0^i will be rejected, if $tw_i > \overline{t}_{k,v,\text{one-sided},\rho_{i0},1-\alpha}$.

The quantiles $\overline{t}_{k,v,\text{one-sided},n_0,n,1-\alpha}$ are tabulated in Table 14. Although not documented, the quantiles and the adjusted p-values can be computed by the SAS function PROBMC (Anonymous, 1995).

According to the ordered mean values, the Williams MCP represents a natural closed stepwise procedure in the balanced case (i.e., starting with $tw_k > \overline{t}_{k,v,\text{one-sided}, 1-\alpha}$ and conditional testing: $tw_{k-1} > \overline{t}_{k-1,v,\text{one-sided},1-\alpha}$, and so on).

b. Closure Principle. The general closure scheme can be restricted to the many-to-one and monotonic order (Hothorn, 1995a) (Fig. 5).

The choice of trend tests is free again (see Sec. III). A simple version consists in using pairwise contrasts $\{C^- \text{ versus } D_{\max}\}$ according

TABLE 14 Selected Quantiles $\overline{t}_{k,v\text{-one-sided},\rho_{i0},1-\alpha=0.95}$

df	$k = 2$	$k = 3$	$k = 4$
5	2.142	2.186	2.209
10	1.908	1.940	1.956
15	1.840	1.868	1.882
20	1.807	1.834	1.847
30	1.776	1.801	1.814
60	1.746	1.770	1.781

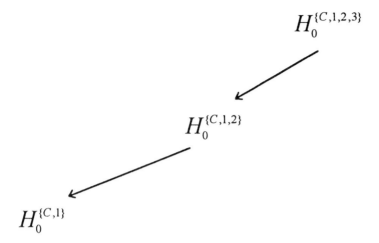

$$H_0^{\{C,1,2,3\}}$$

$$H_0^{\{C,1,2\}}$$

$$H_0^{\{C,1\}}$$

FIGURE 5 Closure system for order-restricted many-to-one comparisons.

to Hothorn and Lehmacher (1991). The application of trend tests for a global test was described by Hothorn (1995a).

Example 7. The data from Example 1 will be used again with a Williams' procedure in a closed step-down version. Start with the global test:

$$tw_k = \frac{\hat{\mu}_k - \overline{X}_0}{\sqrt{\mathrm{MSE}(1/n_k + 1/n_0)}} = \frac{260.43 - 291.44}{\sqrt{243.07 \cdot 2/15}} = -5.45$$

Because the p-value is smaller than 0.05, go to the next step:

$$tw_{k-1} = \frac{\hat{\mu}_{k-1} - \overline{X}_0}{\sqrt{\mathrm{MSE}(1/n_{k-1} + 1/n_0)}} = \frac{276.71 - 291.44}{\sqrt{243.07 \cdot 2/15}} = -2.58$$

With $\bar{t} = \mathrm{PROBMC}(\text{"Williams,"} \ 2.58, ., 56, 2)$ the p-value is 0.0070 and the null hypothesis can be rejected again, and we go to the next step:

$$tw_{k-2}\frac{\hat{\mu}_{k-2} - \overline{X}_0}{\sqrt{\mathrm{MSE}(1/n_{k-2} + 1/n_0)}} = \frac{280.83 - 291.44}{\sqrt{243.07 \cdot 2/15}}$$
$$= -1.864 \text{ and } p = 0.0338$$

Therefore, if we assume a monotonic dose–response relation, all doses show a significant decrease relative to the control. In the following pairwise contrasts as well as an adjusted trend test (Bonferroni-adjusted max[Helmert contrast; reverse Helmert contrast]) will be used employing the closure principle. The global test was already described in Example 1; therefore, we can continue with step 2:

SAS-program

```
proc glm;
class dose;
model bodyw=dose;
contrast 'Helmert contrast' dose -1 -1 2;
contrast 'Reverse Helmert c.' dose -2  1 1;
contrast 'Pairwise contrast' dose -1 0 1 0;
run;
```

SAS-output

Contrast	DF	Contrast SS	Mean Square	F Value	Pr > F
Helmert contrast	1	889.87777778	889.87777778	3.66	0.0608
Reverse Helmert c.	1	1606.97877778	1606.97877778	6.61	0.0128
Pairwise contrast	1	1629.50700000	1629.50700000	6.70	0.0122

The decision of the pairwise contrast is to continue with step 3; the decision of the adjustive trend test is the same, because min(0.0304, 0.0064) < 0.025. Step 3: In the two-sample situation all contrasts are equal. Because the p-value is 0.0338 for the pairwise contrast, the null hypothesis can also be rejected.

2. Nonparametric MCP

a. Simultaneous Procedure According to Shirley (1977). From the k-ranking means $\overline{R}_i$, the correlation coefficients: $\rho_{i0} = \sqrt{n_i/(n_0 + n_i)}$ and the maximum likelihood estimators of the expecting ranking values under the totally ordered alternative: $\hat{R}_i = \max\limits_{1 \le u \le i} \min\limits_{i \le v \le k} \dfrac{\sum_{q=u}^{v} \overline{R}_q}{v - u + 1}$ $i \in$ $(1, \ldots, k)$ (excluding $\overline{R}_0$), the k test statistics can be computed:

$$ts_i = \frac{\hat{R}_i - \overline{R}_0}{\sqrt{(N(N+1)(1/n_i + 1/n_0)/12}} \quad \forall \ i \in (1, \ldots, k)$$

H_0^i will be rejected if: $ts_i > \bar{t}_{k,v=\infty,\text{one-sided},\rho_{i0},1-\alpha}$. The $(1 - \alpha)$ quantiles are shown in Table 15.

Again a closed stepwise procedure can be used in the balanced case here (i.e., starting with $ts_k > \bar{t}_{k,v=\infty,\text{one-sided},1\alpha}$ and conditional testing: $ts_{k-1} > \bar{t}_{k-1,v=\infty,\text{one-sided},1-\alpha}$, and so on) Williams (1986) published a modi-

TABLE 15 Selected Quantiles $ts_i < \bar{t}_{k,v = \infty, \text{one-sided}, \rho_0, 1 - \alpha = 0.95}$

$k = 2$	$k = 3$	$k = 4$	$k = 5$
1.716	1.739	1.750	1.756

fication for stepwise k, $(k - 1)$, $(k - 2)$, . . . ranking; for a randomized block design, House (1986) derived a modification based on Friedman-blocks.

b. Closure Principle. The condition of the closure principle is any level-α test; hence, in analogy with the order-restricted parametric case, this principle can be also used in the nonparametric situation (e.g., any nonparametric contrast test or pairwise u-test). A first version was published by Lüdin (1985).

Example 8. From the data of Example 2, Shirley's closed procedure and a closure based on pairwise u-tests (permutative version) will be demonstrated here. Because the global test according to Shirley was significant, the next step is:

$$ts_2 = \frac{\hat{R}_2 - \overline{R}_0}{\sqrt{N(N + 1)(1/n_2 + 1/n_0)/12}} \propto \bar{t}_{k-1,\infty,1-\alpha}$$

The test statistic $ts_2 = 1.95$, is larger than the quantile $t_{2,\infty,0.95} = 1.716$; therefore, we can go to the next step:

$$ts_1 = \frac{\hat{R}_1 - \overline{R}}{\sqrt{N(N + 1)(1/n_1 + 1/n_0)/12}} \propto \bar{t}_{k-2,\infty,1-\alpha}.$$

Here, the test value 0.43 is smaller than the quantile $t_{2,\infty,0.95} = 1.6449$, the quantile of the gaussian distribution and the procedure stops. The minimum effective dose is D_2. The asymptotic p-values of the u-tests versus control are: $p_{03} = 0.019$, $p_{02} = 0.021$, $p_{01} = 0.25$; hence, the same closure procedure as in the foregoing occurs.

3. MCPs for Dichotomous Endpoints

No many-to-one simultaneous MCP for dichotomous endpoints under order restriction has been published. However, from the closure system (see Fig. 4) simple two-sample tests $\{C^- \text{ versus } D_{\text{max}}\}$; [e.g., Fisher's exact tests (Hothorn and Lehmacher, 1991) or Cochran–Armitage trend tests (Hothorn, 1992) can be used.

TABLE 16   Raw Data: Number of
Revertants in the Ames Assay

Dose/(μg)	Number of revertants				
Control	16	17	17	20	18
5	18	18	19		
15	16	20	20		
50	20	24	23		
150	26	28	20		
500	16	20	16		

C. Many-to-One MCPs with Order Restriction: Principle Order with Possible Downturns at High Doses

In toxicological studies a downturn at high doses sometimes occurs. In such a situation the performance of a trend test can result in a serious loss in power. The use of tests or procedures without order restriction is possible, but a loss in power results if the dose–response is ordered in a monotonic way. Trend tests for the so-called umbrella alternatives were published (e.g., by Chen, 1991). However, the experimental question is to identify increasing effects with possible downturns and not to estimate an umbrella profile. A nonparametric modification of Jonckheere's trend test for downturns was published by Simpson and Margolin (1986), Procedures for partial order or simple tree tests can be used in this situation (e.g., reverse Helmert contrast test; Fligner and Wolfe, 1982).

TABLE 17   MCPs Available in Selected Software

Method	Principle	Conditions
Dunnett, 1955	Parametric, many-to-one	Unbalanced, one/two-sided
Williams, 1971	Parametric, ordered many-to-one	Balanced, one-sided, without PAVA
Koch, 1996	Dichotomous, many-to-one	One-sided, conditional
Koch, 1996	Dichotomous, many-to-one	One-sided, unconditional

TABLE 18   Trend Tests Available in Selected Software

Package	Test	Procedure	Condition
SAS	Linear trend	Proc REG/GLM	Parametric, linearity assumption
	Any contrast	Proc GLM/MIXED, option contrast	Parametric, variance homogeneity
	Adjustive nonparametric test	Macro, Neuhäuser, 1996	Conditional and asymptotic unconditional
	Adjustive dichotomous contrast	Macro, Neuhäuser, 1996	Conditional and asymptotic unconditional
	Adjustive C-A trend test	Macro, Neuhäuser, 1996	Conditional and asymptotic unconditional
	C-A-test	Proc MULTTEST	Asymptotic and exact
SXT	Jonckheere	k-Independent samples/Jonckheere-T	Asymptotic and exact
	C-A-test	Doubly ordered $R \times C$ table	Asymptotic and exact
	Page-test	k-Related samples/page	Asymptotic and exact

The partial ordered procedure (Shaffer, 1986) works as follows: the p-values of the pairwise tests $\{C^- \text{ versus } D_i\}$ are ordered [i.e., $p_{(1)} \leq p_{(2)} \leq \ldots \leq p_{(k)}$]. If $p_{(1)}$ belongs to $\{C^- \text{ versus } D_k\}$ and $p_{(1)} < \alpha/k$ then reject H_0^k and go to the next larger p-value and compare this value with $\alpha/(k-1)$ (Holm procedure). If $p_{(1)}$ belongs to $\{C^- \text{ versus } D_l\}$ for $l < k$ and $p_{(1)} < \alpha/k$ then reject H_0^{li} and ignore all null hypotheses $l + 1$, ..., k. Go to the next larger p value and compare it with $\alpha/(l-1)$. This procedure is based on the p-values, and a similar parametric approach based on linear contrasts was published by Rom et al. (1994).

Example 9. Neuhäuser and Hothorn (1995) demonstrated this principle using the Ames mutagenicity assay data (Table 16).

By using the rank transformation test, according to Brunner and Puri (1997), the p-values are: $p_{5 \ \mu g} = 0.028 < p_{15 \ \mu g} = 0.1175$, $p_{50 \ \mu g} <$

0.0001, $p_{150\ \mu g} < 0.0001$, $p_{500\mu g} = 0.883$. The ordered p-values are $p_{50\ \mu g} = p_{150\ \mu g} = 0.0001 < p_{5\ \mu g} < 0.028 < p_{15\ \mu g} < 0.1175 < p_{500\ \mu g} = 0.883$. Because $p_{50\ \mu g} = p_{150\ \mu g} < \alpha/5$, the null hypotheses for 150 and 50 μg can be rejected (further testing of 500 μg is not necessary), and the next smaller p-value ($p_{5\ \mu g}$) can be compared with $\alpha/2$ level. The conclusion is that the smallest effective dose is 50 μg.

V. SOFTWARE

Standard MCP algorithms are available in most statistics packages. To our knowledge, SAS includes the necessary parametric methods (Tables 17 and 18).

VI. CONCLUSION

Several powerful trend tests and multiple comparison procedures exist in the parametric, nonparametric, and dichotomous situation. The violation of the assumptions of gaussian distribution, variance heterogeneity, possible downturns, and unbalanced data, dramatically reduce the number of useful approaches. Moreover, a uniform, powerful, and robust procedure does not exist. Several approaches are needed and should be implemented in common software (e.g., as SAS-macros).

REFERENCES

Abelson RP, Tukey JW. Efficient utilization of non-numerical information in quantitative analysis: general theory and the case of simple order. Ann Math Stat 34:1347–1369, 1963.

Anonymous. National Archives and Record Service, 10417, 1985.

Anonymous. SAS Technical Report P-229, SAS Institute, Cary NC, 1992.

Anonymous. SAS, Version 6.11. SAS Institute, Cary NC, 1995.

Antonello JM, Clark RL, Heyse JF. Application of the Tukey trend test procedure to assess developmental and reproductive toxicity. I. Measurement data. Fundam Appl Toxicol 21:52–58, 1993.

Armitage P. Tests for linear trends in proportions and frequencies. Biometrics 11:375–386, 1955.

Bailer A, Portier C. Effects of treatment-induced mortality and tumor-induced mortality on tests for carcinogenicity in small sample. Biometrics 44:417–431, 1988.

Barlow RE, Bartholomew DJ, Bremner JM, Brunk HD. Statistical Inference Under Order Restrictions. London: Wiley, 1972.

Bartholomew DJ. A test of homogeneity for ordered alternatives. Biometrika 46:36–48; 328–335, 1959.

Bartholomew DJ. Ordered test in the analysis of variance. Biometrika 48:325–332, 1961.

Berger RL. Multiparameter hypothesis testing and acceptance sampling. Technometrics 24:295–300, 1982.

Bechhofer RE, Dunnett CW. Multiple comparisons for orthogonal contrasts: example and table. Technometrics 24:213–222, 1982.

Benjamini Y. Program and Abstracts of the 1st International Conference on Multiple Comparisons, Tel Aviv, 1996.

Berry JJ. A simulation-based approach to some nonparametric statistic problems. Observations 5:19–26, 1995.

Bieler GS, Williams RL. Ratio estimates, the delta method and quantal response tests for increase carcinogenicity. Biometrics 49:793–801, 1993.

Bolderbuck H, Heimann G, Neuhaus G. Analyzing carcinogenicity assays without cause of death information. Drug Inf J 30:489–507, 1997.

Boos DD. Analysis of dose response data in the presence of extrabinomial variation. Appl Stat 42:173–183, 1993.

Brandt A. Trend Tests für location-scale Alternativen. Ph.D. thesis, University of Hannover 1997.

Brandt A, Hothorn LA. Location-scale trend tests. Report, University of Hannover, 1995.

Brant LJ, Duncan DB, Dixon DO. k-Ratio t tests for multiple comparisons involving several treatments and a control. Stat Med 11:863–873, 1992.

Breslow N. Tests of hypotheses in over-dispersed Poisson regression and other quasi-likelihood methods. J Am Stat Assoc 85:565–567, 1990.

Bristol DR. One-side multiple comparisons of response rates with a control. In: Hoppe FM, ed. Multiple Comparisons, Selection, and Applications in Biometry. New York: Marcel Dekker, 1993, pp 77–96.

Brunner E, Puri ML. Nonparametric methods in design and analysis of experiments. In: Handbook of Statistics, vol. 7, 1997 (in press).

Campbell G, Skillings JH. Nonparametric stepwise multiple comparison procedures. J Am Stat Assoc 80:998–1003, 1985.

Casella G, Berger RL. Statistical Inference. Pacific Grove: Wadsworth & Brooks, 1990.

Capizzi T, Survill TT, Heyse JF, Malani H. An empirical and simulated comparison of some tests for detecting progressiveness of response with increasing doses of a compound. Biometr J 34:275–289, 1992.

Chase GR. On testing for ordered alternatives with increased sample size for a control. Biometrika 61:569–572, 1974.

Chacko VJ. Testing homogeneity against ordered alternatives. Ann Math Stat 34:945–956, 1963.

Chakraborti S, Gibbons JD. One-sided nonparametric comparison of treatments with a standard in the one-way layout. J Qual Tek 23:102–106, 1991.

Chen YI. Notes on the Mack–Wolfe and Chen–Wolfe tests for umbrella alternatives. Biometr J 33:281–290, 1991.

Cheung SH, Holland B. A step-down procedure for multiple tests of treatments versus control in each of several groups. Stat Med 13:2261–2268, 1994.

Cochran WG. Some methods for strengthening the common χ^2 test. Biometrics 10:417–451, 1954.

Collins BJ, Margolin BH, Oehlter GW. Analyses for binomial data, with application to the fluctuation test for mutagenicity. Biometrics 37:775–794, 1981.

Conover WJ, Salsburg DS. Locally most powerful tests for detecting treatment effects when only a subset of patients can be expected to respond to treatment. Biometrics 44:188–196, 1988.

Cuzick J. A Wilcoxon-type test for trend. Stat Med 4:87–90, 1985.

Dunnett CW. A multiple comparison procedure for comparing several treatments with a control. J Am Stat Assoc 50:1096–1121, 1955.

Dunnett CW, Tamhane AC. Step-down multiple tests for comparing treatments with a control in unbalanced one-way layouts. Stat Med 10:939–947, 1991.

Dunnett CW, Tamhane AC. Step-up multiple test procedures. J Am Stat Assoc 87:162–170, 1992.

Dunnett CW, Tamhane AC. Step-up multiple testing of parameters with unequally correlated estimates. Biometrics 51:217–227, 1995.

Fairley D, Fligner MA. Stochastic equivalence of ranking methods. Commun Stat A15:1855–1863, 1986.

Fairweather W, et al. Recommendation for statistical design and analysis of long-term carcinogenicity studies. Drug Inf J (in press), 1997.

Fligner MA, Wolfe DA. Distribution-free tests for comparing several treatments with a control. Stat Neerl 36:119–127, 1982.

Gad S, Weil CS. Statistics and experimental design for toxicologists. Caldwell, NJ: Telford Press, 1986.

Gastwirth JL. On robust rank tests. In: Puri ML, ed. Nonparametric Techniques in Statistical Inference. London: Cambridge University Press, 1970, pp 89–109.

Gastwirth JL. The use of maximin efficiency robust tests in combining contingency tables and survival analysis. J Am Stat Assoc 80:380–384, 1985.

Good PI. Permutation Tests. New York: Springer Verlag, 1994.

Graubard BI, Korn EL. Choice of column scores for testing independence in ordered 2 × k contingency tables. Biometrics 43:471–476, 1987.

Graves TS, Pazdan JL. A permutation test analogue to Tarone's test for trend in survival analysis. J Stat Comput Simul 53:79–89, 1995.

Graves TS. A comparison of test procedures for multidose animal carcinogenicity assays under competing risks. J Biopharm Stat 4:289–320, 1994.

Hauschke D. Testprinzipien bei "Safety" – Studien in der Toxikologie. In: Trampisch HJ, Lange S, eds. Medizinische Forschung Årztliches Handeln. Medizin. Informatik, Biometrie Epidemiologie, vol. 80 München: MVM Medizin Verlag 1995, pp 104–107.

Hauschke D. Statistical proof of safety in toxicological studies. Drug Inf J 30: 197–225, 1997.

Hauschke D, Steinijans VW. Directional decision for a two-tailed alternative. J Biopharm Stat 6:211–213, 1996.

Higazi SMF, Dayton CM. Comparing several experimental groups with a control in the multivariate case. Commun Stat B 13:227–241, 1984.

Hochberg Y. A sharper Bonferroni procedure for multiple tests of significance. Biometrika 75:800–803, 1988.

Hochberg Y, Tamhane AC. Multiple Comparison Procedures. New York: Wiley, 1987.

Hoel DG, Walburg HE. Statistical analysis of survival experiments. J Natl Cancer Inst 49:361–372, 1972.

Holm S. A simple sequentially rejective multiple test procedure. Scand J Stat 6: 65–70, 1979.

Hommel G. A stagewise rejective multiple test procedure based on modified Bonferroni test. Biometrika 75:383–386, 1988.

Horn M, Vollandt R. Multiple Tests und Auswahlverfahren. Stuttgart: Fischer, 1995.

Hotelling H. A generalised T test and measure of multivariate dispersion. Proc 2nd Berkeley Symp Math Stat Prob 1:23–41, 1951.

Hothorn LA. Biometrische Analyse toxikologischer Untersuchungen. In: Adam J, ed. Statistisches Know-How in der medizinischen Forschung. Berlin: Ullstein Mosby, 1992, pp 475–590.

Hothorn LA. Biostatistical analysis of the micronucleus mutagenicity assay based on the assumption of a mixing distribution. Environ Health Perspect 102 (suppl 1):33–38, 1994.

Hothorn LA. Multiple comparisons in long-term toxicity studies. Environ Health Perspect 102 (suppl 1):33–38, 1994a.

Hothorn LA. Biometrie. In: Marquardt H, Schäfer SG, eds. Lehrbuch der Toxikologie. Mannheim: Wissenschaftverlag, 1994b, 15–31.

Hothorn LA. Biostatistical analysis of experimental designs with a positive control group in toxicology. In: Vollmar J, ed. Biometrie in der chemisch-pharmazeutischen Biometrie, vol. 6. Stuttgart: Fischer Verlag, 1994, pp 19–26.

Hothorn LA. Varianten des Abschlußtests zur Auswertung präklinischer Studien. In: Trampisch HJ, Lange S, eds. Medizinische Informatik, Biometrie und Epidemiologie, vol. 80. Munich: MMV Medizin Verlag, 1995a, 117–121.

Hothorn LA, Lehmacher W. A simple testing procedure control versus *k* treatments for one-sided ordered alternatives, with application in toxicology. Biometric J 33:179–189, 1991.

Hothorn LA, Neuhäuser M, Koch H-F. Randomisierte Dosis-Findungs-Studien. Paper Society for Medical Informatics and Statistics, 1996.

Hothorn LA, Neuhäuser M. Stratifizierte Trendtests. Paper presented at the Annual Meeting German IBC, 1997.

Hothorn LA, Lin KK, Hamada C, Rebel W. Recommendations for biostatistics of repeated toxicity studies. Drug Inf J 30:327–334, 1997.

House DE. A nonparametric version of Williams' test for a randomized block design. Biometrics 42:187–190, 1986.

Hsu JC. Multiple Comparisons. London: Chapman & Hall, 1996.

Jacroux M. The A-optimality of block designs for comparing test treatments with a control. J Am Stat Assoc 84:310–317, 1989.

Jonckheere AR. A distribution-free k-sample test against ordered alternatives. Biometrika 41:133–145, 1954.

Koch H-F. Testing strategies for "many-to-one" design with dichotomous data [in German]. Dissertation, Universität Hannover, 1996.

Koziol JA, Reid N. On asymptotic equivalence of two ranking methods f or k-sample linear rank statistics. Ann Stat 5:1099–1106, 1977.

Kropf S, Hothorn LA, Läuter J. Multivariate many-to-one procedures with applications to preclinical trials. Drug Inf J 30:433–447, 1997.

Kruskal WH, Wallis WA. Use rank on one-criterion variance analysis. J Am Stat Assoc 47:583–621, 1952.

Lancaster HO. Significance tests in discrete distributions. J Am Stat Assoc 56: 223–243, 1961.

Lee YJ. Test of monotone trend in k Poisson means. J Qual Techn 17:44–49, 1985.

Lehmann EL. Nonparametrics: Statistical Methods Based on Ranks. San Fransisco: Holden Day, 1975.

Lin KK, Ali MW. Statistical review and evaluation of animal tumorigenicity studies. In: Buncher CR, Tsay J-Y, eds. Statistics in the Pharmaceutical Industry, New York: Marcel Dekker, 1994.

Litt BD, Boyle KE, Myers LE. Statistical analysis of subchronic toxicity studies. In: Krewski D, Franklin C, eds. Statistics in Toxicology. New York: Goron and Breach Science Publishers, 1991, pp 105–125.

Lockhart A, Piegorsch WW, Bishop JB. Assessing overdispersion and dose response in the male dominant lethal assay. Mutat Res 272:35–58, 1992.

Lüdin E. A test procedure based on ranks for the statistical evaluation of toxicological studies. Arch Toxicol 58:57–58, 1985.

Magel RC, Magel KI. A comparison of some nonparametric tests for the simple tree alternative. Commun Stat B 15:435–449, 1986.

Mahrer JM, Magel RC. A comparison of tests for the k-sample, non-decreasing alternative. Stat Med 14:863–871, 1995.

Majumdar D. Optimal repeated measurements designs for comparing test treatments with a control. Commun Stat A 17:3687–3703, 1988.

Mann HB, Whitney DR. On a test of whether one or two random variables is stochastically larger than the other. Ann Math Stat 18:50–60, 1947.

Marcus R, Peritz E, Gabriel KB. On closed testing procedures with special reference to ordered analysis of variance. Biometrika 63:655–660, 1976.

Maurer W, Hothorn LA, Lehmacher W. Multiple comparisons in drug clinical trials and preclinical assays: a priori ordered hypotheses. In: Vollmar J, ed. Biometrie in der chemisch-pharmazeutischen Industrie, vol 6. Stuttgart: Fischer Verlag, 1995, pp 3–18.

McDermott MP, Mudholkar GS. A simple approach to testing homogeneity of order-constrained means. J Am Stat Assoc 88:1371–1379, 1993.

Mehta CR, Patel, NR. A network algorithm for performing Fisher's exact test in *rxc* contingency tables. J Am Stat Assoc 78:427–434, 1983.

Mehta CR, Patel N, Senchaudhuri P. Exact stratified linear rank tests for ordered categorical and binary data. J Comput Graph Stat 1:21–40, 1992.

Meng CYK, Davis SB, Roth AJ. Robust contrast based trend test. ASA Proc Biopharm Sec, 1993, pp 127–132.

Mehta H, Capizzi T, Oppenheimer L. Use of SAS software for trend and sequential trend test analysis. In: Proceedings of the 9th SUGI, SAS Institute, Cary, 1984, pp 794–799.

Mehta C, Patel N. StatXact 3 for Windows. Cambridge: Cytel Software Corp, 1995.

Mukerjee H, Robertson T, Wright FT. Multiple contrast tests for testing against a simple tree ordering. In: Dykstra R, ed. Advances in Order Restricted Statistical Inference. Berlin: Springer, 1986, pp 203–230.

Mukerjee H, Roberston T, Wright FT. Comparison of several treatments with a control using multiple contrasts. J Am Stat Assoc 82:902–910, 1987.

Nam J. A simple approximation for calculating sample size for detecting linear trends in proportions. Biometrics 43:701–705, 1986.

Nelson LS. Tables for testing ordered alternatives in an analysis of variance. Biometrika 64:335–338, 1977.

Nemenyi P. Distribution-free multiple comparisons. Dissertation, Princeton University, 1963. (In German)

Neuhäuser M. [Trend tests for a priori unknown expected value profile]. (In German) Dissertation, University of Dortmund, 1996.

Neuhäuser M, Hothorn LA. Auswertung der Dosis-Wirkungs-Abhängigkeit des Ames Mutagenitätsassay bei direkter Knotrolle des Konsumentenrisikos. In: Trampisch HJ, Lange S, eds. Medizinische Forschung und ärztliches Handeln. Medizin. Informatik, Biometrie und Epidemiologie, vol 80. München: MVM Medizin Verlag, 1995, pp 113–116.

Neuhäuser M, Hothorn LA. Trend tests for dichotomous endpoints. Drug Inf J 30:463–469, 1997.

Neuhäuser M, Hothorn LA. The control of the consumer risk in the Ames assay. Drug Inf J 30:363–367, 1997.

Oluyede BO. Tests for equality of several binomial populations against and order restricted alternative and model selection for one-dimensional multinomials. Biometric J 36:17–32, 1994.

O'Brien PC. Procedures for comparing samples with multiple endpoints. Biometrics 40:1079–1087, 1984.

Ortseifen C, Hothorn LA. Multiple Vergleiche "Kontrolle gegen k Behandlungen" bei Abweichung von den ANOVA-Annahmen. [Multiple comparisons "control versus k treatments under violation of the ANOVA assumptions] [in German] In: Vollmar J, ed. Biometrie in der chemisch-pharmazeutischen Industrie, vol. 6, Sttutgart, Fisher Verlag, 1995, pp 77–100.

Ortseifen C. SAS SUGI. 1996.

Park YC. Kruskal–Wallis trend test for sister-chromatid exchange assay. In: ASA Proceedings Biopharmaceutical Sec. 1987, pp 30–34.

Passing H. Exact simultaneous comparisons with control in an *rxc* contingency table. Biometric J 26:643–654, 1984.

Peto R, Pike M, et al. Guideline for Simple Sensitive Significance Tests for Carcinogenicity Effects in Long Term Animal Experiments. Lyon: IARC Monogr (suppl 2) 1980, pp 311–426.

Piegorsch W. Biometrical methods for testing dose effects of environmental stimuli in lab studies. Environmetrics 4:483–505.

Pigeon JG, Raghavarao D. Crossover designs for comparing treatments with a control. Biometrika 74:321–328, 1987.

Portier C, Hoel D. Type 1 error of trend tests in proportions and the design of cancer screens. Commun Stat A 13:1–14, 1984.

Rhyne AL, Steel RGD. Tables for a treatment versus control multiple comparison sign test. Technometrics 7:293–306, 1965.

Robertson T, Wright FT, Dykstra RL. Order Restricted Statistical Inference. New York: John Wiley & Sons, 1988.

Rom DR, Costello RJ, Connell LT. On closed test procedures for dose response analysis. Stat Med 13: 1583–1596, 1994.

Roth AJ. Multiple comparison procedures for discrete test statistics. In: Benjamini, 1996.

Ruberg SJ. Contrasts of identifying the minimum effective dose. J Am Stat Assoc 84:816–822, 1989.

Rudolph PE. Robustness of multiple comparison procedures: treatment versus control. Biometric J 30:41–45, 1988.

Salsburg DS. Statistics for Toxicologists. New York: Marcel Dekker, 1986.

Shaffer JP. Modified sequentially rejective multiple test procedures. J Am Stat Assoc 81:826–831, 1986.

Shirley EA. A nonparametric equivalent of Williams' test for contrasting increasing dose levels of a treatment. Biometrics 3:386–389, 1977.

Shorack GR. Testing against ordered alternatives in model I analysis of variance: normal theory and nonparametric. Ann Math Stat 38:1740–1753, 1967.

Simes RJ. An improved Bonferroni procedure for multiple test of significance. Biometrika 73:751–754, 1986.

Slivka J. A one-sided nonparametric multiple comparison control percentile test: treatments versus control. Biometrika 57:431–438, 1970.

Steel RGD. A multiple comparison rank sum test: treatments versus control. Biometrics 15:560–572, 1959.

Steel RGD. A multiple comparison sign test: treatments vs. control. J Am Stat Assoc 54:767–775, 1959a.

Storer BE, Kim C. Exact properties of some exact test statistics for comparing two binomial proportions. J Am Stat Assoc 85:146–155, 1990.

Streitberg B, Röhmel J. Exakte Verteilung für Rang- und Randomisationstests im allgemeinen *c*-Stichprobenproblem. [Exact distribution for rank- and randomization test in the general *c*-sample problem] [in German] EDV Med Biol 18:12–19, 1987.

Suissa S, Shuster JJ. Exact conditional sample size for 2 × 2 binomial trials. J R Stat Soc A 148:317–327, 1985.

Tarone RE. Tests for trend in life table analysis. Biometrika 62:679–682, 1975.

Tarone RE. The use of historical control information in testing for a trend in Poisson means. Biometrics 38:457–462, 1982.

Tarone RE. A modified Bonferroni method for discrete data. Biometrics 46:515–522, 1990.

Tarone RE, Gart JJ. On the robustness of combined tests for trends in proportions. J Am Stat Assoc 75:110–116, 1980.

Tamhane AC. Multiple comparison procedures. In: Handbook of Statistics, vol 13. 1996.

Tamhane AC, Dunnett CW, Hochberg Y. Multiple test procedures for dose finding. Biometrics 52:21–37, 1996.

Troendle JF. A stepwise resampling method of multiple hypothesis testing. J Am Stat Assoc 90:370–378, 1995.

Tukey JW. The problem of multiple comparisons (unpublished). 1953.

Tukey JW, Ciminera JL, Heyse JF. Testing the statistical certainty of a response to increasing doses of a drug. Biometrics 41:295–301, 1985.

Yanagawa T, Kikuchi Y, Brown KG. Statistical issues on the no-observed-adverse-effect level in categorical response. Environ Health Perspect 102 (suppl 1):95–101, 1994.

Vollmar J. Biometrie in der chemisch-pharmazeutischen Biometrie, vol 6. Stuttgart: Fischer Verlag 1995.

Weller EA, Ryan LM. Testing for trend with count data. Report Harvard University, 1996.

Westfall PF, Young SS. Resampling Based Multiple Testing. New York: Wiley, 1993.

Wilcoxon F. Individual comparisons by ranking methods. Biometrics 1:80–83, 1945.

Williams DA. A test for differences between treatment means when several dose levels are compared with a zero dose control. Biometrics 27:103–117, 1971.

Williams DA. The comparison of several dose levels with a zero dose control. Biometrics 28:519–531, 1972.

Williams DA. A note on Shirley's nonparametric test for comparing several dose levels with a zero-dose control. Biometrics 42:183–186, 1986.

Williams DA. Dose response models for teratological experiments. Biometrics 43:1013–1016, 1987.

Williams DA. Tests for differences between several small proportions. Appl Stat 37:421–434, 1988.

Wright SP. Adjusted P-values for simultaneous inference. Biometrics 48:1005–1014, 1992.

APPENDIX

TABLE A.1 Body Weight Data

Control	D_{low}	D_{medium}	D_{high}
295.1	287.3	247.5	263.8
277.9	289.5	281.1	255.6
299.4	278.4	284.5	267.2
280.6	281.8	295.0	259.6
285.7	264.9	285.9	238.2
299.2	252.0	273.7	240.4
279.7	284.7	244.1	255.6
277.4	268.9	272.7	255.5
299.2	305.6	262.1	242.5
287.8	295.7	278.8	296.6
292.0	287.6	298.3	246.0
318.8	254.7	298.5	282.7
280.8	292.7	293.5	254.0
292.9	267.9	259.6	280.6
305.2	300.8	275.3	268.2

TABLE A.2 ASAT Data

Control	D_1	D_2	D_3
1.33	2.42	1.53	2.30
1.78	2.22	1.75	1.53
1.53	1.87	2.12	3.17
1.95	1.75	2.83	3.37
1.83	1.80	2.58	2.67
2.17	2.20	2.37	3.25
2.58	1.75	2.92	2.05
2.17	1.97	2.08	3.92
1.97	1.95	3.01	1.25
1.62	1.87	2.99	3.45

5

Subchronic Toxicity Studies

STEVEN BAILEY
Wyeth–Ayerst Research Laboratories, Chazy, New York

I. INTRODUCTION

Subchronic toxicity studies are defined as toxicity studies ranging in length from several days up to 20% of the animal's expected life span. The subchronic toxicity study is one of the first studies done to assess the toxicological effects of repeated dosing with a test compound. Studies are typically designed following guidelines established by the regulatory agencies (DHHS, 1985; FDA, 1987; OECD, 1993); therefore, study design is fairly consistent.

The subchronic study is used to determine the nature of the toxic effects of the test compound and to identify target organs. If designed properly, the study is helpful in determining the no-observed-effect-level (NOEL) and in identifying the lowest dose that elicits a statistically significant response. This information is used to assist in the design of chronic studies and clinical trials.

Although study designs do not differ markedly from sponsor to sponsor, the statistical methods used to analyze these studies vary greatly, depending on the sponsor and the statistical expertise that is available. The traditional statistical approach employed by many sponsors has not changed significantly for several years. Traditional approaches continue to be used because of historical precedent; however, more powerful statistical methods are now available. More sophisticated methods that use recent advances in statistics will be introduced and compared in this chapter.

A few statistical principles will be emphasized repeatedly in this chapter. The reader should pay particular attention to discussions on trend testing, nonnormality of data, skewed data, nonhomogeneous variances, decision tree analysis approach, and one-tailed versus two-tailed tests.

II. TOXICOLOGICAL STUDY DESIGN CONSIDERATIONS

A. Species and Strain Selection

In pharmaceutical development, toxicological studies are done on small animals (rodents) for which economics allows studies with large sample sizes, and in large animals, that have smaller sample sizes, but are more phylogenetically similar to humans. The small animal species commonly used are the rat and mouse, for reasons of economy, availability, and wealth of available historical data. The large animal species commonly used are the dog and monkey. Because of costs, studies conducted with these species have smaller sample sizes, often making a meaningful statistical analysis problematic. However, the similarity between humans and large animal species often enables the toxicologists to glean meaningful information from the individual data values.

Additional problems can exist with monkey studies. First, there is the possibility of contamination of the animals before study initiation. Monkeys that are caught in the wild and, to a lesser extent, first- and second-generation bred monkeys, may have various bacterial organisms and parasites present. Although these may not be detrimental to the animal before study initiation, the assault in combination with test compound treatment may cause important biological effects. This can affect the results in a way such that, combined with the aforementioned small sample sizes, valid statistical results are difficult to achieve. Another problem with monkey studies using wild-caught monkeys is the variable age of the animals. Effects of a test compound vary in magnitude at different stages of an animal's life. Once again, this factor combined with the small sample sizes used in monkey studies can make meaningful analysis difficult to achieve.

B. Route of Exposure

There are various routes used to administer test compound to the study animals: diet, gavage, intravenous, dermal, or inhalation. Ideally, the route of exposure should be analogous with the intended route for humans. The route of exposure chosen can have unwanted problems that can affect the results. For example:

1. Diet: If the diet–test compound mix is unpalatable, decreased food consumption, body weight gain, and related effects may occur. It will be impossible to separate the toxic effect of the test compound and the effect of a decreased food intake owing to unpalatability.
2. Gavage: A gavage study requires a vehicle material that may exert effects of its own. In rodent studies, the procedure can sometimes perforate the esophagus of the animal, causing accidental deaths. Stress from the procedure may also cause effects.
3. Intravenous: Stress from the procedure may cause effects.
4. Dermal: A careful choice of vehicle material is important. Improper choice of vehicle materials could lead to little test compound being absorbed into the animal's system.
5. Inhalation: Inhalation studies are difficult to conduct. Ensuring that the animal receives the proper dose is difficult because of problems in achieving an even concentration of test article in the air of the animal's living environment.

Different routes of exposure may have varying effects because of differences in the metabolic processes. It is important to identify problems with the route and differences in the metabolic process for different routes by conducting studies using more than one route of exposure in each test compound.

C. Dose and Dose Selection

The choice of doses to be used in a subchronic study is one of the most challenging aspects of study design. Information from dose-ranging studies and any prior toxicological studies should be used by the scientist to characterize the anticipated toxic profile of the test compound.

Every toxicological study should contain a concurrent control group in the design. Although there is a wealth of historical information on most study species, comparisons should be made to the maximum extent possible between animals from the same closely defined population. Every study has the possibility of being affected by environmental factors or communicable disease, which could make comparisons to historical controls misleading. All species, particularly inbred laboratory strains, are susceptible to *genetic drift* over time. Animals used as controls should come from the same source and be of a similar age, size, and such as the dosed animals.

There have been several guidelines proposed for choosing doses, but the consensus is to use a high-dose level that will produce a toxicological effect, but not excessive mortality or weight loss compared with control. The low-dose level chosen should produce no toxic effects. At least one other intermediate dose is typically used; this dose level is often 25–50% of the high-dose level.

An alternative method has been proposed by Traina (1983), who recommends using multiples of the anticipated clinical trial doses. For rodents, the recommended doses would be 0, 10, 30, and 100 times the clinical trial dose, and in nonrodents the recommended doses would be 0, 5, 15, and 50 times the clinical trial dose. This method may be applicable for subchronic studies conducted late in the drug development process, but often proposed clinical trial doses are chosen based on results of early subchronic studies.

It is important that the animals receive consistent dosages throughout the study period. To ensure this, the test compound should be periodically sampled and assayed to assess concentration and stability.

D. Test Group Size

Subchronic studies in rodents usually have at least ten animals per sex per dosage group for 1-month studies. Group sizes typically increase as the study duration increases. The most meaningful statistical results, therefore, come from 6-month studies, which have perhaps 25 animals per sex per dosage group and have the animals exposed to the test compound for a longer time, allowing effects to become more evident.

For larger animals, group sizes are often dictated by economic considerations more than statistical considerations. Given the guidelines proposed by Mead (1988), for statistical conclusions to be made from a large-animal study, a minimum of 4 animals per sex per dosage group is required with 5 or more animals per sex per dosage group being preferable. The statistician must be consoled by the fact that for large-animal studies, the toxicologist is often more interested in individual animal values and identifying affected animals in this manner, rather than using statistical techniques to detect dosage group differences. Nonetheless, a statistical analysis is still expected and care must be taken not to place too much emphasis on the results, given the small sample sizes. The relatively few study animals particularly limits the power to detect small or uncommon effects. With this factor in mind, it is recommended by Litt et al. (1991) that for studies with 10 or fewer animals, consideration may be given to p-values up to 0.20 as a basis of statistical inference owing to the low level of study power.

E. Randomization

The effective use of statistics is maximized when the sample of study subjects is divided into comparable groups, by an appropriate method of random allocation, before study initiation. Animals need to be random-ized to dosage groups to balance the variability across animals to the groups. Dosage groups need to be assigned to cages and racks in a manner such that environmental factors that can affect the results will be balanced across the dosage groups.

The sample of animals used in a study contains natural variability for each parameter measured. To minimize this, the simplest approach would be to eliminate unusual animals based on some criterion, usually a function of body weight, and assign the remaining animals to the groups in a random fashion. A directed approach to balance the baseline values of important parameters could be beneficial. If there is a single primary parameter of interest for the study, this could be accomplished by stratifying this parameter. If the study is going to be a general-screening study, the animals are often balanced on body weights, because this is a readily available and reasonably predictive parameter. There is an example of randomization given later that illustrates this stratification procedure. If there is more than one parameter of interest and a desire to balance the allocation over all these parameters, a procedure for two dosage groups has been developed by Taves (1974) and implemented by Jensen (1991) that will balance the allocation to groups across a number of parameters. This procedure can be generalized to more than two dosage groups without much problem. Refer to these articles for details on this procedure.

In addition, the dosage groups should be assigned to cages and racks in such a manner that environmental factors that can affect the results will not be confounded with test compound-related changes. Fac-tors such as heat, light, temperature, and humidity, all affect results. (Andervont, 1944; Ciminera, 1985; Fare, 1965; Hatch et al., 1965; Sigg and Columbo, 1966; Welch and Welch, 1966). Communicable diseases can spread through a portion of the study room and affect a block of study animals. Therefore, a method for assigning dosage groups to the cages and racks that balances the groups within each rack, and within each portion of each rack (top, bottom, front, back, right, left) is required. This is not a difficult task, and there are various possible strategies that would satisfy these requirements. One possible strategy is outlined in the following example.

Example 1. Randomization. Suppose a study is planned with 10 rats per sex per dosage group. The study will contain a control and three dosed groups: 50 male and 50 female rats are received for use in the study. The male rat weights (in grams), sorted by weight, are as follows: 118, 132, 133, 135, 137, 138, 138, 139, 143, 144, 144, 144, 144, 145, 148, 148, 149, 149, 150, 150, 152, 154, 154, 154, 155, 158, 158, 159, 159, 160, 160, 161, 163, 163, 164, 165, 165, 167, 167, 167, 168, 168, 169, 173, 175, 176, 177, 182, 186, 186.

Step 1. Eliminate Outliers. The mean of the foregoing 50 weights is 155.9. Using a criterion of eliminating weights farthest from the mean, the following 10 weights would be eliminated from the sample: 118, 132, 133, 135, 175, 176, 177, 182, 186, 186.

Step 2. Assign Animals to Groups. Create ten stratum of the remaining 40 weights with four animals in each strata. Therefore, the lightest four animals will be assigned to strata 1, the next lightest four to strata 2, and so on. Within each stratum, one animal should be assigned to each dosage group. This should be done in a way such that the lightest animal in each stratum is not assigned to the same dosage group. For example, in strata 1, assign the animals (in order of weight) to groups 1, 2, 3, and 4; in strata 2 use the order 2, 3, 4, 1; in strata 3 use the order 3, 4, 1, 2, and so on. This strategy results in the following group assignments:

Group	Weights	Mean	Standard deviation
1	137,144,148,149,152,159,160,163,165,173	155.0	10.89
2	138,143,148,150,154,155,161,164,167,168	154.8	10.21
3	138,144,144,150,154,158,159,165,167,168	154.7	10.51
4	139,144,145,149,154,158,160,163,167,169	154.8	10.28

Note that the means and standard deviations are balanced reasonably well across all the groups using this strategy. Within each group, the animals with these weights will be assigned sequentially to the cages from the arrangement that is generated in the next step.

Step 3. Assign Groups to Cages and Racks. Assignment of groups to cages and racks often relies on the use of Latin squares. For this example, start with the Latin square

```
1  4  2  3
3  2  4  1
2  3  1  4
4  1  3  2
```

By using a random number sequence, randomly assign doses to the numbers of the Latin square. For the random number sequence 2, 4, 3, 1, the assignment would be 2 = control, 4 = low, 3 = middle, 1 = high. This dose assignment applies to the groups listed in step 2.

By using the Latin square column sequence to fill the front, then the back of the rack (repeating the sequence as needed), along with the weight assignments from step 2, a 4 × 5 rack can now be filled in with group assignments and weights as follows (C = control, L = low, M = middle, H = high-dosage group):

Front of Rack				
H 137	L 144	C 148	M 150	H 152
M 138	C 143	L 145	H 149	M 154
C 138	M 144	H 148	L 149	C 154
L 139	H 144	M 144	C 150	L 154

Back of Rack				
L 158	C 161	M 165	H 165	L 169
C 155	L 160	H 163	M 167	C 168
M 158	H 160	L 163	C 167	M 168
H 159	M 159	C 164	L 167	H 173

This arrangement has a number of desirable properties:

1. Dosage groups are balanced within each column.
2. Dosage groups are as balanced as possible within each row.
3. The end cages on the rack are balanced among dosage groups.
4. Neighboring cages never receive the same treatment.

The same procedure would then be performed for the female animals. This example illustrates a simple procedure for randomization. The procedure ultimately chosen could consider the statistical method that will be used to analyze the study to optimize the randomization. As long as some form of randomization is being performed, the specifics are probably not critical. More complex procedures may add little to the study design and may be so prone to errors that little is gained from the added complexity.

F. Housing and Caging

The number of animals per cage is a factor that should be considered when designing the study. Individual housing for animals leads to improved control over the study because food and water intake can be measured more accurately. Multiply housed animals can also lead to problems owing to aggression and fighting, particularly among male animals.

The types of cages used and the type and amount of bedding material selected can influence the spread of disease and the effect of environmental factors throughout the study population (Fox and Helfrich-Smith, 1980; Keene and Sansone, 1984; Sansone and Fox, 1977; Sansone et al., 1977). This can become particularly important when the test substance affects the animal's immune system.

G. Recovery Studies

Studies are sometimes designed to contain *recovery* animals in some or all dosage groups. This design is used to determine whether test-compound-related effects are reversible once the animals are no longer being dosed with the test compound. Designated animals in each dosage group are typically sacrificed at the end of the dosing period, and the remaining recovery animals are kept in the study for an additional time, without receiving any test compound before being sacrificed. If recovery animals are used, certain parameters that can be collected only at sacrifice (organ weights, terminal blood parameters) will be collected on nonrecovery animals at the end of dosing, and on recovery animals at the end of the recovery period. Therefore, the minimum group sizes specified in Section II. D need to apply independently to the recovery subgroup and the nonrecovery subgroup within each dosage group. These group sizes are required so that valid statistical comparisons can be made at the end of dosing, at the end of recovery, and between the two time periods for these parameters.

H. Statistical Method Specification

Prior selection of statistical methods is an essential component of study design and protocol development. A priori statistical method selection is as important a factor in the design of the study and the preparation of the study protocol as any other factor (as opposed to a post hoc approach). Without a priori method selection, the analysts leave themselves open to the criticism that the statistical methods were chosen in response to the data that were observed. This criticism cannot be refuted, even if it is not true. Many other factors in the study design, such as sample sizes or sampling intervals may depend on the particular methods chosen for analysis. Therefore, it is critical that a statistician be a member of the team responsible for deciding on the study design and developing the protocol.

III. MONITORED PARAMETERS

A. Body Weight

Body weight is perhaps the easiest parameter to collect in a toxicological study, and it is frequently a sensitive indicator of an adverse toxic effect. Also, body weight information on each animal must be kept up to date to perform accurate dose–volume calculations. Consequently, body weight is collected and analyzed on every study.

Often, an analysis of body weights is performed at every week during the study, including predosing (baseline) weeks and recovery weeks, if applicable. If this form of analysis is done, the resulting *p*-values should be used only as a guide, for these tests are not answering specific questions of interest. These tests are analyzing data that is highly correlated from week to week, resulting in *p*-values that do not differ greatly from one week to the next.

An ancillary parameter that is immediately available for analysis is the body weight gain between selected time points. Weight gain is a more sensitive parameter to analyze than body weight. Because each animal acts as its own control, the variability of the data are reduced, making the statistical analysis more sensitive to test–compound-induced differences. If there is a difference between dosage groups in baseline body weights, the gain analysis becomes particularly important, for it would be difficult to make any definitive conclusions from the analysis of raw body weights at subsequent time points.

When analyzing body weights, one must consider trying to reduce the number of analyses and number of p-values that are presented. The typical approach of analyzing body weights at every week results in numerous p-values that come from highly correlated data. One possible alternative analysis strategy would be to perform an analysis at baseline to investigate possible predosing differences, and an analysis of change over selected time periods to investigate possible test–compound-induced differences. This strategy is one possible way of reducing the number of p-values presented without sacrificing the toxicologist's ability to make meaningful conclusions based on the statistical analysis.

B. Food Intake

Food intake is another easily obtainable measurement from toxicological studies. Food intake cannot be measured as accurately as body weight owing to the possibility of food spillage, contamination with urine or feces, and other measurement errors.

If the study involves multiply housed animals, average food intake of the animals in the cage is measured. Average food intake per cage is not as sensitive a measure as individual food intake. If the average food intake per cage is based on different numbers of animals in each cage (e.g., fewer animals owing to death), the variance of these values will differ from cage to cage, violating an assumption required for many of the statistical tests.

Typically, an analysis of food intake is performed every week during the study, including predosing (baseline) weeks and recovery weeks, if applicable. Although the food intake data from week to week are correlated, the problem of performing multiple analyses on correlated data values is not as severe as it is with body weights. Combining food intake over a number of intervals (preferably to correspond to body weight gain intervals) is one possible strategy to reduce the number of p-values presented by the statistical analysis. Once again, the goal is to reduce the number of p-values presented, without sacrificing the toxicologist's ability to make meaningful conclusions based on the statistical analysis.

Body weight gain and food consumption have highly correlated values in control animals. This may not always hold in treated animals if there is a test–compound-related effect that changes the animal's ability to metabolize food, induces diarrhea, or alters the animal's metabolic rate. Hence, an analysis of body weight gain adjusted for food intake over the same period may be of interest. Possible adjusted analyses that could be used in this situation are outlined in Sections VI and VII.

C. Clinical and Laboratory Analyses

To assess the test compound effect over the course of the study, hematological, clinical chemistry, and urine parameters are often periodically monitored. In rodents, owing to the animal's size, periodic blood sampling may induce anemia, with corresponding hematopoiesis that is unrelated to the test compound. Ideally, some type of periodic monitoring of the animal's blood before the initiation of dosing until the conclusion of the study will enhance data validity, as each animal serves as its own control.

Once again, an ancillary parameter that is immediately available for analysis is the change in the value of the analysis parameter over a time period. Change is a more sensitive parameter to analyze than the measured value. Because each animal acts as its own control, the variability of the data are reduced, making the statistical analysis more sensitive to test-compound-induced differences. If there is a difference between dosage groups in the parameter value at baseline, this analysis becomes particularly important because it would be difficult to make any definitive conclusions from the analysis of the parameter values at subsequent time points. The body weight analysis strategy, mentioned earlier, that uses baseline values and change values is applicable for these data as well.

Little effort has yet been made to explore the relations between hematological, clinical chemistry, and urine parameters. As these interrelations are explored in greater detail, more powerful multivariate analyses may become a possibility.

D. Organ Weights

At necropsy, weights are collected on a selected set of organs. The analysis of organ weights is a valuable tool for identifying target organs affected by the test compound.

Some organs have weights that are highly correlated with terminal body weight (e.g., heart). Other organs have weights that have low correlation with terminal body weight (e.g., brain, adrenal). Therefore, for each organ, either unadjusted organ weight, organ weight adjusted for terminal body weight, organ weight adjusted for brain weight, or some combination of the three may be needed to assess test compound effects. The appropriate analysis for a given organ should be decided before a study's initiation and be based on the relation between the organ weight and the terminal body weight or brain weight in historical control animals.

Frequently, the organs of interest (except the brain) in healthy animals change weight relative to the final body weight. There is particular interest in organs for which this relation is not true. Therefore, the analysis adjusting for body weight will be sensitive to this situation, detecting cases in which the organ weight *relative to the body weight* has changed because of the test compound treatment.

The brain weight is thought to be unaffected by test–compound-induced changes in the body weight, as well as unaffected by most test compounds. The brain weight is thought to be highly correlated with how large the animal was at the initiation of treatment. Therefore, the analysis adjusting for brain weight will detect cases for which the organ weight *relative to the "true" size of the animal* has changed because of the test compound treatment.

There is disagreement on how to adjust for the terminal body weight or the brain weight in the analysis. Two common strategies are to analyze the ratio of the organ weight to the chosen adjustor (either the terminal body weight or the brain weight), or to perform a covariance analysis using either the terminal body weight or the brain weight as the covariate in the model. If the ratio approach is used, the ratios would be calculated and these values would be analyzed using a one-way analysis approach, similar to that used for any of the other parameters. Details on the analysis of covariance approach will be outlined in Sections VI and VII.

It is interesting that in the discussion on which of these methods is more appropriate, toxicologists and pathologists usually favor the ratio approach, perhaps because it is easier to understand and visualize, whereas many statisticians favor the analysis of covariance approach, possibly because the mathematical model is more flexible and includes the ratio analysis as a special case. It is easy to make the mistake in thinking that analyzing ratios means that there are no assumptions that should be assessed. In fact, the relation between the organ weight and the adjustor assumed by the ratio analysis is more restrictive than the relation assumed by the covariance model, and this relation should be assessed for validity. The analysis of covariance model assumes that the underlying relation between the organ weight and the adjustor is linear with a slope and an intercept term e.g. the relation can be expressed as

$$Y = a + bX$$

where Y is the organ weight, X is the adjustor value, a is the intercept, and b is the slope. The ratio model assumes that the relation between the response variable and the adjustor is linear, with no intercept (i.e., the relation is proportional). This relation can be expressed as

$$\frac{Y}{X} = b \qquad \text{or equivalently} \qquad Y = bX$$

Therefore, the ratio model is a more restrictive model that is a special case of the analysis of covariance model. Accordingly, it would seem that the added flexibility of the analysis of covariance model should make it the analysis strategy of choice.

E. Histopathology

Histopathological examinations are usually done in subchronic toxicology studies, but the limited duration of the study means that few tumors are found. Thus, histopathology is rarely analyzed in subchronic studies. When histopathology is analyzed, the analysis is identical with the one that is performed for chronic toxicity studies.

F. Other Parameters

On occasion, other parameters are collected on subchronic toxicity studies to answer specific test–compound-related questions. Some examples would be grip strength data on test compounds that are suspected to cause muscle atrophy, or sperm count data on test compounds that target the male reproductive system. These additional parameters need to be evaluated on a case-by-case basis for the best analysis, but the statistical methods that apply to the foregoing data types can usually also be used on these additional parameters.

IV. ANALYTICAL CONSIDERATIONS

In the next few sections, several statistical tests that have been proposed for the analysis of toxicological data will be presented. Some of these tests are better than others; however, all have been presented in the literature as appropriate. No assessment of the relative merits of the tests will be made at this time. The intent is to first present the regularly cited methods for the purpose of completeness. In Section VIII a comparison of the merits of the various tests will be made.

The tests presented in the next few sections are trend tests in that they test for a monotonic response over increasing dosage levels. It is generally accepted that if there is a test–compound-induced response for a given parameter, it will most often be a monotonic response, with larger doses of the test compound causing larger effects. There are various possible test–compound-induced response patterns that all share this property of monotonicity; several of these are illustrated in Fig. 1. The most powerful statistical tests to detect a dose–response of this nature are trend tests (Selwyn, 1995). The tests outlined in the following sections are either trend tests or can be implemented in such a way that the trend hypothesis is tested. Analyses that test the general hypothesis instead of the trend hypothesis have historically been used by many laboratories to analyze all the study data; I will recommend these tests only for the analysis of predosing (baseline) data.

A subchronic toxicity study is designed to answer two questions. First, does the test compound cause an effect for a given parameter? Second, if an effect is found, what is the NOEL? The first question is answered by trend tests, as discussed in the last paragraph. Once an effect has been detected, trend tests are also well suited to determining the NOEL. A strategy designed to answer this question has been outlined by various authors (Tukey et al., 1985; Selwyn, 1988; Selwyn, 1995) and is straightforward in its approach. This strategy is illustrated for four dosage groups (control plus three nonzero dose groups) in Fig. 2. To briefly summarize, if the result from the initial test using all groups is not significant, it is concluded that there is no effect and no further testing is performed. If the result from the initial test is significant, it is concluded that there is an effect at the high-dose level and testing contin-

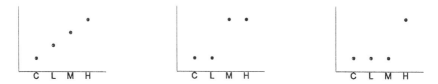

FIGURE 1   Possible dose–response trends.

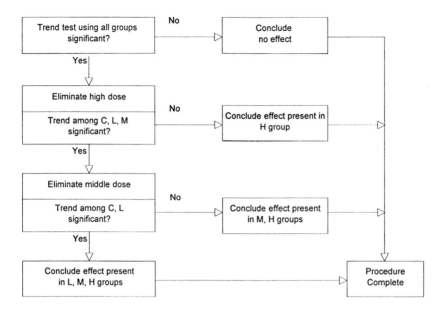

FIGURE 2 Strategy for trend testing (four groups). Key: C, control; L, low dose; M, middle dose; H, high dose.

ues using all the groups except the high-dose group. This process continues until a nonsignificant result is found or it is concluded that an effect is present at the low dose level. When applicable, this procedure will be used to determine the NOEL for the examples in Sections VI and VII.

One approach that will not be presented in detail is what is referred to as the decision tree (or flow chart) approach. In the past many authors have advocated and many laboratories have used the decision tree approach to govern the choice of the statistical test to be used to analyze a given parameter. For example, the data from the parameter would be tested for equality of group variances. If this test was not significant, the data in each dosage group would then be tested for normality. If this test was not significant, then a parametric statistical test would be performed to test for possible test compound effects. If any of the assumptions tests were significant, then alternative methods, such as data transformations or nonparametric tests, would be used. An example of such a decision tree is given in Fig. 3.

There are several reasons why the decision tree approach is not

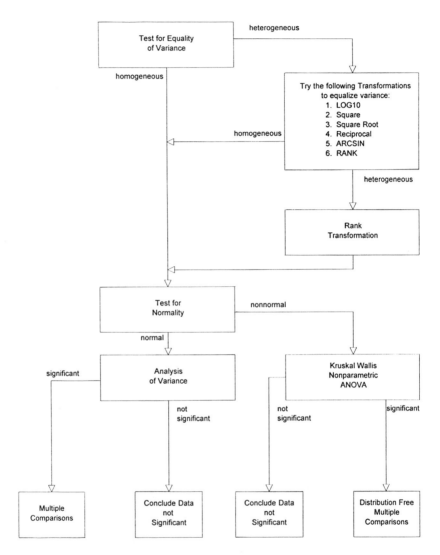

Figure 3   Example of a decision tree approach.

desirable (Selwyn, 1995). First, in a typical 3-month rat study containing four groups, between body weights, food intake, hematology, clinical chemistry, and organ weights, there may be up to 500 analyses, requiring 2000 tests for normality and 500 tests for equality of variance. Given this multitude of tests, what does it mean when one of these tests is significant? Second, if an assumption test is significant and the data is transformed, what does the result of the analysis on data transformed in some unusual way (e.g., by square roots) really mean? Given the multitude of parameters being analyzed, a decision tree approach could lead to confusion over which test was used to analyze a given parameter. Finally, comparisons across time points or across studies for a given parameter may be difficult to assess because different statistical methods may be employed.

Decisions concerning appropriate transformations and decisions about the use of parametric versus nonparametric methods should be based on historical information and should be made before a study's initiation. These decisions should not be based on the data observed for a given parameter in a given study. The decision tree (or flowchart) approach, though historically used for many studies, should be avoided and will not be discussed further.

V. DESCRIPTIVE STATISTICS

Descriptive statistics are used to characterize the features of a data set for a given parameter of interest. These measures are helpful to the scientists trying to make sense out of the p-values that result from the analysis.

The descriptive statistics that have been historically presented in subchronic toxicity studies are the mean, standard deviation (or standard error of the mean), and the sample size. These are well understood descriptors of the data that the toxicological community has been working with for years.

Even at this simple level, there is room for improvement over the commonly used statistics. When the mean and standard deviation are evaluated to characterize the distribution of the data, the way they are used implicitly assumes that the data are symmetric and that the data are distributed close to a normal distribution. For many types of toxicological data, these assumptions are far from the truth. Mitruka and Rawnsley (1977) and Weil (1982) have documented this fact. Also, both the mean and standard deviation are sensitive to outliers in the data.

Some alternate descriptive statistics that are more meaningful in these situations are the median (50th percentile), the interquartile range (the 75th percentile minus the 25th percentile), and the sample size. The median is used as the measure of location (instead of the mean), and the interquartile range is used as the measure of dispersion (instead of the standard deviation). These descriptive statistics do not implicitly assume the data are distributed following any underlying statistical distribution. Also, these measures are not sensitive to outlying values. Skewed data could still be misleading because the interquartile range does not account for skewness in any way. To remedy this problem, one could present the actual values for the 25th and 75th percentiles (the quartiles) instead of the interquartile range, allowing evaluation of both the dispersion and the skewness of the data set.

Example 2. Descriptive Statistics. To illustrate the use of the foregoing descriptive statistics, a random sample of 100 alanine aminotransferase (ALT) values from untreated monkeys (measured in international units per liter; IU/L) were taken from historical control data. A frequency histogram of the data is given in Fig. 4. The descriptive statistics for this data sample are as follows:

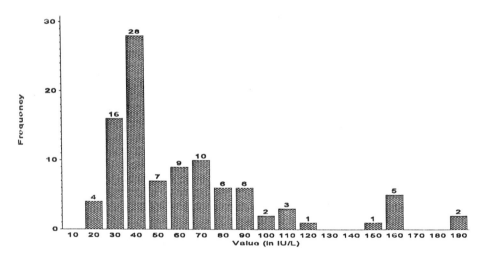

FIGURE 4   Distribution of ALT values in 100 randomly selected monkeys.

Mean	Standard deviation	25th percentile	Median	75th percentile	Interquartile range
62.34	38.81	37.0	46.5	75.0	38.0

It can be seen from the histogram that the data are skewed with a long right tail, and there are many large outlying values. The mean and standard deviation would describe the distribution of a data set well if the data were normally distributed. In this case, statements describing the data that are based on the mean and standard deviation may be misleading. For example, 95% of the data are usually assumed to fall within 1.96 standard deviations of either side of the mean. For these data, this interval would be from -13.73 to 138.41. Because ALT values can never be smaller than 0, it is biologically impossible to observe values in 9% of this interval. There is also a larger than expected number of observed values higher than the upper limit of the interval (8% observed versus 2.5% expected). The median and quartile values, on the other hand, are robust descriptors that are not sensitive to nonnormal or skewed data.

Many biological parameters have skewed distributions, with long right tails. In these cases, the mean and standard deviation, as they are typically used, will not be an accurate description of the data and may lead to misleading conclusions. For these parameters, the median and selected percentiles would more accurately portray the distribution of the data.

There is nothing magical about the 25th and 75th percentiles. One could present the 10th and 90th percentiles as measures of dispersion and symmetry, or even the minimum and maximum values. The farther one moves toward the extremes of the data, the more sensitive the measures become to outlying values, particularly in small data sets. The quartiles (25th and 75th percentiles) have an intuitive appeal and have historically been more widely used than any of the alternatives.

VI. PARAMETRIC STATISTICAL METHODS

Parametric statistical methods are appropriate for data that are measured using a continuous (or approximately continuous) numerical scale and that are distributed, or can be transformed such that they are distributed following a specified (usually normal) distribution. Many toxicological parameters, particularly those for blood chemistry, approximately follow a log–normal distribution. For these parameters, a log transformation would be appropriate to normalize the data for analysis by the following procedures. Once again, discussions on transformations should be made based on historical information and should not be based on preliminary assumptions testing of the study data. Further discussion on transformations will be given in Section X.

A. One-Way Analysis of Variance

Analysis of variance (ANOVA) methods have been used historically to analyze subchronic toxicity data. The one-way ANOVA tests the null hypothesis:

$$H_0 : \mu_1 = \mu_2 = \ldots = \mu_k$$

against the alternative:

$$H_a : \mu_i \neq \mu_j \quad \text{for some } i, j, \text{ where } i \neq j \text{ and } 1 \leq i,j \leq k$$

Details on these calculations can be found in any standard text on data analysis (e.g., see Neter et al., 1985). Any statistical computer package should have an automated procedure to perform the analysis of variance.

If the one-way ANOVA is significant, the conclusion is that a difference among the dosage groups exists; however, conclusions cannot be made for the NOEL, which is the question of interest. To answer this question, some form of a follow-up procedure is needed.

One follow-up method that is commonly used is to perform pairwise t-tests for each dosed group to the control group, using the error mean square from the one-way ANOVA model. This method, although commonly employed, does not account for the ordered structure of the groups and, therefore, is less powerful than a trend test. This method may be the only logical choice in studies that do not have increasing doses of a single test compound (e.g., studies testing several different compounds against a control). In typical toxicological studies involving a control and several increasing dose levels of a single test compound, a trend test is the test of choice.

A more powerful analytical method that could be used when the study contains a control and several increasing doses of a single test compound would be to use statistical contrasts. There are a variety of different approaches using contrasts that can be employed to answer questions about the NOEL. Four commonly suggested strategies for four dosage groups are as follows:

Strategy 1	*Interpretation*
Contrast 1 = $(-1/3, -1/3, -1/3, 1)$	Control, low and middle < high
Contrast 2 = $(-1/2, -1/2, 1/2, 1/2)$	Control and low < middle and high
Contrast 3 = $(-1, 1/3, 1/3, 1/3)$	Control < all doses
Strategy 2 *(orthogonal contrasts)*	
Contrast 1 = $(-1/3, -1/3, -1/3, 1)$	Control, low and middle < high
Contrast 2 = $(-1/2, -1/2, 1, 0)$	Control and low < middle
Contrast 3 = $(-1, 1, 0, 0)$	Control < low
Strategy 3 (linear trend)	
Contrast 1 = $(-3, -1, 1, 3)$	Linear trend for groups 1–4
Contrast 2 = $(-1, 0, 1, 0)$	Linear trend for groups 1–3
Contrast 3 = $(-1, 1, 0, 0)$	Linear trend for groups 1–2
Strategy 4 *(Newman–Kuells)*	
Contrast 1 = $(0, 0, -1, 1)$	Middle < high
Contrast 2 = $(0, -1, 1, 0)$	Low < middle
Contrast 3 = $(-1, 1, 0, 0)$	Control < low

With use of any of these strategies, the test for contrast 1 would be performed first to determine if the high-dose group was affected by the test compound. If this test is significant, the test for contrast 2 would be performed to determine if the middle-dose group was affected by the test compound. Then, if this test is significant, the test for contrast 3 would be performed to determine if the low-dose group was affected by the test compound. This information would then be used to determine the NOEL for the parameter being analyzed.

Note that strategies 1 and 2 have similar interpretations; however, strategy 1 uses information from all the dose groups in every contrast, whereas strategy 2 does not. Strategy 3, after the initial contrast testing for a trend in all groups, is no different than performing pairwise follow-up tests. The initial contrast given in this strategy is the most sensitive to a trend that exhibits a consistent change from group to group. Strategy 4 is simply a series of pairwise comparisons between adjacent groups in the dose ordering.

Example 3. The following neutrophil (NEUT) data were observed in a subchronic rat study:

Group	NEUT value	Mean
1	16.2, 16.6, 21.2, 21.4, 21.9	19.46
2	16.1, 21.9, 23.1, 23.5, 23.8	21.68
3	17.5, 20.2, 21.9, 23.1, 24.1	21.36
4	19.4, 23.1, 24.1, 30.1, 31.0	25.54

These data will be used to illustrate several statistical procedures outlined in this chapter.

Analyzing these data with the one-way ANOVA model results in a p-value of 0.084. Analyzing these data using a one-way model with the trend contrast strategies gives the following results:

	Contrast 1 p-value	Contrast 2 p-value	Contrast 3 p-value
Strategy 1	0.019	0.084	0.078
Strategy 2	0.019	0.686	0.331
Strategy 3	0.021	0.403	0.331
Strategy 4	0.077	0.887	0.331

When using the interpretation as outlined in the foregoing, for any of these strategies, contrast 1 would be examined first to determine if there was a test compound effect present. Note that strategies 1, 2, and 3 all conclude that there is a test compound effect present at the high-dose level, whereas strategy 4 does not detect any test compound effect. The follow-up analysis for strategies 1, 2, and 3 would have us examine the p-value for contrast 2 next, to determine if there was a test compound effect present at the middle-dose level. None of these strategies detected an effect at this level.

B. Linear Trend Test

A test for linear trend with dosage level may be performed based on the model

$$X_{ij} = a + b\,d_i + e_{ij}$$

where

X_{ij} is the jth response at dose d_i.
d_i is the dosage level.
a is the fitted intercept (expected value for control animals).
b is the fitted slope of the regression line.
e_{ij} is a random error term.

This model is a simple linear regression model regressing response on the dosage level. Details on regression models can be found in any basic data analysis text (e.g., see Neter et al., 1985).

Note that the linear trend test is testing for a trend that is linear with dose, because the actual dosage levels are used when fitting the model. Dose–response curves are seldom linear over the wide range of dose levels that are used in a subchronic toxicity study. For some test compounds, the dose–response relation is linear relative to the logarithm of dose. Weil (1972) found the logarithm of dose to be the most effective transformation of dose when modeling the dose–response relation. In these cases, using the logarithm of dose instead of the actual dose level in the foregoing model would improve the validity of the modeling procedure.

This approach is not widely used to analyze subchronic toxicity data. Whether the actual dosage level, the logarithm of the dosage level, or some other transformation of the dosage level is used, the model is dependent on the linearity of the chosen dose–response relation. In reality, many test compounds do not exhibit a linear dose–response relation using either untransformed or transformed values for the dose levels. For example, many test compounds exhibit a threshold effect, during which effects become quite noticeable above a given dosage level, but are almost nonexistent below this level. In these instances, linear regression models do not fit the data well. Also, the limited number of dosage levels used in subchronic toxicological studies combined with the variability of the data do not generate enough information to justify modeling procedures.

A linear trend test approach may have its place later in the drug development process to model the dose–response relation to perform low-dose extrapolation. However, the general questions of interest in a subchronic toxicity study (Is there an effect? If there is, what parameters are affected? What is the NOEL?) require trend-testing methods that will be sensitive to any form of a monotonic dose–response relation.

C. $\bar{t}$ Test (Williams' t-test)

The $\bar{t}$ test (Williams, 1971, 1972) is an order-restricted version of the t-test. It is a series of tests that test the hypothesis:

$$H_0 : \mu_1 = \mu_2 = \ldots = \mu_k$$

against the alternative:

$H_a : \mu_1 \leq \mu_2 \leq \ldots \leq \mu_k$, with at least one inequality being strict.

The idea behind this test is to "amalgamate" means such that they are in nondecreasing order, then calculate the test statistic on the amalgamated values. This amalgamation procedure is important in several tests listed in this section; it is presented in detail in Box 1. Note, that for this test, the control group is excluded from the amalgamation process. (In Williams' 1971 paper, the control group was included in the amalgamation process; however, in the follow-up 1972 paper, the control group was excluded from amalgamation. This presentation uses the more recent 1972 presentation.)

For the $\bar{t}$ test, under H_a the amalgamated means are the maximum likelihood estimates of $\mu_2, \ldots, \mu_k$. The test is used to determine the smallest dosage level that exhibits a difference from the control group, assuming a monotonic ordering of the dose responses. The test is similar in form to the t-test, except that the amalgamated mean values are used instead of the observed mean values in the calculation of the test statistic. If the amalgamation process does not change the means, the test statistics are identical with the t-test. Details on the calculations are given in the Box 2.

This test is superior to pairwise t-tests to determine the NOEL. However, the concerns raised in Box 1 describing the amalgamation procedure are a drawback to this test. Also, in Williams' papers, critical values are presented for only the equal sample size case and only for a limited number of group sample sizes. If critical values for the particular sample sizes in the experiment are desired, calculations similar to those performed by Williams would be required. The need to perform these calculations is another drawback to this procedure.

Box 1 Amalgamation Procedure

Note: This presentation explains the amalgamation procedure using all the groups in the study, because this is how the procedure is commonly used. For the $\bar{t}$ test, the control group would be excluded from the amalgamation procedure.

Suppose the following data is observed:

Group	Mean	Sample size
1	12	10
2	15	10
3	5	10
4	40	10
5	30	20

If we are interested in testing for an increasing trend, the foregoing mean values need to be amalgamated so that they are in nondecreasing order. The method of amalgamation used is referred to as the *pooled adjacent violators algorithm* (Barlow et al., 1972).

To perform this procedure, beginning with group 1, look for the first occurrence of a decreasing mean. In the example data, this occurs between groups 2 and 3. Replace the means for groups 2 and 3 with the following:

Amalgamated mean $= (\bar{x}_2^* w_2 + \bar{x}_3^* w_3)/(w_2 + w_3)$
Amalgamated weight $= w_2 + w_3$

where

$\bar{x}_2, \bar{x}_3$ are the means for groups 2 and 3
w_2, w_3 are the weights for groups 2 and 3

For the example data given in the foregoing, using the sample sizes as the weights ($w_i = n_i$), the values are now the following:

Group	Mean	Sample size (wt)
1	12	10
2-3	10	20
4	40	10
5	30	20

Use these modified data, start the procedure over, and repeat this process until the adjusted means are all in nondecreasing order.

For the example data given in the foregoing, this would result in the following amalgamated values:

Group	Mean	Sample size (wt)
1–2–3	10.667	30
4–5	33.333	30

A Caution Concerning Amalgamation. It is important to use caution when using tests that employ the pooled adjacent violators algorithm to analyze data. There are situations for which extensive pooling would lead to potentially misleading test results. For example, for the data

Group	Mean	Sample size (wt)
1	10	10
2	30	10
3	20	10
4	30	10
5	10	10

If the test is for an increasing trend (using the sample sizes as the weights) the amalgamated values would be

Group	Mean	Sample size (wt)
1	10	10
2–3–4–5	22.5	40

If the test is for a decreasing trend, the amalgamated values would be

Group	Mean	Sample size (wt)
1–2–3–4	22.5	40
5	10	10

These amalgamated values will result in the same p-value for either an increasing or a decreasing trend test. Clearly, this problem is occurring because the monotonicity assumption is violated.

This situation could be avoided by performing a lack-of-fit test to assess how extensively the data have been amalgamated. Although it has been suggested that a test of this type would not be difficult to derive, I am not aware of any widely accepted test that performs this function.

Box 2 The $\bar{t}$ Test (Williams' Test)

Data. The data consist of k random samples. Denote the data in the ith random sample of size n_i by x_{i1}, x_{i2}, . . . , x_{in_i}. Then the data may be arranged as follows:

Sample 1	*Sample 2*	. . .	*Sample* k
$x_{1,1}$	$x_{2,1}$		$x_{k,1}$
$x_{1,2}$	$x_{2,2}$		$x_{k,2}$
. . .	. . .		. . .
x_{1,n_1}	x_{2,n_2}		x_{k,n_k}

Assumptions.

1. All samples are random samples from their respective populations.
2. The observations within each sample are independent, and there is mutual independence among the various samples.
3. The data from each of the k populations are normally distributed.
4. The k population distribution functions have equal variances.

Test Statistic. To calculate the test statistic, first the sample means from all groups except the control group should be amalgamated by using the pooled adjacent violators algorithm explained in Box 1, with the weights being defined as $w_i = n_i$ for groups $i = 2, . . . , k$, where n_i is the group sample size. For the calculation of the test statistic, however, rather than using amalgamated groups, simply replace the corresponding sample means with the amalgamated mean wherever groups were amalgamated.

Therefore, after amalgamation there are still k populations and the subscript i will continue to index the populations. If we define the following terminology:

n_i = sample sizes of the groups ($i = 2, . . . , k$)
n_1 = sample size of group 1 (control)
M_i = corrected mean of group i after amalgamation ($i = 2, . . . , k$)
x_1 = sample mean for group 1 (control)
s^2 = mean square error

The test statistic is

$$\bar{t}_i = (M_i - x_1) \left(\frac{s^2}{n_i} + \frac{s^2}{n_1} \right)^{-1/2}$$

Decision Rule. The critical values at various significance levels for this test statistic in the equal sample size case are presented in Williams' 1972 article. In the unequal sample size case, Williams found that the equal sample size results worked adequately as long as the differences in the sample sizes were moderate. For larger differences in the sample sizes between groups, methods for the generation of critical values are outlined in Williams' 1971 and 1972 papers.

The test is performed sequentially, starting with the highest amalgamated dosed group (i.e., $i = k$). If $\bar{t}_k$ is significant, the test is then performed on the next lowest amalgamated dosed group (i.e., $i = k - 1$), using the M_{k-1} from the original amalgamation of means (do not reamalgamate at each step). This process is repeated until an amalgamated dosage level i is reached that is not significant.

Example 4. The NEUT data outlined in Example 3 will be used to illustrate this test. For neutrophils, the toxicologist has decided that we are interested in an increasing trend only; therefore, the test performed will be a one-tailed test for increasing trend. First, the mean values must be amalgamated to be in nondecreasing order. Therefore, groups 2 and 3 are amalgamated, using the sample sizes as the weights. This results in the following amalgamated mean:

$$\text{Amalgamated mean} = \frac{(\bar{x}_2 * w_2 + \bar{x}_3 * w_3)}{(w_2 + w_3)}$$
$$= \frac{(21.68 * 5 + 21.36 * 5)}{(5 + 5)}$$
$$= 21.52$$

The test statistic calculation will therefore use the following mean values: 19.46, 21.52, 21.52, 25.54.

The initial test statistic for the high-dose group is calculated as follows:

$$\bar{t}_4 = (M_4 - x_1)\left(\frac{s^2}{n_4} + \frac{s^2}{n_1}\right)^{-1/2}$$

$$= (25.54 - 19.46)\left(\frac{12.25}{5} + \frac{12.25}{5}\right)^{-1/2}$$

$$= 2.747$$

From the tables listed in Williams' 1972 paper, this test statistic is significant at the $\alpha = 0.01$ level, but not at the $\alpha = 0.005$ level. The conclusion is that there is a statistically significant increase present at the high-dose level.

Continuing the sequence, the next test statistic is calculated as follows:

$$\bar{t}_3 = (M_3 - x_1)\left(\frac{s^2}{n_3} + \frac{s^2}{n_1}\right)^{-1/2}$$

$$= (21.52 - 19.46)\left(\frac{12.25}{5} + \frac{12.25}{5}\right)^{-1/2}$$

$$= 0.931$$

From the tables listed in Williams' 1972 paper, this test statistic is not significant at the $\alpha = 0.05$ level. Therefore, the conclusion is that there is no evidence of an effect present at the middle dose level and the procedure is complete.

D. $\bar{E}^2$ Test

The $\bar{E}^2$ test (Barlow et al., 1972) is a trend version of the F test. It tests the same trend hypothesis as that just outlined for the $\bar{t}$-test. This test requires the amalgamation of means using the pooled adjacent violators algorithm described in Box 1; however, here all the groups are included in the amalgamation process. Under H_a, the amalgamated means are the maximum likelihood estimates of $\mu_1, \mu_2, \ldots, \mu_k$. The test statistic is based on the between-group sum of squares after amalgamation and the total sum of squares. Details on the calculations are given in Box 3.

This test is also subject to the concerns raised in Box 1 concerning the amalgamation procedure. Although the test statistic calculation is straightforward, the calculation of the corresponding p-value is complex. The need to perform this complex calculation is another drawback to this procedure.

Example 5. The NEUT data outlined in Example 3 will be used to illustrate this test as well. Once again, the interest is in an increasing

Box 3 $\bar{E}^2$ Test

Data. The data consist of k random samples. Denote the data in the ith random sample of size n_i by $x_{i1}, x_{i2}, \ldots, x_{in_i}$. Then the data may be arranged as follows:

Sample 1	*Sample 2*	...	*Sample* k
$x_{1,1}$	$x_{2,1}$		$x_{k,1}$
$x_{1,2}$	$x_{2,2}$		$x_{k,2}$
. . .	. . .		. . .
x_{1,n_1}	x_{2,n_2}		x_{k,n_k}

Assumptions.

1. All samples are random samples from their respective populations.
2. The observations within each sample are independent, and there is mutual independence among the various samples.
3. The data from each of the k populations are normally distributed.
4. The k population distribution functions have equal variances.

Test Statistic. To calculate the test statistic, first the sample means should be amalgamated using the pooled adjacent violators algorithm explained in Box 1, with the weights being defined as $w_i = n_i$ for groups $i = 1, \ldots, k$, where n_i is the group sample size.

Let b represent the number of populations resulting from the amalgamation procedure, and let the subscript a index the amalgamated populations ($a = 1, \ldots, $ b). If we define the following terminology:

n_a = sample sizes of the amalgamated groups
$N = \Sigma_a n_a = \Sigma_i n_i$ is the total sample size
M_a = mean of amalgamated group a
$\bar{X} = \Sigma_{i=1}^{k} \Sigma_{j=1}^{n_i} x_{ij}/N$ is the overall mean

The test statistic is

$$\bar{E}^2 = \frac{\Sigma_{a=1}^{b} n_a (M_a - \bar{X})^2}{\Sigma_{i=1}^{k} \Sigma_{j=1}^{n_i} (x_{ij} - \bar{X})^2}$$

Significance Level. Under H_0, the *p*-value is calculated as follows:

$$\text{Prob}\ (\overline{E}^2 \geq C) = \sum_{d=2}^{k} P(d,k)*$$

$$\text{Prob}\left[F_{d-1,N-d} \geq \frac{(N-d)}{(d-1)} \frac{C}{(1-C)}\right]$$

where $P(d,k)$ is the probability of exactly d groups remaining after the amalgamation, given k groups initially, and $F_{a,b}$ denotes a random variable having an F distribution with a and b degrees of freedom. The expression of the probabilities $P(d,k)$ is not always possible in a simple closed form. Details on methods for calculating these probabilities are given in Barlow et al. (1972).

trend, so the means for groups 2 and 3 will be amalgamated using the sample sizes as the w_i. After amalgamation, the following values will be used for the calculations:

a	Group(s)	M_a	n_a
1	1	19.46	5
2	2, 3	21.52	10
3	4	25.54	5

The test statistic is

$$\overline{E}^2 = \frac{97.218}{293.438} = 0.331$$

The significance level is calculated as

$$\text{Prob}\ (\overline{E}^2 \geq 0.331) = P(2,4) * \text{Prob}\left[F_{1,18} \geq \frac{18}{1} * \frac{0.331}{(1-0.331)}\right]$$

$$+ P(3,4) * \text{Prob}\left[F_{2,17} \geq \frac{17}{2} * \frac{0.331}{(1-0.331)}\right]$$

$$+ P(4,4) * \text{Prob}\left[F_{3,16} \geq \frac{16}{3} * \frac{0.331}{(1-0.331)}\right]$$

$$= (0.458 * 0.0079)$$
$$+ (0.250 * 0.0327)$$
$$+ (0.042 * 0.0847)$$
$$= 0.015$$

The conclusion is that there is evidence of a significant increase present at the high-dose level. By using the strategy outlined in Fig. 2 to determine the NOEL, the test is performed again using data from all the groups except the high-dose group. This results in a test statistic $\overline{E}^2 = 0.124$, which corresponds to a p-value of 0.196. The conclusion is that there is no observed effect at the middle-dose level.

E. Welch Trend Test

All the tests described up to this point assume homogeneous variances. A test was proposed by Welch (1951), and applied to the trend alternative by Roth (1983), that does not require this condition. This procedure tests the same trend hypothesis as that outlined for the last two tests. This test amalgamates the means using the pooled adjacent violators algorithm. However, here, the weights are adjusted for the sample variances. Details on the calculations are given in Box 4.

This test is similar in structure to the $\overline{E}^2$ test, with the exception that this test does not assume homogeneous group variances. Therefore, this test is subject to the same drawbacks as the $\overline{E}^2$ test (i.e., concerns raised about the amalgamation procedure mentioned in Box 1 and difficulty calculating the p-value corresponding to a given test statistic).

Example 6. The NEUT data outlined in Example 3 will again be used. The interest is in an increasing trend, so the means for groups 2 and 3 need to be amalgamated, this time using the n_i/s_i^2 as the weights. Amalgamating groups 2 and 3 we have

$$\text{Amalgamated mean} = \frac{(\overline{x}_2 * w_2 + \overline{x}_3 * w_3)}{(w_2 + w_3)}$$
$$= \left(21.68 * \frac{5}{10.25} + 21.36 * \frac{5}{6.77}\right) /$$
$$\left(\frac{5}{10.25} + \frac{5}{6.77}\right) = 21.49$$

Box 4 Welch Trend Test

Data. The data consist of k random samples. Denote the data in the ith random sample of size n_i by $x_{i1}, x_{i2}, \ldots, x_{in_i}$. Then the data may be arranged as follows:

Sample 1	*Sample 2*	...	*Sample* k
$x_{1,1}$	$x_{2,1}$		$x_{k,1}$
$x_{1,2}$	$x_{2,2}$		$x_{k,2}$
...	...		...
x_{1,n_1}	x_{2,n_2}		x_{k,n_k}

Assumptions.

1. All samples are random samples from their respective populations.
2. The observations within each sample are independent, and there is mutual independence among the various samples.
3. The data from each of the k populations are normally distributed.

Test Statistic. To calculate the test statistic, the sample means should first be amalgamated using the pooled adjacent violators algorithm explained in Box 1, with the weights being defined as $w_i = n_i/s_i^2$ for groups $i = 1, \ldots, k$, where

n_i = group sample size
s_i = group sample standard deviation

Let b represent the number of unique populations resulting from the amalgamation procedure, and the subscript a index the amalgamated populations ($a = 1, \ldots, b$). If we define the following terminology:

n_a = sample sizes of the amalgamated groups
$N = \Sigma_a n_a = \Sigma_i n_i$ is the total sample size
w_a = weights of the amalgamated groups
$W = \Sigma_a w_a = \Sigma_i w_i$ is the sum of the weights
M_a = mean of amalgamated group a
$M = \Sigma_a w_a M_a / W$ is the weighted overall mean

The test statistic is

$$WT = \frac{\Sigma_{a=1}^{b} \, w_a (M_a - M)^2}{(N - b) \, \{1 + 2[(b - 2/(b^2 - 1)] \, \Sigma_a h_a\}}$$

where $h_a = (1 - w_a/W)^2/(n_a - 1)$

Significance Level. Under H_0, the p-value is calculated as follows:

$$\text{Prob}(WT \geq C) = \sum_{\{\mathbf{B} \mid d \geq 2\}} P(\mathbf{B}, k)*$$

$$\text{Prob}\left[F_{d-1, f_B} \geq \frac{N - d}{d - 1} C\right]$$

where

$$f_{\mathbf{B}} = [3\Sigma_a h_a/(d^2 - 1)]^{-1}$$

and $\mathbf{B}$ is the partition of $\{1, 2, \ldots, k\}$ into d subsets that result from the amalgamation. The computation of $P(\mathbf{B}, k)$ is discussed in Roth (1983) and Barlow et al. (1972, pp. 134–145). The computation of the $P(\mathbf{B}, k)$ is defined using a recursive formula that assumes knowledge of $P(r, r)$ for $r = 1, 2, \ldots, k$; however, this can be expressed only in closed form for $k \leq 4$. For $k = 5$, numerical integration is needed to derive an exact answer. For $k > 5$, various approximations can be used, but these are tedious and lose accuracy as k increases. This is a limitation of this procedure. [See Roth (1983) for a more detailed discussion of this topic.]

After amalgamation, the following values will be used for the calculations:

a	Group(s)	M_a	w_a	n_a
1	1	19.46	0.634	5
2	2, 3	21.49	1.226	10
3	4	25.54	0.208	5

Therefore, $W = \Sigma_a w_a = 2.068$, $M = \Sigma_a w_a M_a / W = 21.28$, and $N = \Sigma_a n_a = 20$. Calculating the test statistic we have

$$\sum_a h_a = \sum_a (1 - w_a/W)^2/(n_a - 1) = 0.342$$

therefore,

$$WT = \frac{5.929}{(20 - 3) \{1 + 2[(3 - 2)/(3^2 - 1)] * 0.342\}} = 0.3213$$

The calculation of the corresponding *p*-value can be cumbersome. The following table summarizes the $P(\mathbf{B},k)$ and the $f_\mathbf{B}$ for every element in the set **B**:

B	$P(\mathbf{B},4)$	$f_\mathbf{B}$
{1},{2},{3},{4}	0.052	8.757
{1,2},{3},{4}	0.095	8.130
{1},{2,3},{4}	0.107	7.843
{1},{2},{3,4}	0.073	10.417
{1,2},{3,4}	0.125	17.857
{1,2,3},{4}	0.175	4.926
{1},{2,3,4}	0.149	7.874

The significance level is calculated as

$$\text{Prob}\,(WT \geq 0.3213) = 0.052 * \text{Prob}\left[F_{3,8.757} \geq \frac{16}{3} * 0.3213\right]$$

$$+ 0.095 * \text{Prob}\left[F_{2,8.130} \geq \frac{17}{2} * 0.3213\right]$$

$$\vdots \qquad\qquad \vdots$$

$$+ 0.149 * \text{Prob}\left[F_{1,7.874} \geq \frac{18}{1} * 0.3213\right]$$

$$= 0.067$$

The conclusion is that there is *marginal* evidence of a significant increase present at the high-dose level. By using the strategy outlined in Fig. 2 to determine the NOEL, no further tests are performed because the initial test is not significant at the 0.05 level.

F. Robust Contrast-Based Trend Test

Another test proposed by Meng, Davis and Roth (1993) does not require heterogeneous variances and is robust to nonnormal data. This procedure tests the same trend hypothesis as that outlined for the last three tests. Details on the calculations are given in Box 5.

This test is a good choice for analysis of toxicological data. The test does not require homogeneous variances and is robust to nonnormal data. The critical value calculation is based on the t-distribution, making p-value calculations straightforward.

Example 7.   The NEUT data outlined in Example 3 will again be used. Once again, the interest is in an increasing trend. First, the contrasts C_i must be calculated.

i	n_i	s_i^2	w_i	a_i	C_i	$\bar{x}_i$
0	–	–	–	0	–	–
1	5	7.888	0.634	0.634	-1.143	19.46
2	5	10.252	0.488	1.122	$+0.112$	21.68
3	5	6.768	0.739	1.861	$+0.409$	21.36
4	5	24.083	0.208	2.069	$+0.622$	25.54

Calculating the test statistic we have

$$t_R = \frac{\sum\limits_{i=1}^{k} C_i\bar{x}_i}{\left[\sum\limits_{i=1}^{k} (C_i^2 s_i^2/n_i)\right]^{1/2}} = \frac{4.8075}{(4.177)^{1/2}} = 2.352$$

By using the weighted blend of t-statistics defined in the foregoing, the p-value corresponding to this test statistic is 0.039. The conclusion is that there is evidence of a significant increase present at the high-dose level. With the strategy outlined in Fig. 2 to determine the NOEL, the test is performed again using data from all groups except the high-dose group. This results in a test statistic $t_R = 1.172$, which corresponds to a p-value of 0.153. The conclusion is that there is no observed effect at the middle-dose level.

Box 5 Robust Contrast-Based Trend Test

Data. The data consist of k random samples. Denote the data in the ith random sample of size n_i by $x_{i1}, x_{i2}, \ldots, x_{in_i}$. Then the data may be arranged as follows:

Sample 1	*Sample 2*	...	*Sample* k
$x_{1,1}$	$x_{2,1}$		$x_{k,1}$
$x_{1,2}$	$x_{2,2}$		$x_{k,2}$
...	...		...
x_{1,n_1}	x_{2,n_2}		x_{k,n_k}

Assumptions.
1. All samples are random samples from their respective populations.
2. The observations within each sample are independent, and there is mutual independence among the various samples.
3. The data from each of the k populations are normally distributed.

Test Statistic. The test statistic can be calculated as follows

$$t_R = \frac{\sum_{i=1}^{k} C_i \bar{x}_i}{\left[\sum_{i=1}^{k} (C_i^2 s_i^2 / n_i) \right]^{1/2}}$$

where

$\bar{x}_i$ = sample mean for group i
s_i^2 = sample variance for group i
n_i = sample size for group i

and

$$C_i = \sqrt{a_{i-1}(a_k - a_{i-1})} - \sqrt{a_i(a_k - a_i)}$$

$a_0 = 0$
$a_i = \sum_{j=1}^{i} w_j$
$w_j = n_j / s_j^2$

Decision Rule. The critical value for the test statistic is defined as follows:

$$t' = \frac{\Sigma_{i=1}^{k} \ (C_i^2 s_i^2/n_i)t_i}{\Sigma_{i=1}^{k} \ (C_i^2 s_i^2/n_i)}$$

where t_i is obtained from the t-table for $n_i - 1$ degrees of freedom, and the remaining terms are defined as before. Reject H_0 at the α level if t_R exceeds the critical value t'.

Note: An alternative related test statistic is proposed in Meng and co-workers' 1993 paper. This test statistic was similar to the foregoing, with the exception that the weights w_i were defined as $w_i = n_i$. Given simulation results, the authors recommended the method outlined in detail here. The reader is referred to their paper for further details on the alternate test.

G. Analysis of Covariance

An analysis of covariance model (ANCOVA) can be used to analyze subchronic toxicity data in the presence of one or more confounding factors (covariates). The ANCOVA tests the same hypothesis as the one-way ANOVA model, using an alternative underlying model. Details on the calculations can be found in any standard text on data analysis (e.g., see Neter, et al., 1985). Any statistical computer package should have an automated procedure to perform the analysis of covariance.

The statistical contrasts outlined in the one-way ANOVA section are also applicable using the analysis of covariance model. Refer to the section on the one-way ANOVA for details on the contrast strategies.

Example 8. The following heart and brain weights were observed in a subchronic rat study:

		Weights				
Group	Organ	Animal 1	Animal 2	Animal 3	Animal 4	Animal 5
1	Heart (mg)	919	875	967	879	998
	Brain (g)	1.99	2.08	2.14	1.87	1.90
2	Heart (mg)	857	894	808	919	844
	Brain (g)	1.90	1.85	1.99	1.96	1.96

3	Heart (mg)	859	852	825	686	733
	Brain (g)	1.94	2.10	2.01	1.90	1.97
4	Heart (mg)	750	738	736	743	672
	Brain (g)	1.92	1.84	1.72	1.85	1.76

These data will be used to illustrate statistical procedures that adjust for a covariate variable.

Analyzing these data with an analysis of covariance model to test for a difference in heart weight, using brain weight as the covariate, results in a p-value of 0.002. Analysis of these data, using the covariance model with the trend contrast strategies outlined in the one-way analysis of variance section, gives the following results:

	Contrast 1 p-value	Contrast 2 p-value	Contrast 3 p-value
Strategy 1	0.010	0.001	0.002
Strategy 2	0.010	0.003	0.155
Strategy 3	0.001	0.001	0.155
Strategy 4	0.380	0.038	0.155

When using the foregoing interpretation in the one-way analysis of variance section, for any of these strategies contrast 1 would be examined first to determine if there was a test compound effect present. Strategies 1,2, and 3 all conclude that there is a test compound effect present at the high-dose level, whereas strategy 4 does not detect any test compound effect. The follow-up analysis for strategies 1, 2, and 3 would have us examine the p-value for contrast 2 next, to determine if there was a test compound effect present at the middle-dose level. Strategies 1, 2, and 3 would all conclude that there is a test compound effect present at the middle-dose level. The next step in the follow-up analysis for strategies 1, 2, and 3 would have us examine the p-value for contrast 3 to determine if there was a test compound effect present at the low-dose level. Strategy 1 concludes that there is a test compound effect present at the low-dose level, whereas strategies 2 and 3 detect no test compound effect at the low-dose level.

VII. NONPARAMETRIC STATISTICAL METHODS

Nonparametric statistical analysis is a parallel of the more familiar parametric methods. In nonparametric methods, however, no assumptions about the underlying distribution of the data (e.g., normally distributed) are made. When the data to be analyzed (or a transformation of the data) do not fulfill the necessary assumptions for parametric analysis, the nonparametric methods are usually more powerful than the equivalent parametric test. Even when the data fulfill the assumptions required for the parametric analysis, the nonparametric procedures, although not as efficient as their parametric counterparts, usually perform well.

Nonparametric procedures are increasingly becoming the procedures of choice for toxicological data. Because many of the parameters are not normally distributed [see Mitruka and Rawnsley (1977); Weil (1982)], procedures that do not require distributional assumptions are appealing. Unlike the parametric procedures, the nonparametric procedures are not sensitive to outlying values.

A. Kruskal–Wallis Test

The Kruskal–Wallis test is the nonparametric equivalent of the one-way analysis of variance. The Kruskal–Wallis test has been historically used to analyze subchronic toxicity data; it tests the null hypothesis:

$$H_0{:}\mu_1 = \mu_2 = \ldots = \mu_k$$

against the alternative

$$H_a{:}\mu_i \neq \mu_j \quad \text{for some } i, j, \text{ where } i \neq j \text{ and } 1 \leq i, j \leq k$$

Details for the calculations can be found in any standard text on nonparametric data analysis (e.g., see Hollander and Wolfe, 1973). Most statistical computer packages should have an automated procedure to perform the Kruskal–Wallis test.

Similar to the ANOVA, if the Kruskal–Wallis test is significant, the conclusion is that a difference among the dosage groups exists. To make inferences about the NOEL, some form of a follow-up procedure is needed.

The nonparametric follow-up method that is equivalent to performing pairwise t-tests would be to perform pairwise Mann–Whitney tests of each dosed group to the control group. The Mann–Whitney test is outlined in any basic nonparametric text, but can be easily described as performing a Kruskal–Wallis test on two groups. This method, although often used in practice, does not account for the ordered structure of the groups and does not properly control the overall type I error rate. It is recommended that this particular follow-up method not be used.

Computer packages that provide a procedure to perform the Kruskal–Wallis test do not have the sophisticated options for follow-up contrasts that were described for the parametric ANOVA model. There is a way around these difficulties that combines the advantages of nonparametrics with the flexibility that is available with the one-way ANOVA model in computer packages. This approach will now be described.

B. Rank Transform Analysis of Variance

A commonly employed procedure to perform a nonparametric one-way analysis is to perform the rank transform analysis of variance procedure. This procedure was proposed by Conover and Iman (1981) and has become a commonly accepted alternative to the Kruskal–Wallis test. The test is performed by ranking all the data, then analyzing the ranks using the parametric one-way ANOVA procedures described in the last section. The test statistic generated by this method is a monotonic function of the Kruskal–Wallis test statistic; therefore, the two methods are equivalent.

If this method is used, the pairwise comparisons to control (using the common mean square error) or any of the various trend contrast strategies outlined in Section VI.A for the parametric one-way ANOVA could be used.

Example 9. The NEUT data outlined in Example 3 will be used to illustrate the rank transform analysis of variance.

Analysis of these data with the one-way rank transform analysis of variance model results in a p-value of 0.114. Analysis of these data using the rank transform analysis of variance model, with the trend contrast strategies outlined in Section VI.A, gives the following results:

	Contrast 1 p-value	Contrast 2 p-value	Contrast 3 p-value
Strategy 1	0.050	0.112	0.046
Strategy 2	0.050	0.594	0.160
Strategy 3	0.029	0.244	0.160
Strategy 4	0.176	0.794	0.160

With the interpretation outlined in Section VI.A, for any of these strategies contrast 1 would be examined first to determine if there was a test compound effect present. Strategies 1, 2, and 3 all conclude that there is a test compound effect present at the high-dose level, whereas strategy 4 does not detect any test compound effect. None of the follow-up analyses for strategies 1, 2, and 3 detect a test compound effect present at the middle-dose level.

C. Jonckheere–Terpstra Trend Test

Jonckheere (1954) and Terpstra (1952) independently proposed a trend test that tests the hypothesis:

$$H_0: \mu_0 = \mu_1 = \ldots = \mu_{k-1}$$

against the alternative

$H_a: \mu_0 \leq \mu_1 \leq \ldots \leq \mu_{k-1}$ with at least one inequality being strict.

Details regarding the calculations are given in Box 6.

The Jonckheere's test, as it is commonly known, does not make any assumptions about the distribution of the data; however, the test does assume that the variances of the dosage groups are equal. Note that the calculation of the test statistic does not use information about the actual dose level, it uses only information on the relative ordering of the dosage groups. The Jonckheere's test is most powerful when the underlying (unknown) response levels are strictly ordered and evenly spaced across the groups; however, the test is appropriate to detect any response that is a monotonic increasing (or decreasing) function of the dose level.

Example 10. The NEUT data outlined in Example 3 will be used to illustrate the Jonckheere's test. Once again the interest is in an increasing trend. First the Mann–Whitney counts between pairs of groups need to be calculated. These counts are as follows:

u	v	U_{uv}
1	2	19.5
	3	18.5
	4	22.0
2	3	11.0
	4	18.5
3	4	19.0

Box 6   Jonckheere–Terpstra Test

Data.   The data consist of k random samples. Denote the data in the ith random sample of size n_i by $x_{i1}, x_{i2}, \ldots, x_{in_i}$. Then the data may be arranged as follows:

Sample 1	*Sample 2*	...	*Sample* k
$x_{1,1}$	$x_{2,1}$		$x_{k,1}$
$x_{1,2}$	$x_{2,2}$		$x_{k,2}$
...	...		...
x_{1,n_1}	x_{2,n_2}		x_{k,n_k}

Assumptions.

1. All samples are random samples from their respective populations.
2. The observations within each sample are independent, and there is mutual independence among the various samples.
3. The k population distribution functions have equal variances.

Test Statistic.   To compute the test statistic, first compute the $k(k - 1)/2$ Mann-Whitney counts U_{uv}, $u < v$ as follows:

$$U_{uv} = \Sigma_{i=1}^{n_u} \Sigma_{i'=1}^{n_v} \; \phi(x_{iu}, x_{i'v})$$

where

$$\phi(a,b) = \begin{array}{ll} 1 & \text{if } a < b \\ 0.5 & \text{if } a = b \\ 0 & \text{if } a > b \end{array}$$

Then the test statistic is

$$J = \Sigma_{u<v}^k \; U_{uv} = \Sigma_{u=1}^{k-1} \Sigma_{v=u+1}^k \; U_{uv}$$

Significance Level.   For small samples, this statistic should be compared with tables to find the level of significance [see Lehman (1975) for tables]. For larger samples, define

$$J* = \frac{J - E_0(J)}{[\text{VAR}_0(J)]^{1/2}}$$

Under the null hypothesis, this can be rewritten (Lin, 1976) as follows:

$$J^* = \frac{J - [(N^2 - \Sigma_{i=1}^k n_i^2)/4]}{\left\{\left[\dfrac{N(N-1)}{8}\right]\left[1 - \dfrac{\Sigma_i n_i(n_i - 1)}{N(N-1)}\right]\right.}$$

$$\left[1 - \frac{\Sigma_{h=1}^H d_h(d_h - 1)}{N(N-1)}\right]$$

$$+ \left[\frac{N(N-1)(N-2)}{36}\right]$$

$$\left[1 - \frac{\Sigma_i n_i(n_i - 1)(n_i - 2)}{N(N-1)(N-2)}\right]$$

$$\left.\left[1 - \frac{\Sigma_{h=1}^H d_h(d_h - 1)(d_h - 2)}{N(N-1)(N-2)}\right]\right\}^{1/2}$$

where there are H distinct observations and the hth observation was observed d_h times and we define

$$N = \sum_{i=1}^k n_i$$

Then when H_0 is true, the statistic J^* has an asymptotic $N(0,1)$ distribution. Therefore, at an α level of significance

Reject H_0 if $J^* \geq Z_{(\alpha)}$
Accept H_0 if $J^* < Z_{(\alpha)}$

The Jonckheere–Terpstra test could likewise be used to test for a decreasing trend by reversing the inequalities in the function $\phi(a,b)$.

The test statistic is

$$J = \sum_{u=1}^{k-1} \sum_{v=u+1}^{k} U_{uv} = 108.5$$

Therefore, accounting for ties through the foregoing calculation, $J^* = 2.26$ and the corresponding p-value is 0.012. With this test the conclusion is that there is evidence of a significant increase present at the high-dose level. With the strategy outlined in Fig. 2 to determine the NOEL, the test is performed again using data from all the groups except the high-dose group. This results in a test statistic $J^* = 1.22$, which corresponds to a p-value of 0.111. The conclusion is that there is no observed effect at the middle-dose level.

D. Nonparametric $\bar{E}^2$ Test

The nonparametric version of the $\bar{E}^2$ test is similar to the parametric version; however, the test statistic is based on the ranks of the data. This test was originally introduced by Chacko (1963) and was extended by Shorack (1967). A detailed outline of the test is given in Barlow et al. (1972). It tests the same trend hypothesis as that outlined for the Jonckheere–Terpstra test. This test requires that the means of the ranks of the data be amalgamated using the pooled adjacent violators algorithm described in Box 1. Details for the calculations are given in Box 7.

This test is subject to the concerns raised in Box 1 over the amalgamation procedure. Similar to the $\bar{E}^2$ test, the test statistic calculation is straightforward, but the calculation of the corresponding p-value is complex. The need to perform this complex calculation is a drawback to this procedure.

Example 11.   The NEUT data outlined in Example 3 will be used to illustrate this test. Once again, the interest is in an increasing trend, but in this example the test will be performed on the ranks of the data instead of the raw data values. Ranking the data results in the following:

Group	Rank of NEUT value	Mean rank
1	2, 3, 7, 8, 10	6.0
2	1, 10, 13, 15, 16	11.0
3	4, 6, 10, 13, 17.5	10.1
4	5, 13, 17.5, 19, 20	14.9

Because the interest is in an increasing trend, the means for groups 2 and 3 need to be amalgamated using the sample sizes as the w_i. After amalgamation, the following values will be used for the calculations:

Box 7 Nonparametric $\bar{E}^2$ Test

Data. The data consist of k random samples. Denote the data in the ith random sample of size n_i by $x_{i1}, x_{i2}, \ldots, x_{in_i}$. Then the data may be arranged as follows:

Sample 1	Sample 2	Sample k
$x_{1,1}$	$x_{2,1}$	$x_{k,1}$
$x_{1,2}$	$x_{2,2}$	$x_{k,2}$
. . .	. . .	. . .
x_{1,n_1}	x_{2,n_2}	x_{k,n_k}

Assumptions.

1. All samples are random samples from their respective populations.
2. The observations within each sample are independent, and there is mutual independence among the various samples.
3. The k population distribution functions have equal variances.

Test Statistic. To calculate the test statistic, first all the data should be ranked. Then the sample means of the ranks should be amalgamated using the pooled adjacent violators algorithm explained in Box 1, with the weights being defined as $w_i = n_i$ for groups $i = 1, \ldots, k$, where n_i is the group sample size.

Let b represent the number of populations resulting from the amalgamation procedure and let the subscript a index the amalgamated populations ($a = 1, \ldots, b$). If we define the following terminology:

n_a = sample sizes of the amalgamated groups
$N = \Sigma_a n_a = \Sigma_1 n_i$ is the total sample size
R_a = mean rank of amalgamated group a

The test statistic is

$$\bar{\chi}^2_{\text{rank}} = \frac{12}{N(N + 1)} \sum_{a=1}^{b} n_a \left(R_a - \frac{N + 1}{2} \right)^2$$

Significance Level. Under H_0, the p-value is calculated as follows:

$$\text{Prob} \ (\bar{\chi}_{\text{rank}}^2 \geq C) = \sum_{d=2}^{k} P(d,k) \ \text{Prob}[\chi_{d-1}^2 \geq C]$$

where $P(d,k)$ is the probability of exactly d groups remaining after the amalgamation, given k groups initially and χ_a^2 denotes a random variable having a chi-square distribution with a degrees of freedom. The expression of the probabilities $P(d,k)$ is not always possible in a simple closed form. Details on methods for calculating these probabilities are given in Barlow et al. (1972).

a	Group(s)	M_a	n_a
1	1	6.00	5
2	2, 3	10.55	10
3	4	14.90	5

The test statistic is

$$\bar{\chi}_{\text{rank}}^2 = \frac{12}{20(20 + 1)} \ [5 * (6.0 - 10.5)^2 + 10 * (10.55 - 10.5)^2$$
$$+ 5 * (14.9 - 10.5)^2]$$
$$= 5.659$$

The significance level is calculated as

$$\text{Prob} \ (\chi_{\text{rank}}^2 \geq 5.659) = P(2,4) * \text{Prob}[\chi_1^2 \geq 5.659]$$
$$+ P(3,4) * \text{Prob}[\chi_2^2 \geq 5.659]$$
$$+ P(4,4) * \text{Prob}[\chi_3^2 \geq 5.659]$$
$$= 0.458 * 0.008$$
$$+ 0.250 * 0.015$$
$$+ 0.042 * 0.005$$
$$= 0.028$$

The conclusion is that there is evidence of a significant increase present at the high-dose level. By using the strategy outlined in Fig. 2 to determine the NOEL, the test is performed again using data from all the groups except the high-dose group. This results in a test statistic $\chi^2_{rank} =$ 2.535, which corresponds to a p-value of 0.103. The conclusion is that there is no observed effect at the middle-dose level.

E. Rank Transform Analysis of Covariance

The rank transform procedure, introduced previously for the rank transform analysis of variance, can be used to perform a nonparametric version of the covariance analysis. This procedure was originally outlined by Quade (1967) and was further developed by Conover and Iman (1982).

The method is performed by ranking the response variable and ranking the covariate separately, then analyzing the ranks using the analysis of covariance procedures described in the last section. The approach outlined by Conover and Iman allows for a test for equality of slopes as well as a test for equality of intercepts. The statistical contrasts outlined in Section VI.A are also applicable when using this procedure.

Example 12. The heart and brain weight data outlined in Example 8 will be used to illustrate the rank transform analysis of covariance. Ranking the heart weight and brain weight independently results in the following values for analysis:

		Rank of weight				
Group	Organ	Animal 1	Animal 2	Animal 3	Animal 4	Animal 5
1	Heart	17.5	14	19	15	20
	Brain	15.5	18	20	6	8
2	Heart	12	16	8	17.5	10
	Brain	8	4.5	15.5	12.5	12.5
3	Heart	13	11	9	2	3
	Brain	11	19	17	8	14
4	Heart	7	5	4	6	1
	Brain	10	3	1	4.5	2

An analysis of these ranks with an analysis of covariance model, using the rank of the brain weight as the covariate, results in a p-value of 0.001. Analysis of these ranks using the covariance model with the trend contrast strategies outlined in Section VI.A gives the following results:

	Contrast 1 p-value	Contrast 2 p-value	Contrast 3 p-value
Strategy 1	0.012	0.001	0.001
Strategy 2	0.012	0.003	0.101
Strategy 3	0.001	0.001	0.101
Strategy 4	0.447	0.044	0.101

If we use the interpretation outlined in Section VI.A, for any of these strategies, contrast 1 would be examined first to determine if there was a test compound effect present. Strategies 1, 2, and 3 all conclude that there is a test compound effect present at the high-dose level, whereas strategy 4 does not detect any test compound effect. The follow-up analysis for strategies 1, 2, and 3 would have us examine the p-value for contrast 2 next, to determine if there was a test compound effect present at the middle-dose level. Strategies 1, 2, and 3 would all conclude that there is a test compound effect present at the middle-dose level. The next step in the follow-up analysis for strategies 1, 2, and 3 would have us examine the p-value for contrast 3 to determine if there was a test compound effect present at the low-dose level. Strategy 1 detects a test compound effect at the low-dose level, but strategies 2 and 3 do not detect a test compound effect present at the low-dose level.

F. Nonparametric Trend Testing with a Covariate

The Jonckheere–Terpstra test, the nonparametric $\bar{E}^2$ test, or any other one-way trend test (parametric or nonparametric) can be performed in the presence of a covariate by first generating adjusted values that have the effect of the covariate removed. The adjusted values can then be analyzed using the test of choice.

To perform this procedure, first the data needs to be analyzed using either an analysis of covariance, as described in Section VI.G, or be analyzed with the rank transform analysis of covariance procedure outlined earlier in this section. If a fully nonparametric procedure is desired, the rank transform analysis of covariance should be used. Adjusted values can then be generated for each observation in the original data set by adding the residuals to the corresponding dosage group's least square mean. The trend test of choice (e.g., Jonckheere's test, nonparametric $\bar{E}^2$ test, or other) can then be performed on these adjusted values.

This procedure is subject to the assumptions of both the analysis of covariance model used and the chosen trend test.

Example 13. The heart and brain weight data outlined in Example 8 will be used to illustrate this procedure. For this example, the rank transform analysis of covariance procedure will be used to generate the adjusted values. This model generates the following rank least square means, residuals, and adjusted rank values:

Group	Rank least square mean						
1	16.90	Residual	0.27	−3.40	1.46	−1.60	3.27
		Adjusted value	17.17	13.50	18.36	15.30	20.17
2	12.69	Residual	−0.53	3.71	−5.03	4.67	−2.83
		Adjusted value	12.16	16.40	7.66	17.36	9.86
3	7.38	Residual	5.59	3.05	1.19	−5.21	−4.61
		Adjusted value	12.97	10.43	8.57	2.17	2.77
4	5.03	Residual	2.00	0.47	−0.39	1.37	−3.45
		Adjusted value	7.03	5.50	4.64	6.40	1.58

These adjusted values can then be analyzed using any of the one-way trend tests previously outlined (e.g., Jonckheere's test, nonparametric $\bar{E}^2$ test, or other). The Jonckheere's test for decreasing trend will be performed for this example. An analysis of these adjusted values results in a test statistic $J = 131$, which corresponds to an asymptotic p-value less than 0.001. The conclusion is that there is evidence of a significant decrease present at the high-dose level. With use of the strategy outlined in Fig. 2 to determine the NOEL, the test is performed again using adjusted data from all the groups except the high-dose group. Note that the adjustment procedure is not redone; adjusted values from the adjustment using all groups are used. This results in a test statistic $J = 64$, which corresponds to a p-value of 0.003. Because this test is also significant, the test is performed again using adjusted data from only the control and low-dose groups. This results in a test statistic $J = 20$, which corresponds to a p-value of 0.059. The conclusion is that there is evidence of a significant decrease in the middle-dose level, and *marginal* evidence of a significant decrease at the low-dose level.

VIII. COMPARISON OF METHODS

Several potential statistical tests have been outlined in the last two sections. The question now becomes: Which of these tests are best for the analysis of toxicological data? The criterion used to evaluate these tests will be threefold. First, are the methods applicable to toxicological data; second, are the methods easily implementable; and third, are the methods easy for nonstatisticians to understand and interpret.

The first criterion used to compare the tests is the applicability of the method to toxicological data. The focus of this discussion is the assumptions required by each statistical test and how well toxicological data satisfies these assumptions. The critical assumptions that are often discussed are the assumptions of normality of the data and the equality of group variances.

Toxicological data, particularly hematological and clinical chemistry data, are often either not normally distributed, or not continuous in nature. This fact is documented in Mitruka and Rawnsley (1977) and Weil (1982). An investigation of the normality of hematological and clinical chemistry data, using historical control database, showed statistically significant evidence of nonnormality in 80% of hematological and clinical chemistry parameters in rats at age 7–8 weeks (37/46 parameters tested). This pattern continues into older ages and is consistent in other species. One example of this phenomenon was illustrated back in Example 2 using ALT values. The use of parametric tests that are dependent on the assumption of normally distributed data (one-way analysis of variance, linear trend test, $\bar{t}$ test, $\bar{E}^2$ test, Welch trend test, and analysis of covariance) without correcting for violations of this assumption can lead to misleading results. The one parametric procedure that is robust against nonnormality of the data is the robust contrast-based trend test. None of the nonparametric procedures depend on the assumption of normality of the data.

The second assumption referenced when discussing the analysis of toxicological data is the assumption of homogeneity of group variances. How well this assumption is satisfied on a given study is harder to assess because changes in the group variance are often due to some test compound effect. Many of the tests outlined in the last two sections are dependent on this assumption. The tests that perform well in nonhomogeneous variance situations are the Welch trend test and the robust contrast-based trend test. Both of these tests explicitly adjust for the group sample variance in the calculation of the test statistic. All the nonparametric tests outlined in Section VII list the equality of group variances as an assumption; however, these tests are less sensitive to violations of this assumption than their parametric counterparts, except in the most extreme cases of unequal group variances.

The final topic relative to the applicability of the method to be discussed here is the use of tests that require the amalgamation procedure. The caution on amalgamation mentioned in Box 1 should give reason for concern. Admittedly, the example cited is extreme and is nearly impossible with real data, but because the procedure allows such a possibility causes me to steer away from any tests that use the amalgamation procedure. Many of these procedures are widely used; however, caution should be exercised when using the t-test, the $\bar{E}^2$-test, the Welch trend test, and the nonparametric $\bar{E}^2$-test for this reason.

The next criterion for evaluating the various tests is the ease of implementation using a standard statistical computer package (such as SAS). Some of the tests can be directly obtained from any standard statistical computer package. These tests include the one-way analysis of variance, linear trend test, analysis of covariance, Kruskal–Wallis test, rank transform analysis of variance, and the rank transform analysis of covariance. Of the remaining tests, there are several that require customized programming, but the programming is straightforward and easily manageable. These tests are the robust contrast-based trend test and the Jonckheere test. These tests use readily available statistical distributions for asymptotic significance level calculations. The $\bar{E}^2$-test, Welch trend test, and the nonparametric $\bar{E}^2$-test require customized programming, but in these cases the algorithm used to generate the significance level is based on a complicated iterative equation that does not always have a closed form solution. This makes computer implementation of these tests difficult. The t-test significance level is based on a table look-up, a situation that is unnecessarily limiting in today's computer environment. Finally, generation of adjusted values to perform nonparametric trend testing with a covariate is straightforward to program. Therefore, the ease of implementation of this procedure is dependent on the one-way test chosen to analyze the adjusted values.

The final criterion that will be used to evaluate the tests is their understandability to nonstatisticians. A good understanding of the method and the underlying model is a prerequisite for sensible inference. In general, the methods that are the easiest to implement on the computer are the easiest for toxicologists and pathologists to understand. Methods that can be used on any type of data are preferable because the statistical method used will not need to vary from parameter to parameter. There is an advantage for the toxicologists and pathologists to be interpreting p-values from the same statistical method for all parameters; they become familiar with the method and understand the results when the method is applied to a new type of data. The methods that are the most universally applicable are the robust contrast-based trend test, the Jonckheere test, and nonparametric trend testing with a covariate using one of these two tests.

One final comment that merits discussion is the use of rank-based procedures to analyze data with censored values. There are situations in which hematological or clinical chemistry parameters have data censored owing to values less than or greater than the detection limit of the instrumentation. These values should not be ignored in the analysis, indeed they may be some of the most important data points. Rank-based nonparametric procedures can handle data of this type because a relative rank can be assigned to these values. Parametric procedures that are based on the actual data values do not have a straightforward counterpart for handling censored data of this type.

IX. ANALYTICAL ISSUES

First, when analyzing a study, it is important to test for equality of the parameter values before the initiation of dosing. Because the objective of a subchronic toxicity study is to identify adverse test compound effects, it is critical that parameters that exhibit differences before the initiation of dosing be identified. These differences could have an influence on the interpretation of subsequent analyses. Because dosing had not commenced when these parameters were measured, a statistical test that tests for any difference among groups (an omnibus test) should be used instead of a trend test. If differences are found at baseline, the analysis at subsequent time points should account for this fact. The most common statistical approaches that account for baseline values use the baseline value as a covariate, analyze the change from baseline, or analyze the percentage change from baseline. Note that these analyses are still valid if there is no difference between the dosage groups at baseline. Therefore, a reasonable approach would be to always use the baseline information for all parameters on all studies. This would protect against the possibility of erroneous conclusions that result from differences in the parameters at baseline and not from true test–compound-induced effects.

Once dosing has started, a test–compound-induced response for a given parameter will most often be a monotonic response, with larger doses of the test compound causing larger effects. There are several possible test–compound-induced patterns of response that all share this property of monotonicity, several of these were illustrated earlier in Fig. 1. The most powerful statistical tests to detect a response of this nature will be trend tests. All the tests outlined in Sections VI and VII were either trend tests or could be implemented in such a way that the trend hypothesis would be tested. All statistical tests performed on data collected after the initiation of dosing should test the trend hypothesis.

When using trend tests, a decision should be made for each parameter relative to which direction(s) is of interest in evaluating for test–compound-induced changes (i.e., test–compound-induced increases, decreases, or changes in either direction). For example, only increases may be of interest for neutrophils, decreases for lymphocytes, and changes in either direction for body weights. These decisions should be made before the study is initiated and should be specified in the study protocol. This information would then dictate whether one-tailed or two-tailed statistical tests were performed.

Another important consideration when implementing a statistical analysis strategy is the audience that will ultimately use the statistical results (i.e., the toxicologists and pathologists). This was discussed in the last section, but it is such a critical point it bears repeating. A good understanding of the method and the underlying model is a prerequisite for sensible inference. If the statistical approach becomes too complex, the idiosyncracies of the procedure will not be understood by the biologists. If this happens, when the statistical procedures generate anomalous results, they will not understand what is happening. If you are lucky, you will be asked to explain the unusual results. If you are not so lucky, either the statistical results will be ignored, or erroneous conclusions will be reached. It has been my experience that a straightforward, consistent, and understandable statistical approach will lead to results being more effectively used by the toxicologists and pathologists.

It should be noted that the use of 0.05 as the cutoff point for

statistical significance is purely arbitrary and is mainly based on historical precedent. Most statistical conclusions rely on using the 0.05 level as
a magical cutoff. It is doubtful that the use of 0.05 as a decision rule will
change at any time in the near future; some form of a decision rule is
needed for the toxicologists to be able to make conclusions based on the
statistical results they receive. This paragraph is a plea to report the
actual p-values instead of merely flagging p-values that are significant at
the 0.05 or 0.01 level. Occasionally, there can be important information
contained in a p-value of 0.06; information that is lost if only significant
parameters are flagged.

One area of potential improvement in the statistical analysis that
has not been explored extensively is the use of multivariate analyses. The
methods outlined in this chapter and the methods commonly used to
analyze toxicological data are univariate in that they focus on each parameter independently. Commonly, toxic effects will affect a set of related parameters. For example, increases in alanine aminotransferase
are typically associated with increases in aspartate aminotransferase and
decreases in albumin. The combination of these findings is a strong
indicator of liver damage. Currently, the responsibility for combining
information from the various parameters is left to the toxicologist interpreting the statistical results. If the statistical analysis were to make
use of the relations and correlations between parameters so that sets
of parameters were analyzed using multivariate methods, the statistical
approach will be one step closer to analyzing the underlying biological
mechanisms. Although many of these relations are well understood by
the toxicologists, little attempt has been made by the statisticians to
employ this information in the analysis of toxicological data. This is an
area that has great possibilities in the improvement of the statistical
analysis of toxicological data for the future.

X. EXAMPLE STRATEGIES FOR ANALYSIS

In this section, three recommended strategies for analysis are presented.

A. Strategy 1: Nonparametric

The nonparametric strategy relies completely on nonparametric tests.
When a parameter would satisfy the assumptions for a parametric approach, the statistical power is reduced, but this reduction is minor. The
advantages of this strategy are that the approach is consistent for all

parameters in all studies, and it does not depend on the assumption of normally distributed data.

The tests used would be as follows:

1. Kruskal–Wallis test (or rank transform analysis of variance) to analyze baseline data
2. Jonckheere test to analyze dosing period data
3. Jonckheere test with a covariate to analyze any dosing period data that has a covariate variable

The iterative strategy to determine the NOEL outline in Section IV would be used with the trend tests.

B. Strategy 2: Parametric or Nonparametric Based on Historical Control Data

This strategy chooses whether a parametric or nonparametric test will be performed based on assumption tests for the normality of the data, which are performed on historical control data. The result of these assumption tests determine which approach is used for a given parameter, and these decisions are made before the study's initiation. The decision *does not depend* on the data observed in the study. This strategy improves the statistical power over strategy 1 for parameters that historically have normally distributed data. The disadvantage of this strategy is that the statistical approach varies from parameter to parameter in the study. A dilemma occurs in choosing what strategy to use when the historical data from a given parameter violates the assumptions at one age, but does not violate the assumptions at a different age. A decision needs to be made on which strategy to use for new parameters that have little or no historical data available.

The tests used would be as follows:

1. Parametric

1. One-way analysis of variance to analyze baseline data
2. Robust contrast-based trend tests to analyze dosing period data
3. Robust contrast-based trend test adjusted for a covariate to analyze any dosing period data that has a covariate variable

2. Nonparametric

1. Kruskal–Wallis test (or rank transform analysis of variance) to analyze baseline data
2. Jonckheere test to analyze dosing period data

3. Jonckheere test with a covariate to analyze any dosing period data that has a covariate variable

The iterative strategy to determine the NOEL outlined in Section IV would be used with the trend tests.

C. Strategy 3: Parametric, Transformed Parametric, or Nonparametric, Based on Historical Control Data

This strategy is similar to Strategy 2, except that if historical data from a given parameter does not meet the assumptions required for a parametric analysis, meaningful transformations (e.g., the log transformation) would be tried on the historical data to attempt to satisfy the assumptions. If a transformation can be identified, the transformation would be used on the study data. If not, then the nonparametric approach would be used for that parameter. Once again, all these decisions would be made before a study's initiation, and the decisions *do not depend* on the data observed in the study. This strategy improves the statistical power over Strategies 1 and 2 for parameters that historically have normally distributed data or transformations that lead to normally distributed data. The disadvantage of this strategy is that the statistical approach and the transformations used vary from parameter to parameter in the study, even more so than Strategy 2. Allowing this many possible options could make it difficult to remember how a given parameter was analyzed and confusing for the biologists to interpret the results. Dilemmas occur in choosing a transformation when the transformed historical data from a given parameter does not violate the assumptions at one age, but the transformed data violates the assumptions at a different age.

The tests used would be as follows:

1. Parametric (Data Values or Transformed Data Values, as Appropriate)

1. One-way analysis of variance to analyze baseline data
2. Robust contrast-based trend tests to analyze dosing period data
3. Robust contrast-based trend test adjusted for a covariate to analyze any dosing period data that has a covariate variable

2. Nonparametric

1. Kruskal–Wallis test (or rank transform analysis of variance) to analyze baseline data
2. Jonckheere test to analyze dosing period data

3. Jonckheere test with a covariate to analyze any dosing period data that has a covariate variable

The iterative strategy to determine the NOEL outlined in Section IV would be used with the trend tests.

XI. CONCLUSION

The statistical methods that are available to analyze subchronic toxicity study data have advanced dramatically in the last 10 years. There are now trend tests available that perform well in the presence of nonnormal and heteroscedastic data. In particular, the robust contrast-based trend test and the Jonckheere's test are easily implemented, easily understood tests that are universally applicable to subchronic toxicity study data. Any analysis of a subchronic toxicity study should rely on tests such as these that test the trend hypothesis and that are not sensitive to these assumptions.

The parameters that are measured in a subchronic toxicity study have numerous relations, both across time for a given parameter and between related parameters. More analyses that perform adjustments for possible covariates or baseline values should be used in the analysis of subchronic toxicity studies. That these adjustments are still valid (if meaningless) if there is no covariate or baseline effect on a given study makes it possible to routinely adjust for these possible effects.

We hope that the next 10 years will see further advances in the statistical methodology that is available to analyze subchronic studies. A better understanding of the relations between parameters will lead to the use of directed multivariate statistics that allow summarization of study results with far fewer p-values than is currently possible.

REFERENCES

Andervont HB. Influence of environment on mammary cancer in mice. J Natl Cancer Inst 4:579–581, 1944.

Armitage P. Statistical Methods in Medical Research. New York: Wiley, 1971.

Arnold DL. Subchronic toxicity testing. In: Krewski D, Franklin C, eds. Statistics in Toxicology. New York: Gordon and Breach Science, 1991, pp 91–104.

Bailey SA. Calculating the Jonckheere–Terpstra test statistic using the SAS system under VMS. In: 1990 SAS Users Group International Conference Proceedings. SAS Institute, 1990, pp 1327–1330.

Barlow RE, Bartholomew DJ, Bremner JM, Brunk HD. Statistical Inference Under Order Restrictions. New York: Wiley, 1972.

Chacko VJ. Testing homogeneity against ordered alternatives. Ann Math Stat 34:945–956, 1963.

Ciminera JL. Some issues in the design, evaluation, and interpretation of tumorigenicity studies in animals. In: Proceedings of the Symposium on Long-Term Animal Carcinogenicity Studies: A Statistical Perspective. Biopharmaceutical Section of the American Statistical Association, 1985, pp 26–35.

Conover W. Practical Nonparametric Statistics. New York: Wiley, 1971.

Conover W, Iman R. Rank transformations as a bridge between parametric and nonparametric statistics. Am Stat 35:124–129, 1981.

Conover W, Iman R. Analysis of covariance using the rank transformation. Biometrics 38:715–724, 1982.

DHSS: United States Department of Health and Human Services. Guide for the Care and Use of Laboratory Animals. Bethesda, MD: National Institutes of Health, 1985.

Fare G. The influence of number of mice in a box on experimental skin tumour production. Br J Cancer 19:871–877, 1965.

FDA: US Food and Drug Administration. Guideline for the Format and Content of the Nonclinical Pharmacology/Toxicology Section of an Application. Washington, DC: 1987.

Fox JG, Helfrich-Smith ME. Chemical contamination of animal feeding systems: evaluation of two caging systems and standard cage washing equipment. Lab Anim Sci 30:967–973, 1980.

Franklin CA. Current challenges in toxicity testing. In: Krewski D, Franklin C, eds. Statistics in Toxicology. New York: Gordon and Breach Science, 1991, pp 3–10.

Friedman L. Symposium on the evaluation of the safety of food additives and chemical residues: II. The role of the laboratory animal study of intermediate duration for evaluation of safety. Toxicol Appl Pharmacol 16:498–506, 1969.

Gad SC, Weil CS. Statistics for toxicologists. In: Hayes AW, ed. Principles and Methods of Toxicology, 2nd ed. New York: Raven Press, 1989, pp 435–483.

Gad SC. Practical statistical analysis. In: Gad SC, ed. Product Safety Evaluation Handbook. New York: Marcel Dekker, 1988.

Gad SC, Weil CS. Statistics and Experimental Design for Toxicologists. Caldwell, NJ: Telford Press, 1988.

Hatch A, Wiberg G, Zawidzka Z, Can M, Airth J, Grice H. Isolation syndrome in the rat. Toxicol Appl Pharmacol 7:737–745, 1965.

Hollander M, Wolfe D. Nonparametric Statistical Methods. New York: Wiley, 1973.

Jensen C. A computer program for randomizing patients with near-even distribution of important parameters. Comput Biomed Res 24:429–434, 1991.

Johnson J. Past and present regulatory aspects of drug development. In: Peace K, ed. Biopharmaceutical Statistics for Drug Development. New York: Marcel Dekker, 1988, pp 1-20.

Jonckheere AR. A distribution free k-sample test against ordered alternatives. Biometrika 41:133-145, 1954.

Keene JH, Sansone EG. Airborne transfer of contaminants in ventilated spaces. Lab Anim Sci 34:453-457, 1984.

Krewski D, Bickis M. Statistical issues in toxicological research. In: Krewski D, Franklin C, eds. Statistics in Toxicology. New York: Gordon and Breach Science, 1991, pp 11-41.

Lehman EL. Nonparametrics: Statistical Methods Based on Ranks. San Francisco: Holden-Day, 1975.

Lin FO, Haseman JK. A modified Jonckheere test against ordered alternatives when ties are present at a single extreme value. Biom Z Bd 18:623-631, 1976.

Litt BD, Boyle KE, Myers LE. Statistical analysis of subchronic toxicity studies. In: Krewski D, Franklin C, eds. Statistics in Toxicology. New York: Gordon and Breach Science, 1991, pp 105-125.

Mead R. The Design of Experiments. New York: Cambridge University Press, 1988.

Meng C, Davis S, Roth A. Robust contrast based trend tests. In: 1993 Proceedings of the Biopharmaceutical Section, 1993, pp 127-132.

Mitruka BM, Rawnslay HM. Clinical Biochemical and Hematological Reference Values in Normal Experimental Animals. New York: Masson, 1977.

Mosberg AT, Hayes AW. Subchronic toxicity testing. In: Hayes AW, ed. Principles and Methods of Toxicology, 2nd ed. New York: Raven Press, 1989, pp 221-236.

Neter J, Wasserman W, Kutner M. Applied Linear Statistical Models, 2nd ed. Homewood IL: Richard Irwin, 1985.

OECD: Organization for Economic Cooperation and Development. OECD Guidelines for Testing of Chemicals. Paris: OECD, 1993.

Quade D. Rank analysis of covariance. J Am Stat Assoc 62:1187-1200, 1967.

Reed A, Henry R, Mason W. Influence of statistical method used on the resulting estimate of normal range. Clin Chem 17:275-284, 1971.

Roth A. Robust trend tests derived and simulated: analogs of the Welch and Brown-Forsythe tests. J Am Stat Assoc 78:972-980, 1983.

Ruberg S. Dose response studies: analysis and interpretation. J Biopharm Stat 5: 15-42, 1995.

Salsburg D. Statistics for Toxicologists. New York: Marcel Dekker, 1986.

Sansone EB, Fox JG. Potential chemical contamination in animal feeding studies: evaluation of wire and solid bottom caging systems and gelled feed. Lab Anim Sci 27:457-465, 1977.

Sansone EB, Losikoff AM, Pendelton RA. Potential hazard from feeding test chemicals in carcinogen bioassay research. Toxicol Appl Pharmacol 39: 435-450, 1977.

Selwyn M. The use of trend tests to determine a no-observable-effect level in animal safety studies. J Am Coll Toxicol 14:158–168, 1995.

Selwyn M. Preclinical safety assessment. In: Peace K, ed. Biopharmaceutical Statistics for Drug Development. New York: Marcel Dekker, 1988, pp 231–272.

Shorack GR. Testing against ordered alternatives in model I analysis of variance; normal theory and nonparametric. Ann Math Stat 38:1740–1753, 1967.

Sigg E, Day C, Columbo C. Endocrine factors in isolation-induced aggressiveness in rodents. Endocrinology 78:679–684, 1966.

Snedecor GW, Cochran WG. Statistical Methods. 6th ed. Ames, IO: Iowa State University Press, 1967.

Taves D. Minimization: a new method of assigning patients to treatment and control groups. Clin Pharmacol Ther 15:443–453, 1974.

Terpstra TJ. The asymptotic normality and consistency of Kendall's test against trend, when ties are present in one ranking. Indagationes Math 14:327–333, 1952.

Traina V. The role of toxicology in drug research and development. Med Res Rev 3:43–72, 1983.

Tukey JW, Ciminera JL, Heyse JF. Testing the statistical certainty of a response to increasing doses of a drug. Biometrics 41:295–301, 1985.

Weil CS. Statistical analysis and normality of selected hematologic and clinical chemistry measurements used in toxicologic studies. Arch Toxicol Suppl 5: 237–253, 1982.

Weil CS. Statistics vs. safety factors and scientific judgement in the evaluation of safety for man. Toxicol Appl Pharamacol 21:454–463, 1972.

Welch BL. On the comparison of several mean values: an alternative approach. Biometrika 38:330–336, 1951.

Welch BL, Welch AS. Graded effect of social stimulation upon d-amphetamine toxicity, aggressiveness and heart and adrenal weight. J Pharmacol Exp Ther 151:331–338, 1966.

Williams DA. The comparison of several dose levels with a zero dose control. Biometrics 28:519–531, 1972.

Williams DA. A test for differences between treatment means when several dose levels are compared with a zero dose control. Biometrics 27:103–117, 1971.

6

Safety Assessment in Toxicological Studies: Proof of Safety Versus Proof of Hazard

DIETER HAUSCHKE
Byk Gulden Pharmaceuticals, Konstanz, Germany

LUDWIG A. HOTHORN
University of Hannover, Hannover, Germany

I. INTRODUCTION

Before administration of the first dose of a new compound to human subjects, a toxicological safety assessment has to be performed. Statistical analysis plays a fundamental part in the interpretation of the corresponding experiments. Usually, the traditional null hypothesis of no difference in the effect between the treatment and a vehicle or negative control group is tested. Failure to reject the null hypothesis (e.g., if the corresponding p-value is greater than 0.05), often leads to the conclusion of evidence in favor of safety. The major drawback of this indirect procedure is what is controlled by the prespecified level is the probability of erroneously concluding hazard (producer risk). However, the primary concern of safety assessment is the control of the consumer risk, that is limiting the probability of erroneously concluding safety. Thus, the adequate test problem should be formulated by reversing the null hypothesis and the alternative and incorporating an a priori- or a posteriori-defined threshold. This direct approach will be demonstrated for the two-sample and k-sample many-to-one problem relative to nonmonotonic and monotonic response relations.

II. TWO-SAMPLE SITUATION

A. Proof of Hazard

Let X_{ij} represent the observation of the primary toxicological endpoint for the jth experimental unit (e.g., animal, plate, or cell) in the ith group ($i = 0, 1$ and $j = 1, \ldots, n_i$). Suppose that these random variables are mutually independent and have a continuous distribution function from a location parameter family, that is $F_i(x) = F(x - \mu_i)$ with μ_0 denoting the effect for the control and μ_1 that for the treatment group. Suppose further that, independent of any examination of the data, it is a priori known that $\mu_0 \leq \mu_1$, indicating the appropriateness of a one-sided alternative. The corresponding test problem for the proof of hazard is formulated as follows:

$$H_0^h : \mu_1 - \mu_0 \leq 0 \text{ (compound is safe under test conditions)} \qquad (1)$$

$$H_1^h : \mu_1 - \mu_0 > 0 \text{ (compound is hazardous under test conditions)}.$$

Failure to reject the null hypothesis by a statistical test at level α_h (e.g., Student's t-test or Wilcoxon test) traditionally leads to the conclusion that the compound has no deleterious effect in the underlying toxicological experiment. A p-value greater than α_h might indicate that there is no harmful effect of the treatment. However, because of inadequately small sample sizes or large variability, a toxicologically important effect may be present, but not statistically significant.

In toxicological studies, the sample size is often determined by regulatory guidelines. For example, in a repeated toxicity study, male and female animals should be used, there should be at least ten animals in each group. In Fig. 1, the power curves of the Student t-test are shown for $F_i(x) = \Phi[(x - \mu_i)/\sigma]$, where $\Phi(\cdot)$ denotes the cumulative distribution function of the standard normal distribution and σ^2 the unknown variance. For $\alpha_h = 0.05$, $2n_0 = 2n_1 = n = 20$, various coefficients of variation ($CV_0 = 100\sigma/\mu_0\%$), and values from the alternative $\mu_1 - \mu_0 > 0$, which are presented relative to the control mean μ_0, the figure gives an impression of the power achieved. As the CV_0 increases and the specific value from the alternative approaches the limit of the null hypothesis, the power decreases dramatically. Hence, only large effects can be detected with a sufficiently high probability for variabilities to occur in repeated toxicological studies (Chanter et al., 1987).

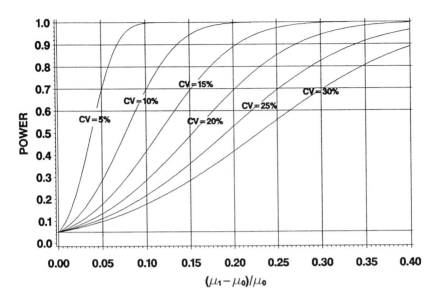

FIGURE 1 Hazard approach [see Eq. (1)]: power of the t-test; $\alpha_h = 0.05$, $2n_0 = 2n_1 = n = 20$, and $CV_0 = 5, 10, \ldots, 30\%$. (From Hauschke, 1997.)

However, from an ethical, scientific, and regulatory point of view, a toxicological study must have a reasonable chance of detecting a relevant treatment effect. Consequently, the sample size should be based on the type I and type II error, the underlying variability, and the specific size of effects considered appropriate by the toxicologist. The sample sizes from regulatory guidelines are not based on a formal power calculation, and any interpretation of the experiment should take this into account. The sample size issue was also subject of a draft guideline for toxicity tests provided by the Food and Drug Administration (FDA) (1993) which postulated that "a power calculation should be provided for tests that failed to reject the null hypothesis, particularly to justify the adequacy of the sample size."

It is obvious that the prospective use of power analysis provides a direct way to design an experiment precise enough to detect effects of toxicological importance. Retrospective power calculation, on the other hand, can be only an indirect way to reach the conclusion of no treatment effect. Furthermore, criteria for judging that a retrospectively determined power is adequate are rarely fixed in advance in the study protocol.

A significant statistical result could provide evidence for the conclusion that there is a toxicological effect of the treatment. On the other hand, good laboratory practice with a large sample size and little experimental variation may lead to the problem that a toxicologically unimportant difference will be declared statistically significant. This phenomenon often occurs in mutagenicity studies, when the individual cell is considered the experimental unit instead of the animal, and thus very large sample sizes result (Hauschke et al., 1997).

Summing up, proof of hazard is an indirect approach and often leads to the problem that statistical significance does not necessarily mean toxicological relevance and that statistical nonsignificance does not necessarily mean toxicological irrelevance. The major reason for these difficulties is the choice of the null hypothesis and the alternative. In statistical hypothesis testing, the null and alternative hypotheses are not treated equally. One demonstrates the likelihood of the alternative by measuring the strength of evidence against the null hypothesis. A way of directly concluding that a treatment has no harmful effect is the proof of safety, which requires that the test problem should be formulated by reversing the null hypothesis and the alternative and incorporating a threshold.

These issues were discussed by Bross (1985) and Millard (1987) on the question of whether an environment is safe or hazardous, and the authors noted that the proof of safety requires larger sample sizes than the proof of hazard. Therefore, Holland and Ordoukhani (1990) recommended consideration of higher levels in the proof of hazard and equating type I and type II error. Recently, Erickson and McDonald (1995), Hauschke (1995, 1997), and Stallard and Whitehead (1996) contributed to this topic in the field of toxicology. Erikson and McDonald focused on the determination of the threshold values and presented tables of these values for various sample sizes, number of treatments, and coefficients of variation. Unfortunately, they erroneously named the safety approach as a "test for bioequivalence of control media and test media in studies of toxicity." However, it should be noted that the term *bioequivalence* refers to pharmacokinetics and is defined as the equivalence of different formulations of the same drug substance relative to rate and extent of absorption. Stallard and Whitehead reviewed and illustrated the safety approach using long-term animal carcinogenicity studies. As an alternative to the Peto test, which is the standard method of analysis for carcinogenicity studies, they used a parametric multistate model and proposed a test for equivalence for the comparison of a single-dose group with the control group. Hauschke (1995, 1997) published general statistical aspects of the safety approach, which will be presented next.

B. Proof of Safety

1. One-Sided Test Problem

Regulatory requirements for new drug development allow the sponsor to proceed along the lines indicated by the fundamental assumptions that compounds are considered nonefficacious until proved otherwise, and that they are considered safe until proved otherwise (Peace, 1993). Therefore, conventional statistical testing directly controls the consumer risk for demonstrating efficacy, but only the producer risk for demonstrating safety.

However, in safety studies the primary concern of regulatory agencies should be the control of the consumer risk (erroneously accepting safety). Consequently, the adequate test problem for toxicological studies should be formulated as a proof of safety, providing consistency of the consumer risk for approval based on both efficacy and safety:

$$H_0^s : \mu_1 - \mu_0 \geq \delta \text{ (compound is hazardous under test conditions)}$$

$$H_1^s : \mu_1 - \mu_0 < \delta \text{ (compound is safe under test conditions)}, \qquad (2)$$

where δ, $\delta > 0$, denotes the minimally relevant safety difference and $(-\infty, \delta)$ the safety range.

This shifted null hypothesis can be tested by two-sample test procedures, and current methods can be used for sample size determination. It should be noted that the concept of shifted hypotheses was presented by Victor (1987) in the field of clinical trials. Testing a nonzero null hypothesis, that is incorporating a shift parameter δ, permits the assessment of the clinical relevance of an observed treatment difference. Figure 2 gives the corresponding power curves for the test problem [Eq. (2)] assuming a safety range of $(-\infty, \delta) = (-\infty, 0.2\mu_0)$.

In practice, there is often a reluctance to define δ a priori. If δ can be specified only a posteriori, the statistical method should be based on confidence intervals; that is, concluding safety at nominal level α_s if the upper limit of the one-sided $100(1 - \alpha_s)\%$ confidence interval for $\mu_1 - \mu_0$ is lower than δ. Specification of δ requires that the statisticians and toxicologists think about what constitutes a minimally relevant difference; ideally, this should happen at the planning stage of the experiment,

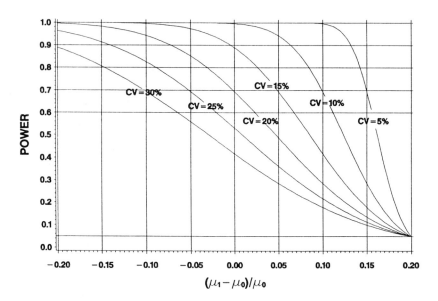

FIGURE 2 Safety approach [see Eq. (2)]: power of the t-test; $\delta = 0.2\mu_0$, $\alpha_s = 0.05$, $2n_0 = 2n_1 = n = 20$, and $CV_0 = 5, 10, \ldots, 30\%$.

but no later than after statistical analysis, when point estimates and confidence intervals have been calculated and the results are to be discussed. When neither an a priori nor an a posteriori definition of the minimally relevant difference can be given, an objective evaluation of toxicological results becomes difficult.

2. Two-Sided Test Problem

The one-sided formulation of the test problem makes sense for most toxicological studies. Nevertheless, in particular experiments, the following two-sided alternative might be more appropriate:

$$H_0^s: |\mu_1 - \mu_0| \geq \delta \text{ (compound is hazardous under test conditions)}$$
$$H_1^s: |\mu_1 - \mu_0| < \delta \text{ (compound is safe under test conditions)}, \quad (3)$$

where the interval $(-\delta, \delta)$ defines the safety range. A split into two one-sided hypotheses results in:

$$
\begin{array}{ccc}
H_{01}^s: \mu_1 - \mu_0 \leq -\delta & & H_{02}^s: \mu_1 - \mu_0 \geq \delta \\
H_{11}^s: \mu_1 - \mu_0 > -\delta & \text{and} & H_{12}^s: \mu_1 - \mu_0 < \delta.
\end{array} \quad (4)
$$

According to the intersection–union principle (Berger, 1982), H_0^s is rejected in favor of H_1^s (safety) at level α_s if both hypotheses H_{01}^s and H_{02}^s are rejected at nominal α_s. For example, assuming $F_i(x) = \Phi[(x - \mu_i)/\sigma]$, with an unknown but common σ^2, H_{01}^s is rejected, if

$$t_{11} = \frac{[\overline{X}_1 - \overline{X}_0 + \delta]}{[\hat{\sigma}\sqrt{(1/n_1 + 1/n_0)}]} \geq t(\alpha_s, n_0 + n_1 - 2)$$

and H_{02}^s is rejected, if

$$t_{12} = \frac{[\overline{X}_1 - \overline{X}_0 - \delta]}{[\hat{\sigma}\sqrt{(1/n_1 + 1/n_0)}]} \leq -t(\alpha_s, n_0 + n_1 - 2) \qquad (5)$$

where $\overline{X}_0$ and $\overline{X}_1$ denote the sample means of the control and treatment group, $\hat{\sigma}^2$ the pooled estimator of σ^2 and $t(\gamma, \nu)$ the upper γ percentile of the central t-distribution with ν-degrees of freedom. This decision procedure (Schuirmann, 1987) is equivalent to the inclusion of the ordinary two-sided $100(1 - 2\alpha_s)\%$ confidence interval for $\mu_1 - \mu_0$ in the range $(-\delta, \delta)$:

$$[\overline{X}_1 - \overline{X}_0 \pm t(\alpha_s, n_0 + n_1 - 2)\hat{\sigma}\sqrt{1/n_1 + 1/n_0}] \subset (-\delta, \delta). \qquad (6)$$

The following nonparametric method using Wilcoxon rank sum statistics for hypothesis testing and confidence interval construction was published by Hauschke et al. (1990): let $R_{1j}(\delta)$ denote the rank of $X_{1j} - \delta$ in the combined sample

$$X_{11} - \delta, \ldots, X_{1n_1} - \delta, X_{01}, \ldots, X_{0n_0} \qquad (7)$$

and let $R_1(\delta) = \Sigma_j R_{1j}(\delta)$, that is $R_1(\delta)$ is the sum of the ranks assigned to the shifted observations in the treatment group. H_{01}^s is rejected, if $R_1(-\delta) \geq r(\alpha_s, n_0, n_1)$, where $r(\gamma, n_0, n_1)$ is the upper γ percentile of the Wilcoxon's rank statistic $R_1(-\delta)$, and H_{02}^s is rejected, if $R_1(\delta) \leq n_1(n_0 + n_1 + 1) - r(\alpha_s, n_0, n_1)$. As with the parametric method, the following relation between the two one-sided tests and the confidence interval holds true (Hauschke and Steinijans, 1991; Chow and Liu, 1992). Rejecting H_{01}^s and H_{02}^s by Wilcoxon tests at nominal level, α_s is equivalent to the inclusion of the corresponding nonparametric $100(1 - 2\alpha_s)\%$ confidence interval for $\mu_1 - \mu_0$ in the safety range $(-\delta, \delta)$.

The calculation of this confidence interval according to Moses (Hollander and Wolfe, 1973) can be performed as follows. Let $D(1) \leq \ldots \leq D(n_0 n_1)$ denote the ordered values of the $n_0 n_1$ differences $X_{1j} - X_{0j^*}$ ($j = 1, \ldots, n_1$ and $j^* = 1, \ldots, n_0$). The median of these pairwise differences serves as the Hodges–Lehmann estimator (Hodges and Lehmann, 1963) and the lower and upper limits of the $100(1 - 2\alpha_s)\%$ confidence interval for $\mu_1 - \mu_0$ are given by

$$L = D(l) = D[C(\alpha_s)] \qquad \text{and}$$
$$U = D(u) = D[n_0 n_1 + 1 - C(\alpha_s)] \qquad (8)$$

where

$$C(\alpha_s) = \frac{n_1(2n_0 + n_1 + 1)}{2} + 1 - r(\alpha_s, n_0, n_1)$$

The values l/u corresponding to those of the ranked differences $X_{1j} - X_{0j^*}$ that form the 90% confidence limits are presented in Table 1 for total sample sizes of $n = n_0 + n_1 = 6, \ldots, 30$. For large n_0 and n_1, $C(\alpha_s)$ may be approximated by

$$C(\alpha_s) = \frac{n_0 n_1}{2} - z(\alpha_s) \sqrt{\frac{n_0 n_1 (n_0 + n_1 + 1)}{12}} \qquad (9)$$

where $z(\gamma)$ denotes the upper γ percentile of the standard normal distribution.

Hence, the safety assessment based on parametric or nonparametric confidence intervals can be used if a threshold δ is defined a posteriori.

3. A Numerical Example

The most common design for repeated toxicity studies includes a control group and three dose groups at low, medium, and high levels of the new compound. For an adequate safety assessment, it is also important to know whether a particular response is reversible. To examine the reversibility, the toxicologist may decide to include extra animals in the control and high-level group. These animals are removed from the compound after the treatment period, observed for an additional recovery period, and then subjected to the same toxicological analyses as those sacrificed after the dosing period. In Table 2 the individual terminal body weights of the male rats from the recovery groups are given. Table 3 gives the parametric and nonparametric point estimator and the corresponding 90% confidence intervals. By assuming a range $(-\delta, \delta)$ of ± 40 g, reversibility can be concluded at level 5% for both approaches. Application of the large-sample approximation [see Eq. (9)] results in $[-35.5, 19.4]$, which is nearly identical with the exact one.

TABLE 1 Values l/u for the Construction of the Nonparametric 90% Confidence Interval for $\mu_1 - \mu_0$

n_0	$n_1 = 3$	4	5	6	7	8	9	10	11	12	13	14	15
3	1/9	1/12	2/14	3/16	3/19	4/21	5/23	5/26	6/28	6/31	7/33	8/35	8/38
4	1/12	2/15	3/18	4/21	5/24	6/27	7/30	8/33	9/36	10/39	11/42	12/45	13/48
5	2/14	3/18	5/21	6/25	7/29	9/32	10/36	12/39	13/43	14/47	16/50	17/54	19/57
6	3/16	4/21	6/25	8/29	9/34	11/38	13/42	15/46	17/50	18/55	20/59	22/63	24/67
7	3/19	5/24	7/29	9/34	12/38	14/43	16/48	18/53	20/58	22/63	25/67	27/72	29/77
8	4/21	6/27	9/32	11/38	14/43	16/49	19/54	21/60	24/65	27/70	29/76	32/81	34/87
9	5/23	7/30	10/36	13/42	16/48	19/54	22/60	25/66	28/72	31/78	34/84	37/90	40/96
10	5/26	8/33	12/39	15/46	18/53	21/60	25/66	28/73	32/79	35/86	38/93	42/99	45/106
11	6/28	9/36	13/43	17/50	20/58	24/65	28/72	32/79	35/87	39/94	43/101	47/108	51/115
12	6/31	10/39	14/47	18/55	22/63	27/70	31/78	35/86	39/94	43/102	48/109	52/117	56/125
13	7/33	11/42	16/50	20/59	25/67	29/76	34/84	38/93	43/101	48/109	52/118	57/126	62/134
14	8/35	12/45	17/54	22/63	27/72	32/81	37/90	42/99	47/108	52/117	57/126	62/135	67/144
15	8/38	13/48	19/57	24/67	29/77	34/87	40/96	45/106	51/115	56/125	62/134	67/144	73/153

TABLE 2   Terminal Body Weights (g) of Male Rats

	Control–recovery	High-dose–recovery
	519.8	465.0
	535.7	492.2
	491.7	466.3
	508.7	555.5
	565.5	528.1
	485.8	483.8
	520.7	502.8
	507.5	468.1
	428.9	519.2
	466.0	500.2
n	10	10
Mean	503.0	498.1
Median	508.1	496.2
Standard deviation	37.9	29.6

4. Sample Size Determination

The problem of power calculation and sample size determination was addressed in a series of articles dealing primarily with bioequivalence studies (Phillips, 1990; Diletti et al., 1991; Liu and Chow, 1992; Hauschke et al., 1992). However, with minor modifications, the method can also be applied to the problem of safety assessment. The probability of correctly accepting H_1^s, in this case safety, is called the power of the test procedure and can be calculated for the balanced design; that is, $n_0 = n_1 = n/2$, as follows:

$$P[t_{11} \geq t(\alpha_s, n - 2) \wedge t_{12} \leq -t(\alpha_s, n - 2) \,|$$
$$-\delta < \mu_1 - \mu_0 < \delta, \sigma]$$
$$= Q_f[-t(\alpha_s, f), \Delta_2, 0, \psi] - Q_f[t(\alpha_s, f), \Delta_1, 0, \psi] \quad (10)$$

TABLE 3   Point Estimate and 90% Confidence Interval for $\mu_1 - \mu_0$

Statistical procedure	Point estimate	90% confidence interval
Parametric	−4.9	[−31.3, 21.5]
Nonparametric	−7.8	[−36.0, 19.8]

where

$$Q_f(t, \Delta, 0, \psi) = [\sqrt{2\pi}/[\Gamma(f/2)2^{f/2-1}]]$$

$$\int_0^\psi \Phi\left(\frac{ty}{\sqrt{f}} - \Delta\right) y^{f-1} \Phi'(y)\, dy$$

$$\Phi'(y) = \frac{1}{\sqrt{2\pi}} \exp(-y^2/2), \quad f = n - 2, \quad \psi = \frac{A_1 - A_2}{A_1 - A_2}$$

$$\Delta_i = \frac{[\mu_1 - \mu_0 - (-\delta)^i]}{[\sigma\sqrt{4/n}]}, \quad A_i = \frac{t_i}{\sqrt{f}}$$

$$i = 1, 2, \quad t_2 = -t_1 = -t(\alpha_s, f)$$

Expressing the safety range, the difference in means and σ as a percentage of the control mean:

$$\delta = \pm\nabla\mu_0, \quad \nabla > 0, \quad -\delta < \mu_1 - \mu_0 = \theta\mu_0 < \delta, \quad \sigma = CV_0\mu_0$$

simplifies the presentation of the noncentrality parameters:

$$\Delta_1 = \frac{(\theta + \nabla)}{[CV_0\sqrt{4/n}]} \quad \text{and} \quad \Delta_2 = \frac{(\theta - \nabla)}{[CV_0\sqrt{4/n}]} \tag{11}$$

The exact form of these integrals and an algorithm for their calculation has been provided by Owen (1965). Hence, the sample size calculation can be performed by specifying the power $1 - \beta_s$, the type I error α_s, the coefficient of variation CV_0, the safety range $(-\nabla\mu_0, \nabla\mu_0)$ and a value $\theta\mu_0$ from the alternative. In Fig. 3, the power curves for the decision procedure based on two one-sided t-tests are presented for particular sample sizes and a safety range of $(-\delta, \delta) = (-0.2\mu_0, 0.2\mu_0)$. For $n_0 = n_1 = n/2 = 10$ a maximum power of about 80% is achieved. The calculation of the power is mathematically complex and computational difficult; for that reason, the total sample size (n) to achieve a power of $1 - \beta_s$ at nominal level α_s can be calculated according to the following approximate formulas:

if $\theta = 0$ 　　　　　$\Rightarrow n \geq 4[t(\alpha_s, n - 2)$

$$+ t(\beta_s/2, n - 2)]^2 \left[\frac{CV_0}{\nabla}\right]^2$$

if $0 < \theta < \nabla$ 　　　$\Rightarrow n \geq 4[t(\alpha_s, n - 2)$

$$+ t(\beta_s, n - 2)]^2 \left[\frac{CV_0}{\nabla - \theta}\right]^2$$

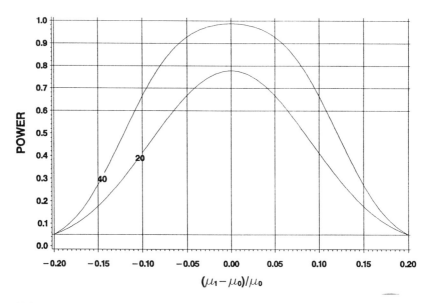

FIGURE 3   Safety approach [see Eq. (3)]: power of the procedure based on two one-sided t-tests; $(-\delta, \delta) = (-0.2\mu_0, 0.2\mu_0)$, $\alpha_s = 0.05$, $CV_0 = 15\%$, and $2n_0 = 2n_1 = n = 20, 40$.

$$\text{and if } -\nabla < \theta < 0 \Rightarrow n \geq 4[t(\alpha_s, n - 2)$$
$$+ \ t(\beta_s, n - 2)]^2 \left[\frac{CV_0}{-\nabla - \theta} \right]^2 \tag{12}$$

Table 4 gives the sample sizes to attain a power of at least 0.80 for $|\theta| = 0.05, \ldots, 0.15$ and various CV_0. For the corresponding configuration, the exact sample sizes are given in the first line and the approximate ones in the second line, the latter only if they deviate from the exact ones. Because an even number of subjects is needed, calculated odd sample size have been rounded up.

For small absolute values of θ (i.e., $|\theta| < 0.05$ and $\theta \neq 0$), the sample size determination by the approximate formula may result in irregularities. This occurrence is due to the step from $t(\beta_s, n - 2)$ for $\theta \neq 0$) to $t(\beta_s/2, n - 2)$ for $\theta = 0$ in the foregoing equations. Here the exact formula should be used.

TABLE 4   Exact (First Line) and Approximate (Second Line) Total Sample Sizes (n), $\alpha_s = 0.05$, $\beta_s = 0.20$ and the Safety Range is $(-\delta, \delta) = (-0.2\mu_0, 0.2\mu_0)$

	$|\theta|$			
CV_0	0.00	0.05	0.10	0.15
0.05	6	6	8	28
	—	—	10	—
0.10	12	14	28	102
	—	—	—	—
0.15	22	28	58	224
	—	—	—	226
0.20	36	48	102	398
	—	46	—	—
0.25	56	72	156	620
	—	—	158	—
0.30	80	102	224	892
	—	—	226	—

C. Relation Between Proof of Safety and Proof of Hazard

The proponents of the classic approach (e.g., Ng, 1995) sometimes justify their method with the argument that, under the assumption of normality with known variance, both approaches coincide, provided the error rates and the sample sizes are adequately chosen. However, Hauschke and Steinijans (1996) disproved this as follows. Let X_{ij} be mutually independent and normally distributed with known common variance: X_{ij} i.i.d $\sim F(x) = \Phi[(x - \mu_i)/\sigma]$, $i = 0, 1$ and $j = 1, \ldots, n_0 = n_1 = n/2$, and let η denote the actual difference $\mu_1 - \mu_0$. The decision procedure at nominal level α_s in favor of safety (H_1^s) is based on the inclusion of the classic two-sided $100(1 - 2\alpha_s)\%$ confidence interval for $\mu_1 - \mu_0$ in the safety range $(-\delta, \delta)$. The approximate Eq. (12) can also be applied with minor modifications for the case of known variance and for the specification of the safety range in absolute values. The test problem for proof of hazard is formulated as follows:

$$H_0^h:\mu_1 - \mu_0 = 0$$
$$H_1^h:\mu_1 - \mu_0 \neq 0, \tag{13}$$

and the decision procedure at nominal α_h in favor of difference (H_1^h) is based on the exclusion of the value 0 from the two-sided $100(1 - \alpha_h)\%$ confidence interval for $\mu_1 - \mu_0$. The sample size can be determined by specifying the power at $1 - \beta_h$ for $\eta = \mu_1 - \mu_0$ and is given by the well-known equation:

$$n \geq 4\left[z\left(\frac{\alpha_h}{2}\right) + z(\beta_h)\right]^2 \left[\frac{\sigma}{\eta}\right]^2 \tag{14}$$

One can easily verify that failing to reject H_1^h is equivalent to rejecting H_0^s if one chooses $\alpha_s = \beta_h$, $\beta_s = \alpha_h$, and calculates the corresponding confidence interval using the sample size determined at $\eta = 0$ for the safety approach and at $\eta = \delta$ for the hazard approach. However, when $\alpha_s = \beta_h$, $\beta_s = \alpha_h$, but $-\delta < \eta < \delta$, $\eta \neq 0$, the sample size calculated by the hazard approach $(\eta = \delta)$ obviously differs from the value calculated for the safety approach $(\eta \neq 0)$. For example, if $\sigma = \delta = 1$, $\alpha_s = \beta_h = 0.05$, $\beta_s = \alpha_h = 0.20$, and $\eta = 0$, $n = 18$ results for both approaches; however, if $\eta = 0.5$, $n = 18$ results in the hazard approach and $n = 50$ in the safety approach. The larger sample size for the safety approach is indicative of the lack of sensitivity of the proof of hazard, rather than the result of the proposed new method. By analogy, the same relation holds true if the variance has to be estimated and also if there is a one-sided test problem.

III. k-SAMPLE MANY-TO-ONE SITUATION

A. Nonmonotonic Response Relation

The following one-way layout represents a typical experimental design for toxicological studies:

$$\{\text{Control, treatment}_1, \text{treatment}_2, \ldots, \text{treatment}_k\} \tag{15}$$

where the k treatment groups may be different substances or combinations of substances. This design is sometimes extended by the inclusion of a positive control group: administering a compound of known toxic, teratogenic, mutagenic, or carcinogenic potential, the sensitivity of the test system (e.g., animal species or bacterial strain) can be validated within the actual experiment itself. The appropriate statistical analysis for the inclusion of a positive control group was published by Hothorn (1995). Let X_{ij} denote the observation for the jth experimental unit in the ith treatment group and suppose that X_{ij} i.i.d $\sim F(x - \mu_i)$, $i = 0, 1$,

$\ldots$, k and $j = 1, \ldots, n_i$. The relevant safety parameters are the k differences $\mu_i - \mu_0$, $i \geq 1$. Let H_{0i}^s be the null hypothesis that the ith treatment does not meet the safety criterion and H_{1i}^s the alternative that it does. The following cases of global and partial safety are of particular interest.

1. Global Safety

In the situation of global safety, it must be shown that all k treatments have no harmful effect. The test problem can be formulated either one-sided

$$H_0^{gs}{:}\mu_i - \mu_0 \geq \delta \qquad \exists\ i \in (1, \ldots, k)$$
$$H_1^{gs}{:}\mu_i - \mu_0 < \delta \qquad \forall\ i \in (1, \ldots, k) \tag{16}$$

or two-sided

$$H_0^{gs}{:}|\mu_i - \mu_0| \geq \delta \qquad \exists\ i \in (1, \ldots, k)$$
$$H_1^{gs}{:}|\mu_i - \mu_0| < \delta \qquad \forall\ i \in (1, \ldots, k) \tag{17}$$

The statistical analysis can be performed according to the intersection–union priciple; that is rejection of H_0^{gs} in favor of H_1^{gs} (safety) at level α if all k hypotheses H_{0i}^s, $i = 1, \ldots, k$, are rejected at level α.

    a. One-Sided Test Problem. Assuming $F_i(x) = \Phi[(x - \mu_i)/\sigma]$, with unknown, but common, σ^2, H_0^{gs} is rejected for the one-sided situation [see Eq. (16)], if

$$t_i = \frac{[\overline{X}_i - \overline{X}_0 - \delta]}{\hat{\sigma}\ \sqrt{(1/n_i + 1/n_0)}} \leq -t(\alpha, v) \quad \forall\ i \in (1, \ldots, k), \tag{18}$$

where $\overline{X}_0$ and $\overline{X}_i$ denote the sample means of the control and ith treatment group, $\hat{\sigma}^2 = \dfrac{1}{v} [\Sigma_i \Sigma_j (X_{ij} - \overline{X}_{i.})^2]$ the pooled estimator of σ^2 with $v = \Sigma_i n_i - (k + 1)$ and $t(\gamma, v)$ the upper γ percentile of the univariate central t-distribution with v-degrees of freedom. When δ is determined a posteriori, global safety can be concluded if all upper limits of the one-sided $100(1 - \alpha)\%$ confidence intervals for $\mu_i - \mu_0$ are lower than δ; that is

$$\left(-\infty,\ \overline{X}_i - \overline{X}_0 + t(\alpha, v)\hat{\sigma} \sqrt{\frac{1}{n_i} + \frac{1}{n_0}}\ \right] \subset (-\infty, \delta)$$
$$\forall\ i \in (1, \ldots, k). \tag{19}$$

For the nonparametric approach the method of pairwise ranking is applied, that is $R_{ij}(\delta)$ denotes the rank of $X_{ij} - \delta$ in the combined sample of size $n_0 + n_i$. H_0^{gs} is rejected, if $R_i(\delta) \leq n_i(n_0 + n_i + 1) - r(\alpha, n_0, n_i)$ for all $i \in (1, \ldots, k)$, where $R_i(\delta) = \Sigma_j R_{ij}(\delta)$.

The calculation of the nonparametric one-sided $100(1 - \alpha)\%$ confidence interval for $\mu_i - \mu_0$ is based on the ordered values $D(1) \leq \ldots \leq D(n_0 n_i)$ of the $n_0 n_i$ differences $X_{ij} - X_{0j^*}$ ($j = 1, \ldots, n_i$ and $j^* = 1, \ldots, n_0$):

$$(-\infty, U_i] = (-\infty, D[n_0 n_i + 1 - C_i(\alpha)]] \tag{20}$$

where

$$C_i(\alpha) = \frac{n_i(2n_0 + n_i + 1)}{2} + 1 - r(\alpha, n_0, n_i)$$

and global safety is inferred if $(-\infty, U_i) \subset (-\infty, \delta)$ for all $i \in (1, \ldots, k)$.

b. Two-Sided Test Problem. Under the assumption of normality with common variance, H_0^{gs} is rejected for the two-sided test problem [see Eq. (17)], if

$$t_{i1} = \frac{[\overline{X}_i - \overline{X}_0 + \delta]}{[\hat{\sigma}\sqrt{(1/n_i + 1/n_0)}]} \geq t(\alpha, v)$$

and

$$t_{i2} = \frac{[\overline{X}_i - \overline{X}_0 - \delta]}{[\hat{\sigma}\sqrt{(1/n_i + 1/n_0)}]} \leq -t(\alpha, v) \quad \forall i \in (1, \ldots, k) \tag{21}$$

which is equivalent to the inclusion of the two-sided $100(1 - 2\alpha)\%$ confidence intervals for $\mu_i - \mu_0$ in the safety range:

$$\left[\overline{X}_i - \overline{X}_0 \pm t(\alpha, v)\hat{\sigma}\sqrt{\frac{1}{n_i} + \frac{1}{n_0}}\right] \subset (-\delta, \delta)$$

$$\forall i \in (1, \ldots, k) \tag{22}$$

A single test procedure for global safety was provided by Bofinger and Bofinger (1993) and Giani and Strassburger (1994). Bofinger and Bofinger considered the largest absolute different $\eta^* = \max_i |\mu_i - \mu_0|$, defined global safety by postulating $\eta^* \leq \eta_0$ and based their decision procedure on the upper confidence bound for η^*. Giani and Strassburger characterized global safety in a standardized form (i.e., η^*/σ rather than η^*) and proposed a test based on a two-sided many-to-one statistic.

However, the major disadvantage of both methods consists of the complex computation of the upper confidence bound and the critical values of the test procedure, respectively.

Following the nonparametric approach, H_0^{gs} is rejected, if $R_i(-\delta)$ $\geq r(\alpha, n_0, n_i)$ and $R_i(\delta) \leq n_i(n_0 + n_i + 1) - r(\alpha, n_0, n_i)$ for all $i \in (1, \ldots, k)$. The lower and upper limits of the $100(1 - 2\alpha)\%$ confidence interval for $\mu_i - \mu_0$ are given by

$$L_i = D[C_i(\alpha)], \qquad U_i = D[n_0 n_i + 1 - C_i(\alpha)] \qquad (23)$$

and safety is concluded if $[L_i, U_i] \subset (-\delta, \delta)$ for all $i \in (1, \ldots, k)$.

2. Partial Safety

The criterion of global safety holds true only if all treatments fulfill the safety criterion. This is a very strong condition; therefore, it might be useful to consider only partial safety. The corresponding test problem can be formulated either one-sided

$$H_0^{ps}:\mu_i - \mu_0 \geq \delta \qquad \forall \; i \in (1, \ldots, k)$$
$$H_1^{ps}:\mu_i - \mu_0 < \delta \qquad \exists \; i \in (1, \ldots, k) \qquad (24)$$

or two-sided

$$H_0^{ps}:|\mu_i - \mu_0| \geq \delta \qquad \forall \; i \in (1, \ldots, k)$$
$$H_1^{ps}:|\mu_i - \mu_0| < \delta \qquad \exists \; i \in (1, \ldots, k) \qquad (25)$$

This is the union–intersection problem according to Roy (1953) (i.e., H_0^{ps} is rejected if *at least one* individual hypothesis H_{0i}^s is rejected).

a. One-Sided Test Problem. Provided that the assumptions of homogeneous variances and normality are met, the many-to-one comparison, based on the multivariate t-distribution (Dunnett, 1955), can be performed, which controls the familywise error rate (i.e., the probability of at least one erroneous rejection of a null hypothesis H_{0i}^s, $i = 1, \ldots, k$). Consider first the problem of testing $H_{0i}^s:\mu_i - \mu_0 \geq \delta$ versus the one-sided alternative $H_{1i}^s:\mu_i - \mu_0 < \delta$; the t-statistics are given by

$$t_i = \frac{[\overline{X}_i - \overline{X}_0 - \delta]}{[\hat{\sigma} \sqrt{(1/n_i + 1/n_0)}]} \qquad 1 \leq i \leq k \qquad (26)$$

Given H_0^{ps}, the statistics $t_1, \ldots, t_k$ have a k-variate t-distribution with v degrees of freedom and correlation matrix P_k with corresponding coefficients given by $\rho_{ij} = \lambda_i \lambda_j$, $1 \leq i \neq j \leq k$, where $\lambda_i = \sqrt{n_i/(n_i + n_0)}$ (Dunnett and Tamhane, 1991). The hypotheses H_{0i}^s are rejected if $t_i \geq t(\alpha, k, v, P_k)$, where $t(\gamma, l, v, P_l)$ denotes the upper γ percentile of the distribution of max $\{t_1, \ldots, t_l\}$ under H_0^{ps}, which is a l-variate t-distribution with v degrees of freedom and correlation matrix P_l.

Given the closed testing procedure (Marcus et al., 1976), Dunnett and Tamhane (1991) provided a more powerful step-down procedure. The statistics are ordered in an ascending manner (i.e., $t_{(1)} \leq t_{(2)} \leq \ldots \leq t_{(k)}$, and $H_{0(1)}^s, \ldots, H_{0(k)}^s$ denote the corresponding hypotheses). $H_{0(i)}^s$ is rejected for $i = k, \ldots, 1$ if $t_{(i)} \geq t(\alpha, i, v, P_i)$ and $H_{0(i+1)}^s, \ldots, H_{0(k)}^s$ have been rejected, otherwise $H_{0(1)}^s, \ldots, H_{0(i)}^s$ are retained. Dunnett and Tamhane (1992, 1995) also proposed an analogous step-up procedure; however, a statistical proof for the condition that this method controls the familywise error is still missing for the unequal correlation structure.

A more general and easier method to apply is the well-known Bonferroni adjustment, which uses level α/k for every single test problem H_{0i}^s; that is, replacing the critical values $t(\alpha, k, v, P_k)$ by $t(\alpha/k, v)$. For large k, this method is very conservative and can be improved by a step-down test procedure (Holm, 1979) in which the p-values of the single tests are ordered by their magnitude [i.e., $p_{(1)} \leq \ldots \leq p_{(k)}$], with the corresponding hypotheses $H_{0(1)}^s, \ldots, H_{0(k)}^s$. The Holm procedure rejects $H_{0(l)}^s$ if and only if all $H_{0(i)}^s$ have been rejected, $i < l$, and $p_{(l)} \leq \alpha/(k - l + 1)$. In some special situations (e.g., independence of the statistics), the Bonferroni procedure and the Holm modification can be further improved (Simes, 1986; Hochberg, 1988; Hommel, 1988; Rom, 1990).

The simultaneous parametric $100(1 - \alpha)\%$ one-sided confidence intervals for $\mu_i - \mu_0$ are given by

$$\left(-\infty, \overline{X}_i - \overline{X}_0 + t(\alpha, k, v, P_k)\hat{\sigma}\sqrt{\frac{1}{n_i} + \frac{1}{n_0}} \right] \quad 1 \leq i \leq k \qquad (27)$$

and can be used in an a posteriori definition of the minimally relevant difference, and safety is concluded for ith treatment, $1 \leq i \leq k$, if the upper limit of the foregoing confidence interval is lower than δ.

So far, a specific parametric distributional model was assumed. Steel (1959) proposed a nonparametric many-to-one procedure for which it is assumed that $n_1 = \ldots = n_k = m$ and m may be different from the sample size of the control n_0. The hypotheses H_{0i}^s are rejected, if $R_i(\delta) \leq m(n_0 + m + 1) - r(\alpha, k, n_0, m)$, where $r(\gamma, k, n_0, m)$ is the upper γ

percentile of the distribution of $\max\{R_1(\delta), \ldots, R_k(\delta)\}$ under H_0^{ps}. Exact critical values were provided by Steel for the constellation $k = 2, 3$ and $n_0 = m = 3, 4, 5$, and large sample size approximations were given by Hochberg and Tamhane (1987) and Hsu (1996).

The corresponding nonparametric simultaneous $100(1 - \alpha)\%$ one-sided confidence intervals for $\mu_i - \mu_0$ are given by Hochberg and Tamhane (1987):

$$(-\infty, U_i] = (-\infty, D[n_0 m + 1 - C_i(\alpha)]] \tag{28}$$

where

$$C_i(\alpha) = \frac{m(2n_0 + m + 1)}{2} + 1 - r(\alpha, k, n_0, m)$$

and can be used for the partial safety assessment in an analogous manner.

b. Two-Sided Test Problem. In the following, the problem of testing $H_{0i}^s: |\mu_i - \mu_0| \geq \delta$ versus the two-sided alternative $H_{1i}^s: |\mu_i - \mu_0| < \delta$ is considered. A split into two one-sided hypotheses results in

$$\begin{array}{cc}
H_{01i}^s: \mu_i - \mu_0 \leq -\delta & H_{02i}^s: \mu_i - \mu_0 \geq \delta \\
H_{11i}^s: \mu_i - \mu_0 > -\delta & \text{and} \quad H_{12i}^s: \mu_i - \mu_0 < \delta
\end{array} \quad 1 \leq i \leq k. \tag{29}$$

H_{0i}^s is rejected, if H_{01i}^s and H_{02i}^s can be rejected, i.e.,

$$t_{i1} = \frac{[\overline{X}_i - \overline{X}_0 + \delta]}{[\hat{\sigma} \sqrt{(1/n_i + 1/n_0)}} \geq t(\alpha/k, v)$$

and

$$t_{i2} = \frac{[\overline{X}_i - \overline{X}_0 - \delta]}{[\hat{\sigma} \sqrt{(1/n_i + 1/n_0)}} \leq -t(\alpha/k, v) \tag{30}$$

The Bonferroni adjustment implies the control of the familywise error rate; that is, the probability of at least one erroneous conclusion of safety. This method can be improved by the following step-down procedure: let $p_i = \max\{p_{i1}, p_{i2}\}$, where p_{i1} and p_{i2} denote the p-values of the test statistics t_{i1} and t_{i2}, respectively. Again, the values p_i are ordered by their magnitude and the corresponding hypotheses $H_{0(1)}^s$, $\ldots$, $H_{0(k)}^s$ can be tested by the Holm procedure rejecting $H_{0(l)}^s$ if and only if all $H_{0(i)}^s$ have been rejected, $i < l$, and $p_{(l)} \leq \alpha/(k - l + 1)$.

In analogy to Eq. (30), simultaneous two-sided $100(1 - 2\alpha)\%$ confidence intervals for $\mu_i - \mu_0$ are given by

$$\left[\overline{X}_i - \overline{X}_0 \pm t(\alpha/k, v)\hat{\sigma} \sqrt{\frac{1}{n_i} + \frac{1}{n_0}} \right] \qquad 1 \le i \le k \qquad (31)$$

The Bonferroni adjustment can also be applied for the nonparametric test procedure and the corresponding confidence intervals.

Recently, Bofinger and Bofinger (1995) constructed, for the special case of balanced treatment groups (i.e., $n_1 = \ldots = n_k = m$) expanded simultaneous confidence intervals of the form

$$\left(\left(\overline{X}_i - \overline{X}_0 - c_k\hat{\sigma} \sqrt{\frac{1}{m} + \frac{1}{n_0}} \right)^-, \right.$$

$$\left. \left(\overline{X}_i - \overline{X}_0 + c_k\hat{\sigma} \sqrt{\frac{1}{m} + \frac{1}{n_0}} \right)^+ \right] \qquad (32)$$

where $y^- = \min\{0, y\}$, $y^+ = \max\{0, y\}$ and c_k are special critical points from the multivariate t-distribution, specified by the authors. Given these confidence intervals, the hypotheses H_{0i}^s are rejected while controlling the familywise error, if

$$\left(\left(\overline{X}_i - \overline{X}_0 - c_k\hat{\sigma} \sqrt{\frac{1}{m} + \frac{1}{n_0}} \right)^-, \right.$$

$$\left. \left(\overline{X}_i - \overline{X}_0 + c_k\hat{\sigma} \sqrt{\frac{1}{m} + \frac{1}{n_0}} \right)^+ \right] \subset (-\delta, \delta). \qquad (33)$$

The authors demonstrated that the effective lengths are shorter for these intervals than Dunnett's classic, two-sided simultaneous confidence intervals, which could also be used in testing H_{0i}^s:

$$\left[\overline{X}_i - \overline{X}_0 \pm |t| \, (\alpha, k, v, P_k)\hat{\sigma} \sqrt{\frac{1}{n_i} + \frac{1}{n_0}} \right] \qquad 1 \le i \le k \qquad (34)$$

where $|t|$ (α, k, v, P_k) denotes the critical point for the two-sided situation (Dunnett, 1955).

3. A Numerical Example

In 1989, Bedotto et al. published the paper *Cardiac Hypertrophy Induced by Thyroid Hormone Is Independent of Loading Conditions and beta-Adrenoceptor Blockade*. The authors investigated in a pharmacological experiment whether left-ventricular hypertrophy induced by thyroid hormone (T_4) in the rat is inhibited by treatment with captopril, hydralazine, propranolol, and a combination of captopril and propranolol. Their conclusion was based on a statistical test for difference in the sense of proof of hazard. But supposing that the experiment had been designed to demonstrate that the left-ventricular hypertrophy induced by T_4 is not further enhanced by simultaneous administration of the active treatments, proof of safety would have been a more appropriate method. The relevant part of the results necessary for the safety approach is given in Table 5.

The pooled estimator of the standard variation $\hat{\sigma} = 0.1538$ with 93 degrees of freedom for calculation of the upper confidence limit was provided by Dunnett and Tamhane (1991). If one assumes that the increase in effect for T_4 and (T_4 plus drug) is considered pharmacologically unimportant up to at most 1 empirical standard deviation (i.e., $\delta = \hat{\sigma} = 0.1538$), safety can be concluded only for the group with coadministration of captopril.

B. Monotonic Response Relation

Many toxicological drug studies involve the investigation of a dose-response relation. The substance is administered in increasing doses D_1, $D_2, \ldots, D_k$ to k groups of experimental units, and a response, such as body weight loss of animals, is measured at a specific time. The mean responses for each dose group are $\mu_1, \ldots, \mu_k$ and the mean response is a nondecreasing function of the dose level (i.e., $\mu_1 \leq \ldots \leq \mu_k$). It is

TABLE 5   Sample Means, Sizes for the Endpoint Left-Ventricular Weight/Body Weight (mg/g)[a] and Upper 95% Simultaneous Confidence Limits [Eq. (27)] for the Comparisons with T_4

Treatment group	Sample mean	Sample size	Upper confidence limit
Negative control	2.21	11	—
T_4	2.52	10	—
T_4 + captopril	2.49	9	0.125
T_4 + propranolol	2.60	12	0.224
T_4 + hydralazine	2.54	10	0.171
T_4 + propranolol + captopril	2.56	10	0.191

Source: [a]Dunnett and Tamhane, 1991.

customary to include a zero dose to serve as negative or vehicle group and if μ_0 denotes the control mean, the effect of the compound at dose i is measured by the difference $\mu_i - \mu_0$, $1 \le i \le k$.

1. Proof of Hazard

The conventional approach is to find the no-observed-adverse-effect level (NOAEL), that is the highest dose at which there is no statistically significant increase in $\mu_i - \mu_0$. However, the NOAEL represents a statistical no-effect level that depends on the power of the study. Hence, a less sensitive toxicological experiment with a small sample size results in higher "safe" doses than the corresponding study with a larger sample size and lower variability.

Consider the following hypothetical example (Table 6) provided by Gaylor (1983) in which the proportions of diseased animals are the same at each dose level in two experiments with different sample sizes.

The conventional statistical analysis of the experimental results is performed by the Cochran–Armitage test using ordinal dose scores and including all groups in the first step; a discussion about the choice of optimal dose scores was given by Podgor et al. (1996) and Neuhäuser and Hothorn (1997). For a significant result (i.e., p-value ≤ 0.05), the test is repeated in the second step without the highest dose. If it is again significant, the test is repeated in the third step without the highest and the medium dose. A nonsignificant test result (i.e., p-value > 0.05) will be used for declaring the highest dose in the corresponding test as the NOAEL. In Table 7 the corresponding exact p-values are presented. In addition, the asymptotic power of the Cochran–Armitage test is calculated according to Nam (1987) on the basis of the control, low, and medium dose.

TABLE 6   A Hypothetical Example

	Proportion of diseased animals	
Treatment group	Experiment 1	Experiment 2
Control	0/20	0/60
Low-dose D_1	1/20	3/60
Medium-dose D_2	2/20	6/60
High-dose D_3	10/20	30/60

Source: Gaylor, 1983.

TABLE 7   Exact p-Values of the Cochran–Armitage Test

Treatment group	Proportion	Experiment 1	Experiment 2
Low-dose D_1	0.05	—	0.121
Medium-dose D_2	0.10	0.144 (0.28)[a]	0.009 (0.75)[a]
High-dose D_3	0.50	<0.001	<0.001

[a]Asymptotic power.

In the first experiment, the highest nonsignificant dose is D_2 and in the second study the NOAEL is the low-dose D_1. However, looking at the power value of 0.28 it is obvious that smaller sample sizes result in higher "safe" doses, which is exactly the opposite of what is desired.

The statistical determination of the NOAEL has been dealt with in a series of papers (e.g., Williams, 1971, 1972); Shirley, 1977; Tukey et al., 1985; Rom et al., 1994; see also Chap. 4). However, all of the proposed original methods defined the NOAEL as the highest experimental dose at which there is no statistical increase in the underlying toxicological endpoint; hence, they have the statistical deficiencies described in the foregoing. Brown and Erdreich (1989) and Yanagawa et al. (1994, 1995) emphasized that applying the conventional approach implies that the smaller the sample sizes, the larger the doses selected as the NOAEL and the less toxic a compound is likely to appear. Brown and Erdreich recommended the a posteriori calculation of the power to detect a difference of interest before drawing a conclusion, and if this probability is low, then the statistical evidence should only be inconclusive. Yanagawa et al. observed that these calculations may be cumbersome; therefore, they explored the use of the Akaike information criterion for the determination of the NOAEL.

2. Proof of Safety

According to the principle of the proof of safety, the adequate definition of the NOAEL is as follows:

$$\text{NOAEL} = D_i, \text{where } i = \max\{i: \mu_i - \mu_0 < \delta\} \tag{35}$$

In other words, safety of dose D_i (i.e., $\mu_i - \mu_0 < \delta$) has to be formulated as the alternative. Neuhäuser and Hothorn (1995) and Hauschke (1995) described the following sequentially rejecting procedure, controlling the familywise error for the determination of the highest safe dose. Starting with the lowest dose, the hypothesis

$$H_{01}^s : \mu_1 - \mu_0 \geq \delta$$
$$H_{11}^s : \mu_1 - \mu_0 < \delta$$

is tested by two-sample test (e.g., a pairwise contrasts test (Tamhane et al., 1996)). If H_{01}^s is rejected at level α, the problem

$$H_{02}^s : \mu_2 - \mu_0 \geq \delta$$
$$H_{12}^s : \mu_2 - \mu_0 < \delta$$

is tested. For a nonsignificant result, the procedure stops. In general, H_{0i}^s *is rejected at level* α *if and only if all* H_{0l}^s have been rejected at level α, $l < i$, $i = 1, \ldots, k$. The NOAEL is the highest dose for which H_{0i}^s: $\mu_i - \mu_0 \geq \delta$ was rejected in favor of $H_{11}^s : \mu_i - \mu_0 < \delta$ (safety).

If δ can be specified only a posteriori, the statistical method can be based on the upper limits of the corresponding one-sided $100(1 - \alpha)\%$ confidence intervals. In toxicological experiments, the assumption of a parametric dose–response model is usually not appropriate; therefore, the usual confidence bounds for $\mu_i - \mu_0$ are presented, that is,

$$\left(-\infty, \overline{X}_i - \overline{X}_0 + t(\alpha, \nu)\hat{\sigma} \sqrt{\frac{1}{n_i} + \frac{1}{n_0}} \right] \qquad 1 \leq i \leq k \qquad (36)$$

Frequently, the assumption of a nondecreasing dose–response curve is fulfilled; hence, this information can be used to provide better estimates. Schoenfeld (1986) introduced the calculation of nonsimultaneous isotonic confidence bounds for the parameters μ_i by inverting the corresponding likelihood ratio test. These bounds provide a substantial improvement over the usual confidence limits when the dose–response curve does not increase rapidly. Recently, Lee (1996) published a generalization of the simultaneous isotonic confidence intervals for μ_i (Korn, 1982). However, both methods are based on the studentized maximum modulus and the application of this procedure for the differences $\mu_i - \mu_0$ is not appropriate. Further research by us on simultaneous isotonic and nonsimultaneous isotonic confidence intervals for the differences $\mu_i - \mu_0$ is in progress.

3. A Numerical Example

Table 8 presents the summary statistics of serum ASAT values (μmol/L) for three dose levels of a new compound and one control group in a 6-month toxicological study on female Wistar rats (Hothorn, 1991).

According to the sequentially rejecting approach only the lowest

TABLE 8 Sample Means, Standard Deviations, Sizes for the Endpoint ASAT-Values (μmol/L) and *p*-Values for the Safety Comparisons with the Zero Control Assuming $\delta = 0.5\mu$mol/L

Dose group (mg/kg)	Sample mean	Standard deviation	Sample size	*p*-value
0	2.087	0.569	19	—
20	2.064	0.304	16	0.0012
200	2.514	0.722	17	0.3683
1000	2.753	0.831	13	0.7466

Source: Hothorn, 1991.

dose can be declared as the NOAEL, and the probability of erroneously declaring 20 mg/kg as a safe dose is at most 0.05.

The comparisons with the control were performed by pairwise *t*-tests using the pooled estimator of the standard deviation for the control and the corresponding dose group. Because of reduction to two-sample tests, the Welch modification can be applied without any problem in variance heterogeneity.

IV. CONCLUSION

The traditional proof of hazard is only an indirect way of reaching the decision that a treatment has no effect and often leads to the problem of inequivalence between statistical significance and toxicological relevance. One major reason for this logical difficulty is clearly described by Fisher (1935): "the null hypothesis is never proved or established, but is possibly disproved in the course of experimentation. Every experiment may be said to exist only in order to give the facts a chance of disproving the null hypothesis."

Proof of safety provides consistency of the consumer risk for approval of a new compound based on efficacy as well as on safety. This paper demonstrated that current statistical methodology can be applied for safety ranges defined both a priori and a posteriori.

REFERENCES

Bedotto JE, Gay RG, Graham SD, Morkin E, Goldman S. Cardiac hypertrophy induced by thyroid hormone is independent of loading conditions and beta-adrenoceptor blockade. J Pharm Exp Ther 248:632–636, 1989.

Berger RL. Multiparameter hypothesis testing and acceptance sampling. Technometrics 24:295–300, 1982.

Bofinger E, Bofinger M. Equivalence of normal means compared with a control. Commun Stat Theory Methods 22:3117–3141, 1993.

Bofinger E, Bofinger M. Equivalence with respect to a control: stepwise tests. J R Stat Soc B 57:721–733, 1995.

Bross ID. Why proof of safety is much more difficult than proof of hazard. Biometrics 41:785–793, 1985.

Brown KG, Erdreich LS. Statistical uncertainty in the no-observed-adverse-effect level. Fundam Appl Toxicol 13:235–244, 1989.

Chanter DO, Tuck MG, Coombs DW. The chances of false negative results in conventional toxicology studies with rats. Toxicology 43:65–74, 1987.

Chow S-C, Liu J-P. Design and Analysis of Bioavailability and Bioequivalence Studies. New York: Marcel Dekker, 1992.

Diletti E, Hauschke D, Steinijans VW. Sample size determination for bioequivalence assessment by means of confidence intervals. Int J Clin Pharmacol Ther Toxicol 29:1–8, 1991.

Dunnett CW. A multiple comparison procedure for comparing several treatments with a control. J Am Stat Assoc 50:1096–1121, 1955.

Dunnett CW, Tamhane AC. Step-down multiple tests for comparing treatments with a control in unbalanced one-way layout. Stat Med 10:939–947, 1991.

Dunnett CW, Tamhane AC. A step-up multiple test procedure. J Am Stat Assoc 87:162–170, 1992.

Dunnett CW, Tamhane AC. Step-up multiple testing of parameters with unequally correlated estimates. Biometrics 51:217–227, 1995.

Erickson WP, McDonald LL. Tests for bioequivalence of control media and test media in studies of toxicity. Environ Toxicol Chem 14:1247–1256, 1995.

Fisher RA. The Design of Experiments. London: Oliver and Boyd, 1935.

Food and Drug Administration. Toxicological principles for the safety assessment of direct food additives and color additives used in food. Draft, 1993.

Gaylor DW. The use of safety factors for controlling risk. J Toxicol Environ Health 11:329–336, 1983.

Giani G, Strassburger K. Testing and selecting for equivalence with respect to a control. J Am Stat Assoc 89:320–329, 1994.

Hauschke D. Testprinzipien bei Safety-Studien in der Toxikologie. In: Trampisch HJ, Lange S, eds. Medizinische Forschung-Ärztliches Handeln. München: MMV Medizin Verlag, 1995, pp 104–107.

Hauschke D. Statistical proof of safety in toxicological studies. Drug Inf J 31: 357–361, 1997.

Hauschke D, Steinijans VW. Ein verteilungsfreies Verfahren zur statistischen Auswertung von Bioäquivalenzstudien. In: Vollmar J, eds. Biometrie in der chemisch-pharmazeutischen Industrie. Stuttgart: Gustav Fisher, 1991, pp 69–89.

Hauschke D, Steinijans VW. A note on conventional null hypothesis testing in active control equivalence studies [letter]. Controlled Clin Trials 17:347–349, 1996.

Hauschke D, Hayashi M, Lin KK, Lovell DP, Robinson WD, Yoshimura I. Recommendations for biostatistics of mutagenicity studies. Drug Inf J 31: 323–326, 1997.

Hauschke D, Steinijans VW, Diletti E. A distribution-free procedure for the statistical analysis of bioequivalence studies. Int J Clin Pharmacol Ther Toxicol 28:72–78, 1990.

Hauschke D, Steinijans VW, Diletti E, Burke M. Sample size determination for bioequivalence assessment using a multiplicative model. J Pharmacokinet Biopharm 20:557–561, 1992.

Hochberg Y. A sharper Bonferroni procedure for multiple tests of significance. Biometrika 75:800–802, 1988.

Hochberg Y, Tamhane AC. Multiple Comparison Procedures. New York: Wiley, 1987.

Hodges JL, Lehmann EL. Estimates of location based on rank tests. Ann Math Stat 34:598–611, 1963.

Holland, B, Ordoukhani NK. Balancing type I and type II error probabilities: further comments on proof of safety vs proof of hazard. Commun Stat Theory Methods 19:3557–3570, 1990.

Hollander M, Wolfe DA. Nonparametric Statistical Methods. New York: Wiley, 1973.

Holm S. A simple sequentially rejective multiple test procedure. Scand J Stat 6: 65–70, 1979.

Hommel G. A stagewise rejective multiple test procedure based on a modified Bonferroni test. Biometrika 75:383–386, 1988.

Hothorn LA. General statistical principles in testing of toxicological studies. In: Hothorn LA, ed. Statistical Methods in Toxicology. Berlin: Springer, 1991, pp 111–131.

Hothorn LA. Biostatistical analysis of the control vs k treatments design including a positive control group. In: Vollmar J, ed. Testing Principles in Clinical and Preclinical Studies. Stuttgart: Gustav Fischer Verlag, 1995, pp 19–26.

Hsu JC. Multiple Comparisons. London: Chapman & Hall, 1996.

Korn EL. Confidence bands for isotonic dose–response curves. Appl Stat 31:59–63, 1992.

Lee C-IC. On estimation for monotone dose–response curves. J Am Stat Assoc 91:1110–1119, 1996.

Liu J-P, Chow S-C. Sample size determination for the two one-sided tests procedure in bioequivalence. J Pharmacokinet Biopharm 20:101–104, 1992.

Marcus R, Peritz E, Gabriel KR. On closed testing procedures with special reference to ordered analysis of variance. Biometrika 63:655–660, 1976.

Millard SP. Proof of safety vs proof of hazard. Biometrics 43:719–725, 1987.

Nam J. A simple approximation for calculating sample sizes for detecting linear trends in proportions. Biometrics 43:701–705, 1987.

Neuhäuser M, Hothorn LA. Auswertung der Dosis-Wirkungs-Abhängigkeit des Ames Mutagenitätsassay bei direkter Kontrolle des Konsumentenrisikos. In: Trampisch HJ, Lange S, eds. Medizinische Forschung-Ärtzliches Handeln. München: MMV Medizin Verlag, 1995, pp 113–116.

Neuhäuser M, Hothorn LA. Trend tests for dichotomous endpoints with application to carcinogenicity studies. Drug Inf J 31:463–469, 1997.

Ng T-H. Conventional null hypothesis testing in active control equivalence studies. Controlled Clin Trials 16:356–358, 1995.

Owen DB. A special case of a bivariate non-central t-distribution. Biometrika 52:437–446, 1965.

Peace KE. Design and analysis considerations for safety data, particularly adverse events. In: Gilbert GS, ed. Drug Safety Assessment in Clinical Trials. New York: Marcel Dekker, 1993, pp 305–316.

Phillips KF. Power of the two one-sided tests procedure in bioequivalence. J Pharmacokinet Biopharm 18:137–144, 1990.

Podgor MJ, Gastwirth JL, Metha CR. Efficiency robust tests of independence in contingency tables with ordered classifications. Stat Med 15:2095–2105, 1996.

Rom DM. A sequentially rejective test procedure based on a modified Bonferroni inequality. Biometrika 77:663–665, 1990.

Rom DM, Costello RJ, Connell LT. On closed test procedures for dose–response analysis. Stat Med 13:1583–1596, 1994.

Roy SN. On a heuristic method of test construction and its use in multivariate analysis. Ann Math Stat 24:220–238, 1953.

Schoenfeld DA. Confidence bounds for normal means under order restrictions, with application to dose–response curves, toxicology experiments, and low-dose extrapolation. J Am Stat Assoc 81:186–195, 1986.

Schuirmann DJ. A comparison of the two one-sided tests procedure and the power approach for assessing the equivalence of average bioavailability. J Pharmacokinet Biopharm 15:657–680, 1987.

Shirley E. A non-parametric equivalent of Williams' test for contrasting increasing dose levels of a treatment. Biometrics 33:386–389, 1977.

Simes RJ. An improved Bonferroni procedure for multiple tests of significance. Biometrika 73:751–754, 1986.

Stallard N, Whitehead A. An alternative approach to the analysis of animal carcinogenicity studies. Regul Toxicol Pharmacol 23:244–248, 1996.

Steel RGD. A multiple rank sum test: treatments versus control. Biometrics 15:560–572, 1959.

Tamhane AC, Hochberg Y, Dunnett CW. Multiple test procedures for dose finding. Biometrics 52:21–37, 1996.

Tukey JW, Ciminera JL, Heyse JF. Testing the statistical certainty of a response to increasing doses of a drug. Biometrics 41:295–301, 1985.

Victor N. On clinically relevant differences and shifted null hypotheses. Methods Inf Med 26:109–116, 1987.

Williams DA. A test for differences between treatment means when several dose levels are compared with a zero dose control. Biometrics 27:103–117, 1971.

Williams DA. The comparison of several dose levels with a zero dose control. Biometrics 28:519–531, 1972.

Yanagawa T, Kikuchi Y. Determination of the no-observed-adverse-effect level by the AIC. Sankhya B 57:285–297, 1995.

Yanagawa T, Kikuchi Y, Brown KG. Statistical issues on the no-observed-adverse-effect level in categorical response. Environ Health Perspect 102 (suppl 1):95–101, 1994.

7

The Design of Long-Term Carcinogenicity Studies

R. JOHN WEAVER AND MARSHALL N. BRUNDEN*

Pharmacia & Upjohn, Inc., Kalamazoo, Michigan

I. INTRODUCTION

It has been estimated that the pharmaceutical industry as a whole conducts or contracts for about 72–84 long-term carcinogenesis screens each year, with each study costing from 2 to 8 million dollars (1). This large expenditure makes it prudent to conduct each study in a manner as efficient as possible. Study design, therefore, is an extremely important component of the overall process of conducting these studies.

The major objective of the long-term carcinogenicity study is to identify those compounds that are probable human carcinogens. A *probable human carcinogen* is defined as an agent that has the ability to (a) cause an increased incidence of tumor types that are also seen in control animals, (b) cause an earlier appearance of tumors than in the control, (c) cause tumor types not seen in control animals, or (d) cause an increased multiplicity of tumors in individuals. Studies in animals are important, as the International Agency for Research on Cancer (2) notes "in the absence of adequate data on humans, it is biologically plausible and prudent to regard agents for which there is sufficient evidence of

---

*Retired.

carcinogenicity in experimental animals as if they presented a carcinogenic risk to humans." The relevance of these studies is demonstrated by the fact that nearly all of the known human carcinogens have been carcinogenic in one or more species of rodents. Furthermore, of the 20 pharmaceuticals that are considered to be human carcinogens, there is an 85% concordance in the organs affected (3).

Although studies in animals to assess potential human toxicity date back to the early 20th century, it has only been in the last four decades that long-term assays for carcinogens have evolved to what we see today. In the 1960s, the National Cancer Institute (NCI) started to develop procedures to evaluate large numbers of chemicals for potential carcinogenicity. During the next decade, continued improvements and standardizations were made to study protocols. By 1971, a standard evaluation procedure was in place that used two species of rodents, typically rats and mice, in studies that approximated the life spans of these animals. These study designs are summarized in the well-known guidelines issued in 1976 (4). Procedures became even more formalized with the development of the National Toxicology Program (NTP) in the 1980s. In the past two decades, the NCI and the NTP between them have conducted more than 450 of these carcinogenicity studies at a total cost of over 650 million dollars. Additional guidelines have issued from the Food and Drug Administration (FDA) in the famous *Red Book* in 1982, revised in 1993 (5), the Environmental Protection Agency (EPA) in 1987, (6), and the International Agency for Research in Cancer (1).

The evolution of these guidelines was partly motivated by the growing appreciation of the importance of study design. Poorly designed studies are less efficient, harder to analyze and interpret, less reproducible, and may not yield the required information. In any scientific discipline, designing an experiment requires a well-thought-out process or sequence of steps that ensures that the information to be collected is relevant to the problem at hand. In addition, there are concerns specific to carcinogenicity studies that need to be addressed. Typical questions that might be asked when designing a carcinogenicity study are the following:

1. What species is appropriate for the study?
2. What characteristics are to be measured and analyzed?
3. What dose levels should be used?
4. How long should the study be?
5. How many replications of the basic experiment should be used?

6. Are there factors other than the drug(s) that may influence (bias) the results?

In this chapter we will discuss some general concepts in experimental design, then discuss in some detail the foregoing questions and other issues specific to these studies.

II. GENERAL CONCEPTS IN EXPERIMENTAL DESIGN

A. Introduction

This section will discuss some general concepts in experimental design that apply not only to long-term carcinogenicity studies, but also to essentially any experimental situation. When planning an experiment, it is hoped that the design employed will lead to a savings in time and expense, with resultant gains in information owing to the use of valid and efficient analytical procedures. Employing these concepts will increase the likelihood of achieving these goals.

Even with an optimal experimental design, it should be remembered that correctly applied statistical analysis methods never allow anything to be proved. Instead, what takes place is the ascertainment of the likelihood of error in any statement of confidence made about an experimentally derived value. For example, in a carcinogenicity study, we might want to determine the effect of drug on hepatocellular tumor incidence in rodents. The experimental results may indicate that the drug increases the incidence of hepatocellular carcinomas from 2% in controls to 12% in the high-dose group. This in itself offers no proof that in repeated experimentation a similar increase would be observed. The use of a suitably designed experiment followed by statistical analysis of the results allows the researcher to give only a value to the reliability of his or her results. What can be demonstrated is that under certain assumptions, increases as extreme as those obtained in the experiment might arise less than 1 : 100 times if the drug had no effect. The researcher is then quite safe in discounting that the drug has no effect on hepatocellular carcinoma incidence and conclude instead that it causes increased incidence. In addition to inferring the existence of the drug effect, the well-planned experiment will also allow one to place limits within which the true values for the incidence of hepatocellular carcinoma will almost certainly lie. For example, in the foregoing experiment, the true increase in hepatocellular carcinoma when exposed to high doses of the drug may be calculated to lie almost certainly (with a high degree of probability) between 9 and 15%.

B. Principles Used in Experimental Design

Most elementary texts on experimental design, from the early writings of Kempthorne (7), Quenouille (8), and Cochran and Cox (9), to the more recent books by Winer (10) and Montgomery (11), all have in common some discussion of (a) the scientific method, (b) the importance of a statement of the experimental objectives, and (c) the basic principles to be used in experimentation. In the following, we will give a brief discussion of some of the basic principles, including the experimental unit, experimental variation and its control, and replication.

1. The Experimental Unit

At first glance, the concept of an experimental unit seems clear-cut. A study is conducted with 50 animals, so there are naturally 50 experimental units. Correct? This is usually a correct statement, but not always, because most statistical tests used in the analysis of data from toxicological studies require independence among the basic sampling units. The experimental unit is that unit to which a single treatment (possibly a combination of two or more factors) is applied in one replication of the basic experiment, and it should take into account all attributes of that unit.

Consider, for example, cages containing multiply housed animals receiving drug through dietary intake from a common source in the cage. The cage is the unit to which the treatment is applied, so the cage is the experimental unit. Now, consider the similar situation of multiply housed animals receiving the same treatment, but with each animal treated individually. Can the animals now be considered as responding independently, or are their responses dependent on the influences of their particular cage and common environment? If the former is true the individual animal is the correct experimental unit, if the latter is true, it is still the cage. Because the experimenter usually does not know for certain, to assure the validity of the statistical approach, the cage should still be considered the experimental unit.

The same reasoning applies to other attributes of the sampling unit. Attributes can be groups of cages of individual animals arranged in racks with all animals of a treatment group placed together, animals from the same litter receiving the same treatment, different technicians examining different treatment groups, and so on. In all of these examples, the critical factor is not whether the attribute plays a dominant role in influencing the measured responses, but if it plays any role at all. If it does, then the attribute should be considered the experimental unit. Generally, if a larger attribute or grouping of the sampling units distinguishes the units relative to treatment, then the larger attribute would more appropriately be considered the experimental unit.

2. Sources of Experimental Variation

The sum of those effects that influence experimental precision are referred to by the statistician as the *experimental error*. This term might be more properly referred to as the sum of sources of variability. In a particular experimental setting *error* reflects the normal variation in biological response in animals, variation in the experimental procedures, unavoidable errors of measurement, and the combined effects of all other extraneous factors that influence the study. The precision of the experiment increases if we decrease the experimental error.

In general, if any such sources of variability can be identified, the design should be constructed to remove, or at least control for them. The failure to consider these factors at the design stage can result in the variability becoming confounded with treatment effects or, even worse, introducing bias into the tests for treatment effect.

Some sources of variability can be easily controlled by the experimenter. Using the same supplier for all animals on study, using the same food and water sources throughout the course of the experiment, using the same personnel and maintaining consistency in all procedures, are simple, but extremely important aspects of a well-run study. Other potential factors are harder to identify and control. A good discussion of factors that have been identified as potential sources of variability is given by Haseman et al. (12).

One of the more important factors to be considered is the animal room environment. Toxicological studies involve the caging of animals at differing locations within the confines of an atmospherically controlled room or rooms. Within such an environment there are potentials for differences between rooms, and for temperature, light, and other gradients within rooms that may affect the experimental outcomes. Although these factors should be addressed in any study, the consequences could be more pronounced in long-term studies. There is evidence that nonneoplastic eye lesions are associated with row level in a rack, with increased incidences observed in the top rows that are closer to the light source (13,14). Associations of tumor prevalence with cage position are less clear. There are reports of room effects for hepatocellular neoplasms in mice (15,16), pancreatic acinar tumors in rats (17), and reticuloendo-thelial tumors in mice (18). Other authors question the existence of these effects (19). Although it is uncertain if these effects truly exist, the systematic assignment of treatment groups to contiguous cage positions, while logistically practical, should be avoided. In some cases, a small uniformity trial can be run to assess the effects of height and lateral position of the animal cages on critical experimental measures.

3. Control of Experimental Variation

Experimental variation is typically handled in two ways: randomization and blocking. Randomization is used to control for unknown or unsuspected sources, whereas blocking can be used to control for or remove known or suspected sources of variation. Well-planned experiments always employ randomization, but also often employ blocking.

Randomization is used to balance or even out between treatment groups unknown or unsuspected sources of variability. A proper randomization is one in which nothing distinguishes the treatment groups other than the treatment itself. This will assure that any unknown factors do not bias the statistical tests. The most important use of randomization is in the assignment of treatments to experimental units. As mentioned previously, housing animals systemically by treatment group should be avoided. In addition to possible environmental influences, other problems can result from this housing scheme. The authors are aware of an example for which components of an automatic watering system failed, causing several racks of animals to be deprived of water for several days. These racks happened to contain only control animals, and the resulting losses in body weight induced what appeared to be a significant treatment effect. A common argument against complete randomization is that it increases the possibility of dosing errors. Although this may be true, the benefits of randomization outweigh the risk of dosing errors. If dosing errors do occur, with a properly randomized study they would most likely be at random and to individual animals. A systematic housing scheme increases the possibility that several animals or even an entire group could be misdosed.

Randomization should also be used at various other stages of experimentation, such as the selection of animals for tests, the order in which blood samples and necropsies are performed, or any other situation that might induce variation into the observations.

Blocking is used to control for known or suspected sources of variation in an experiment. Blocks can represent attributes of the animal, such as body weight, age, litter, and such, or can represent environmental influences, such as cage location. These sources of variation are sometimes called "nuisance parameters," for they are not of primary interest to the investigator. If these sources of variation exist, then a well-planned blocking scheme combined with an appropriate statistical analysis allows the variation caused by these source(s) to be estimated and removed from the experimental error. This can greatly increase the precision of the experiment. The use of blocking will be illustrated in the next section (see Sec.II.C) on specific experimental designs. The results of a uniformity trial can provide vital information on sources of variation and how blocking can be employed to decrease experimental variability.

4. Replication

To have adequate precision, the experimenter must calculate the number of replications of the experimental unit that are necessary to adequately assess the reproducibility of results and to detect what the experimenter considers a significant difference. An increase in the number of experimental units will decrease the estimated experimental error and increase the precision. The proper designation of the experimental unit and the use of blocking will affect the number of replications required. If blocking is successful, substantial reductions in the sample size required can be achieved.

Sample size requirements are usually stated in terms of power for detecting specified alternatives. *Power* refers to the probability of declaring a specified alternative significant if, in fact, the alternative is true. There are several commercially available software packages available to calculate sample sizes required for stated levels of power for the various designs.

C. Experimental Designs

Various experimental designs for toxicology have been described in the literature. In the text by Gad and Weil (20), *Statistics and Experimental Design for Toxicologists*, the authors state that there are four basic experimental design types used in toxicology. These are randomized block, Latin square, factorial design, and nested design. Bickis and Krewski (21) also consider the statistical design of long-term carcinogenicity studies within Chapter 6 of the first volume of a two-volume book.

The experimental designs considered by these authors are the completely randomized design and restricted randomized design (equivalent to the randomized block).

In actuality, there is no such thing as a factorial design (22). Instead, the term *factorial* refers to the special way in which treatment combinations are formed when more than one factor is being administered at more than one level to the experimental units within the study. In fact, the factorial treatment layout may be used with either a completely randomized or randomized block design. It could even be used with the Latin square design, although this design usually uses only one factor at more than one level.

In what follows we will discuss briefly three experimental designs and two treatment layouts. The designs considered are the completely randomized, randomized block, and Latin square. Treatment layouts considered are the single-factor and factorial. Examples of the six combinations of study design and treatment layout are given.

1. Completely Randomized Design

The most commonly used design for long-term carcinogenicity studies and other toxicological studies is the completely randomized design. This is a design in which the treatments are assigned completely at random to the experimental units. The design imposes no restrictions (such as blocking) on the allocation of treatments to the experimental units, although a balance on the number of experimental units used per treatment group is usually sought. This design should be used in the case of nearly homogeneous experimental units and when no identifiable sources of external variability are present. If either of these conditions exist, then blocking should be used to increase the design efficiency.

2. Randomized Block Design

The randomized block design is used to control for a single identified or suspected source of variation. In a randomized block design the experimental units are allocated to blocks, such that the experimental units within a block are relatively homogeneous and the number of experimental units within a block is equal to the number of treatments being investigated. The treatments are then assigned at random to the experimental units within each block. Typical blocking variables were discussed in Section II.B.3.

With an appropriate statistical analysis, the effect of this type of blocking is the removal of the variability associated with the blocks from the experimental error.

3. *Latin Square Design*

The Latin square design permits the investigator to assess treatment effects when a double-blocking restriction is used on the experimental units, controlling for two sources of variation. This is a logical extension of the randomized block design. Within the Latin square design the number of row blocks, number column blocks, and number of treatment groups are equal. The randomization of the treatments to the experimental units is restricted, such that each row block and each column block has all of the treatments represented.

Additional replicates of experimental units is accomplished through replication of the squares. The effect of this type of blocking is the removal of the variability associated with the row and column blocks from the experimental error. Blocks can represent sources of variation as described in the previous section. When the rows and columns represent the physical location of the cage, then the effects of environmental gradients can be controlled.

D. Treatment Layouts

1. *Single-Factor Layout*

This is the most common treatment layout used in carcinogenicity studies. Here the treatment is represented by only one factor administered at more than one level. *Factors* are things the investigator is interested in making inferences about, in contrast with blocks, which are not of primary interest. In the context of carcinogenicity studies, a *single factor* usually refers to a single drug and *level* corresponds to dosage.

2. *Factorial Layout*

In a factorial layout, the treatments comprise all possible combinations of two or more factors, each at two or more levels. Examples of combinations of factors can be (a) different drugs, each administered at more than one level, (b) sex and a single drug at several levels, (c) two or more strains of animal and a single drug at several levels, or some other combination. The notation used for factorial treatment allocations is the product of the factor levels. A 2×2 factorial arrangement indicates the use of all combinations of two factors, each at two levels. A 2×3

arrangement is the use of all combinations of two factors, the first at two levels and the second at three levels, and so on.

E. Examples of Designs with Treatment Layouts

1. Completely Randomized Design with Single-Factor Layout

Suppose that the study is to have as a single-factor drug A at four doses (where the doses are designated as 1, 2, 3, and 4). Animals are placed at random into racks of cages. In our example a rack of cages contains five rows and eight columns, with each cage containing one animal. The experimental unit is the cage–animal. Random number sequences for placing animals in cages and assigning treatments to the cages can be generated using PROC PLAN of SAS (23). After a complete randomization of the treatments to the cages ($n = 10$ subjects per drug level) we could have results similar to that illustrated within Fig. 1.

2. Completely Randomized Design with Factorial Layout

Suppose that we want to study the effects of the combination of two drugs, each at two levels. The factors are drug A with doses designated by 1 and 2 and drug B with doses also designated by 1 and 2. The study has a factorial treatment layout and is called a 2 × 2 factorial. For simplicity, the treatment combinations will be designated 1,1; 1,2; 2,1; and 2,2; with the first digit representing the level of drug A, the second

1	4	4	1	2	4	2	3
2	1	2	1	3	4	4	2
2	1	4	1	1	3	1	2
3	3	3	3	2	4	4	3
1	2	1	4	2	3	3	4

FIGURE 1   Completely randomized design (one factor). Treatments 1, 2, 3, and 4.

the level of drug B. Again we have racks containing five rows and eight columns of cages, each containing one animal placed in the cage at random. The experimental unit is again the cage–animal. After a complete randomization of the treatment combinations to the cages ($n = 10$ subjects per drug–dose combination) we would have results similar to that illustrated within Fig. 2.

3. Randomized Block Design with Single-Factor Layout

Suppose again that the study is to have as a single factor drug A at four doses. When the animals arrive, it is noticed that there is substantial variability in pretest body weights. We might wish to control for this in our study design. This can be accomplished by blocking on body weight. Animals of similar body weights are placed together in blocks of size four, and each block placed in the cages of a column of the 5 × 8 rack, leaving the bottom row empty. The blocks can be formed by ranking animals, based on increasing body weight, and taking consecutive groups of four. If extra animals were included in the acclimation period, animals at each extreme of body weight can be eliminated before study assignment. The experimental unit is the cage–animal within a block. After a randomization of the treatments to the cages ($n = 8$ subjects per drug level) within each column we would have results similar to that illustrated within Fig. 3.

2,2	1,1	1,1	2,2	1,2	1,1	1,2	2,1
1,2	2,2	1,2	2,2	2,1	1,1	1,1	1,2
1,2	2,2	1,1	2,2	2,2	2,1	2,2	1,2
2,1	2,1	2,1	2,1	1,2	1,1	1,1	2,1
2,2	1,2	2,2	1,1	1,2	2,1	2,1	1,1

FIGURE 2 Completely randomized design (two factor). Treatments 1,1; 1,2; 2,1; and 2,2.

1	2	3	4	2	2	4	1
4	3	4	3	4	3	1	3
3	1	1	2	3	4	3	2
2	4	2	1	1	1	2	4
X	X	X	X	X	X	X	X

FIGURE 3 Randomized block design (one factor). Columns on blocks. Treatments 1, 2, 3, and 4.

4. Randomized Block Design with Factorial Layout

By letting dose 1 represent the two-factor low-dose combination 1,1 and similarly letting dose 2 represent the combination 1,2, dose 3 represents the combination 2,1, and dose 4 represents the high-dose combination 2,2 it is possible to change a one-factor randomized block design into a 2 × 2 factorial randomized block design. Blocking and randomization would then proceed as in the previous section.

5. Latin Square Design with Single-Factor Layout

Figure 4 gives an example of a Latin square design with a single-factor treatment layout. The rows and columns correspond to the blocks used in the experiment. If there is a suspected effect owing to cage location, rows and columns can be used to control for horizontal and vertical environmental gradients, and the squares can correspond to different rooms used in the study.

6. Latin Square Design with Factorial Layout

By using a schema similar to that discussed in section II.E.4 the single-factor Latin square design is easily configured as a 2 × 2 factorial Latin square design.

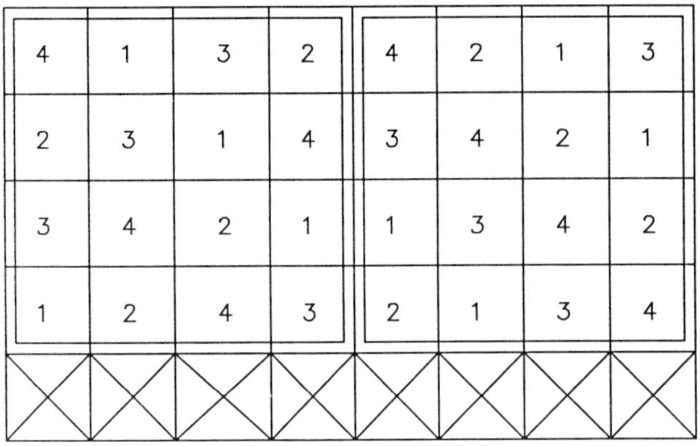

FIGURE 4 Latin square design (one factor); two replicate squares. Treatments 1, 2, 3, and 4.

III. ANIMALS: CHOICE OF SPECIES AND STRAIN

A. Introduction

Much like medieval food testers for the king or canaries in coal mines, animals serve as surrogates for humans in the search for carcinogens. Ideally, the animal species chosen for a carcinogenicity assessment should be similar to humans in physiology, biochemistry, and metabolism of xenobiotics. In reality, no species of animals meets all these criteria, and the choice relies more on practical considerations.

Because an ideal animal model does not exist, the IARC recommends that the compound be tested in at least two species (2). Mice and rats have historically been the species of choice because of their size, cost, ready availability, ease of handling, and abundance of background or historical information. Syrian golden hamsters have sometimes been used, and they are particularly appropriate for studies on respiratory and urinary tract carcinogens (24). Occasionally, other species may be indicated by metabolic or pharmacokinetic data, susceptibility to a class of carcinogen or route of administration. Nonrodent species, such as ferrets, marmosets, miniature pigs, and others have been investigated, but are generally not accepted as alternatives. It is unlikely that the rodent will be replaced any time soon as the animal of choice for carcinogenicity studies.

B. Genetic Considerations

Genetic variations in the response of the study animals to the chemical should be a very important consideration when designing an assay (25). Within each species, the genotype of the animal may strongly influence its susceptibility to a drug. Many authors have found strain differences in response to carcinogens. A good example is diethylstilbestrol (DES). The ACI strain of rat is highly sensitive to DES, with greater than 70% incidence of mammary adenocarcinomas, whereas the Sprague–Dawley strain is quite resistant, with incidences near zero (26). Similar differences in DES susceptibility have been reported between some strains of mice (27). Examples of strain sensitivity to other compounds appear throughout the literature (28,29).

There are three general genetic types of laboratory animals commonly used in research: inbred strains, F_1 hybrids, and outbred stock. These labels refer to breeding methods, and there is some overlap in the official definitions. A characterization that may be less ambiguous is isogenic or nonisogenic (30). *Isogenic* animals are genetically identical, whereas *nonisogenic* animals are not.

1. Inbred Strains

An *inbred strain* is one in which each individual is genetically identical (isogenic) and homozygous at all loci (apart from a few, owing to recent mutations). Inbred animals are ancestors of a single breeding pair, followed by 20 or more generations of brother–sister mating. Inbred strains have essentially no genetic variability, and thus show much less variability in their responses to drugs. This uniformity means that using inbred strains requires fewer animals to ascertain treatment effects (increased statistical precision). Inbred strains remain genetically constant for long periods, making historical control data from the same laboratory more reliable for a longer time.

2. F_1 Hybrids

An F_1 *hybrid* is a first-generation cross of two inbred strains. It is also isogenic (i.e., all individuals are genetically identical), but the individuals are heterozygous at all loci where the parental strains differ. The phenotypic variability is reported to be the least in F_1 hybrids, even less than in inbred strains (31). Because the individuals are heterozygous at some loci, they do not breed true. In fact, F_2 hybrids, derived from mating F_1 hybrids, are extremely heterogeneous genetically, even more so than outbred strains. Hybrid strains are typically more vigorous than their parental inbred strains.

3. Outbred Stock

Any stock that does not fit into the foregoing two categories is considered to be an outbred stock. These animals typically come from closed colonies that use random or haphazard mating schemes, although sometimes breeding schemes that avoid brother–sister mating are used. Each individual is genetically distinct (i.e., nonisogenic). Although these strains have more genetic variability than inbred strains, they can still involve a good deal of inbreeding. Genetic segregation will occur, with the sporadic appearance of abnormal young. Outbred stocks are widely used, and include Wistar, Sprague–Dawley, and Long–Evans rats and Swiss, Swiss–Webster, CD-1, CFW, and CF-1 mice. A complication is that, at present, it can be difficult to tell some of these stains apart. In fact, there are no genetic markers to distinguish between Wistar and Sprague–Dawley rats. The supplier must be trusted. There is little genetic monitoring or quality control, with possible selection and genetic drift resulting in a less stable strain. Background or historical data is relevant for a much shorter time.

4. Choice of Strain

There has been much debate on whether it is better to use inbred, outbred, or hybrid strains in carcinogenicity studies. The debate centers around extrapolation to humans. Nonisogenic outbred strains have been recommended by some because their genetic variability more closely resembles the human population. The isogenic inbred and hybrid strains, on the other hand, control for genetic variability and produce more precise results. Even though inbred and hybrid strains offer many advantages, using them has been compared with running a clinical trial with one human and his clones or twins. The inference to the entire population is then much more difficult to make. Currently, both isogenic and nonisogenic strains are used and will continue to be used in long-term studies.

Even in outbred strains, the amount of genetic variation is substantially less than in humans. DNA fingerprinting has been used to investigate the genetic variation in six outbred stocks of rats; the degree of band sharing was 84–95%, indicating a very high degree of genetic uniformity (32). In contrast, inbred strains have essentially 100% band sharing within a strain, and $34 \pm 15\%$ band sharing between strains.

The variability between strains is roughly of the degree expected in random samples of the human population.

Since approximately 1970, the NCI–NTP carcinogenesis bioassays have employed the inbred Fisher F244N rat and the F_1 hybrid B6C3F1 mouse as the standard strains. Although the choice of these strains has been debated for years, they have been repeatedly determined to be appropriate, or at least the best of the alternatives. These strains have not been without problems, however. The mice, especially the males, are highly prone to spontaneous liver tumors, and the rats are characterized by high rates of endocrine neoplasms, mononuclear cell leukemia, and fibrosarcoma of subcutaneous tissue.

4. Multistrain Factorial Designs

A possible compromise in the choice of strain is to use more than one genetically independent strain in the experiment, and employ a strain by drug factorial treatment layout. This has been proposed for over 20 years (27,33,34). The basic idea is that instead of using 50 animals of a single isogenic strain per treatment group, we would use two strains with 25 animals each, or five strains of 10 animals each, or some such combination. The total number of animals used is approximately the same, but the number of genotypes represented would increase. Experiments with this design have been carried out (35), so they are technically feasible.

There are several advantages to such a design. The use of several strains would decrease the chance of having randomly chosen a resistant strain. With normally distributed data, the multistrain factorial is more powerful, more comprehensive, and has a wider inductive basis than a design using just one strain (36). With dichotomous data, it has been shown by simulation that in terms of the Mantel–Haenszel test, the multistrain factorial design is usually also more powerful than the standard design, and often substantially so (33). The differences between strains in conjunction with pharmacokinetic data may provide insight into carcinogenetic mechanisms. It might even be possible to identify genetic loci associated with susceptibility.

There are also drawbacks to these designs. The major one is that the maximum tolerated dose (MTD) for a particular compound may differ between strains (see the next section for the precise definition of MTD). The different strains would either have to be dosed at different levels, or the minimum MTD from the various strains could be used for all strains. The target organs may differ between strains. For example

A/J mice primarily develop lung tumors, whereas B6C3F1 mice nearly always develop liver tumors, no matter what the carcinogen.

The multistrain factorial treatment layout has not been used to a great extent, but it does have potential usefulness in decreasing animal usage and costs.

C. Concordance Between Rats and Mice

The NCI–NTP bioassays offer a good database for examining the concordance between rats and mice in carcinogenicity testing. In the 284 experiments using isogenic strains, 206 (73%) gave results consistent between rats and mice (37). There were 78 studies that found compounds to be carcinogens in only one of the species. Some of these are probably due to false-positive results, whereas others may be due to nonsusceptible stains being used. Overall, they suggest that the use of both species is probably still necessary.

D. Other Considerations

Whatever species and strain is chosen for the carcinogenicity study, it is important that the animals be as close as possible to each other in age and weight. If there is some variation in age or body weights, a randomized block design should be considered. All animals should originate from the same supplier. They should have a brief acclimation period, during which they are observed for general health and signs of disease. Because sex differences in susceptibility have been noted, equal numbers of males and females are generally included in the study design.

There has been some recent literature (38) that has suggested using only one sex of each species, cutting the total number of animals used in half. A retrospective analysis indicated that 86–92% of rodent carcinogens identified by the full protocol would have also been identified by this reduced protocol. With continued pressure to reduce the use of laboratory animals, these reduced protocols should be investigated and might become more common in the future.

IV. DOSE SELECTION

A. Introduction

The selection of doses, particularly the high dose, is one of the most complex and controversial aspects of study design. This is evident by the fact that the International Life Sciences Institute (ILSI) has listed and reviewed 27 different published sets of guidelines for dose selection in chronic toxicity or carcinogenicity studies (39). The historical philosophy behind the selection of doses is that, because we are using a limited number of animals and extrapolating the millions of humans, the study should include high-dose levels to give the test article the greatest chance of expressing its inherent carcinogenicity. Assuming that high-dose levels produce more of the same tumors as low doses, increasing dose levels increases the sensitivity of the assay (40). Pharmacokinetic differences between humans and rodents necessitate higher doses to achieve equivalent pharmacological effects. For most compounds, equivalent blood levels in rats require eight times the human dose, on a milligram per kilogram basis (41). There is a practical limit however to how high a dose can be. In feeding studies, the high dose is often limited to 5% (50,000 ppm), as doses higher than this level may affect the nutrition of the animals. The high-dose level should not adversely affect the longevity of the animals, other than that associated with tumor induction. Excessive toxicity and mortality in the high-dose group can seriously compromise the results of the study. Doses high enough to cause indirect carcinogenesis, such as tumors associated with mineralization in the urinary tract, or nonspecific toxicity, characterized by reparative proliferation of cells, can complicate the interpretation of results and may be the underlying cause of discordant results between strains or species. In these cases, the finding of carcinogenicity may be more related to the specific test system than to the properties of the compound.

B. Maximum Tolerated Dose

The longtime approach has been to use the *maximum tolerated dose* as the high-dose level. The results of subchronic studies can help estimate a MTD, most often defined as "the dose that causes no more than a 10% body weight decrement, as compared to appropriate control groups, and does not produce mortality, clinical signs of toxicity, or pathologic lesions (other than those related to a neoplastic response) that would be predicted (in the long-term bioassay) to shorten the animal's natural lifespan" (4). The MTD is not a nontoxic dose, and will produce some level of toxicity in the test animals. Interestingly, in Europe, the MTD is defined as the minimal toxic dose.

Various authors have argued that the MTD is usually too high for the top dose. Pharmaceutical agents in carcinogenicity studies have generally been screened previously for toxicity, and agents reaching this stage of the development process probably do not have extreme toxicity. As a result the estimated MTD for a pharmaceutical agent can be extremely high. Other authors have proposed an upper limit on the high dose: 1000 mg kg^{-1} has been proposed as an upper limit (42), whereas other research stated that all human carcinogens to which humans are exposed orally would have been detected using high doses below 43 mg kg^{-1} or 880 ppm in the diet. As a compromise, upper limits of 500 mg kg^{-1} for gavage studies and 1% for drug-in-diet studies have been proposed (43).

C. Toxicokinetic Considerations

Some alternatives to the MTD have been explored. A primary task of the ICH-2 was the development of a pharmacokinetic, systemic–exposure-based alternative to the MTD in carcinogenicity studies for pharmaceutics (44). These guidelines are likely to be adopted in the future.

The current ICH proposal used five criteria, any one of which can be used to set the high dose (45). The first consideration is whether there are dose-limiting pharmacodynamic effects that preclude using doses above some level. Second, the standard MTD approach can be used. Third, the relative *systemic exposure ratio* can be used. This is defined as the ratio of the plasma area under the concentration–time curve (AUC) of the drug and major metabolites in the rat at the MTD to the human plasma AUC at the anticipated maximum recommended daily dose (MRD). The guidelines specify a ratio as high as 25 being acceptable, although between 1 and 3 are more likely ratios. Fourth, if there is saturation of absorption, then doses above this level should not be used. Finally, there may be a maximum feasible dose, as in feeding studies.

Nonlinearity of pharmacokinetic parameters is also a concern with higher doses, and possibly bioaccumulation with long-term dosing. Many of the physiological and biochemical processes that affect the disposition of chemicals in the body are capacity-limited (saturable). If any of these absorption, distribution, metabolism, or elimination pathways become saturated, the animals exposure to the compound is altered from what the investigator expects. Disproportionate increases or decreases in drug concentration will occur if the detoxification pathways or metabolic activation pathways, respectively, become saturated, and this can have effects on the toxicity and carcinogenicity. There is evidence that metabolic or elimination pathways in rodents may become saturated even at relatively low multiples of the human dose (46). Also important are possible changes in metabolism as the animals ages. The periodic pharmacokinetic monitoring of groups of satellite animals during the duration of the study would address these concerns.

D. Number of Dose Groups

The number of dose groups used in a study depends on the objectives of the study. The standard design developed in the early 1970s by the NCI was to use three groups, control, ½ MTD, and the MTD, with each group containing 50 animals per sex. These studies were designed basically for qualitative risk estimation. Later, when interest was more quantitative, including low-dose extrapolation, the NTP used studies that included an additional dose group. This allowed a better characterization of the dose response curve, and additionally provided a safety measure in case of substantial mortality in the high-dose group. If there are orders of magnitude between the MTD and the human exposure level, then the mid-dose may be as low as 1/10 MTD. The low dose should approximate the human exposure. Many carcinogenicity studies have used twofold spacing, which also has certain optimality properties (47). The ICH-2 guidelines dictate that the middle and low doses be in the linear region of the dose–response curve, that human exposure and therapeutic dose be considered, that the pharmacodynamic response in rodents be compared with humans, that alterations in the rodents physiology be evaluated, that mechanistic information for potential threshold effects be taken into account, and that the lack of predictability of progression of toxicity in short-term studies be taken into account by adjusting the spacing of dose levels in the long-term study (44). Subchronic studies, of 3 months duration or longer, can provide this useful information on the expected dose response and aid in the selection of the lower-dose levels.

E. Route of Administration

The route of administration should as closely as possible mimic the intended route of administration in humans. The bioavailability of the test compound by the chosen route should be determined, using single and multiple dose pharmacokinetic studies, before the long-term study.

The three main routes of exposure for humans are oral, skin absorption, and inhalation. In laboratory animals the oral administration occurs by mixing the compound in the food, in the water, or by oral gavage. Oral gavage has the advantage that the exact dose administered is known to the investigator. It also has several serious disadvantages. It is time-consuming, the high levels of the compound can sometimes cause local injury to the upper digestive tract, and physical dosing errors can be common, sometimes resulting in the deaths of the animals. Determining the MTD is more difficult for a gavage study, and retrospective examination of the NTP–NCI bioassays indicate that it was often exceeded in these studies (40). Choice of vehicle can also influence the study. There is evidence that corn oil gavage in itself results in increases in pancreatic acinar hyperplasia and hypertrophy and possibly pancreatic adenomas. Corn oil also has known promotional effects in liver, pancreas, and breast. Generally, the gavage route is used only if the test article is volatile, unpalatable, or unstable. Because of these and other difficulties the NTP began to limit the number of new gavage studies in the mid-1980s, and fewer and fewer of these studies are being conducted.

There are several considerations when the drug is administered in the diet, especially at the high-dose level. Most compounds do not add calories; therefore, consumption must be increased to maintain the normal caloric intake. If the compound does add calories, then the intake of protein, vitamins, and minerals may proportionally decrease. The test compound may decrease food consumption by decreasing the diets' palatability. Any of these could compromise the study if they occur to a great extent. Possible actions include the addition of micronutrients to the diet, reducing dose levels, or going to an alternative route of administration. Another potential solution, if investigations show it to be feasible, would be to use a purified diet with the test article substituted for a nonessential macroingredient.

V. STUDY DURATION

Exposure to the test compound should begin a few weeks after weaning and continue for a good portion of the animals' life span. Although some studies are designed to continue until a specified percentage of the animals, say 25%, remain alive, the most common design is scheduled termination. Current guidelines generally set the duration of rodent studies at 24 months, although it is not uncommon to have 18-month studies in mice. An obvious argument for extending this is that some carcinogenic effects may appear only after 24 months, which has validity in some cases. Cadmium chloride, for example exhibits a carcinogenic effect after about 27 months in rats. However, there is also the problem of geriatric changes and disease complicating the assessment of carcinogenicity in longer studies. Numerous studies have demonstrated an association between age and the incidence of neoplasms. Spontaneous tumor incidence increases dramatically after about 18–24 months, thus decreasing the precision of the assay.

On the other hand, there is also substantial support for decreasing the duration of these tests. Data on 179 chemicals have shown that in 95% of the cases, the carcinogenic effect was evident by 18 months, and in all cases evident by 24 months (48). Other authors have recommended an 18-month assay, with 12–15 months of treatment followed by 3–6 months of observation (49). The current consensus is that unless there is an overriding reason, 24 months should be adequate for the carcinogenicity screen.

In certain special situations, an experiment might be terminated before the recommended study duration. The main reason for early termination is to have enough animals from each group for a thorough pathological evaluation. When survival in the control or low dose group reaches 20–25%, then consideration should be given to terminating the entire experiment. If survival in the high dose animals alone decreases to 20–25%, then that group might be terminated, leaving the other groups on study.

VI. OBSERVATIONS: ENDPOINTS OF TOXICITY AND CARCINOGENICITY

A. Introduction

As in all toxicological studies, it is essential to have a well-written, detailed protocol before study initiation in which all observations to be made are clearly outlined. This protocol should be a collaboration between the study director and other study personnel, including the chemists, toxicologists, laboratory animal specialists, pathologists, and statisticians. The study protocol must be adhered to as much as possible, with any changes made only after consultation with the appropriate personnel, and such changes should be well documented in protocol addenda.

The actual observations and endpoints measured depend on the particular objectives of the specific study protocol. Previous shorterterm studies of the drug may have identified suspected target organs, and this should be taken into account when deciding what data to collect. In the absence of such specific information, there are general guidelines on data collection that apply to most carcinogenicity studies.

With the widespread use of computer technology, it is desirable that all data collected during a study be stored in a electronic format that is readily assessable and easy to transfer to other parties, such as to the regulatory agencies. There are some fairly standard formats used by various parties, the STUDIES format of the EPA (50) being an example.

In addition to the actual endpoints, there is a certain amount of background data that should be included with each study observation. Experiment number, animal number, group, and sex are important to record, In addition, good laboratory practice (GLP) regulations require the recording of the data collected, time of input, and identification of the responsible person. This information is required of all raw data entries in a GLP-regulated study.

B. In-Life Phase

A physical examination of each animal should be conducted on a regular basis, preferably daily. Any clinical observations should be recorded, noting the date first observed and the date last observed, if applicable, so that the duration of the continuous time period for which the specific clinical observation was noted can be calculated. It should also be noted whether the observation was or was not a palpable mass. Opthalmological examinations should also be conducted, at least in the control and high-dose groups, and in all groups if abnormalities are detected.

Body weights of the animals should be recorded individually. The IARC recommends that weights be taken every week for the first couple of months, then every 4 weeks for the duration of the study.

For drug-in-diet studies, it is important to measure food consumption to monitor the drug intake for each animal. For other routes of administration, food consumption can be measured on a subset, say 20, of the animals in each group. The usual way of summarizing food consumption is grams per animal per day measured over several days, usually a week.

Water consumption is sometimes measured, particularly if the drug is administered in the water. It can also be important if the urinalysis endpoints are considered important to the interpretation of the study results.

C. Clinical Chemistry

Repeated sampling of blood is usually not necessary, and may adversely affect the interpretation of the results. If interim measurements are needed, it may be better to obtain these from satellite groups of animals.

Blood samples are commonly taken at study termination. Measurements typically made at the terminal blood draw include hematology endpoints; hematocrit, hemoglobin; counts of leukocytes, erythrocytes, reticulocytes, and platelets; differential leukocyte counts; MCH, MCV, MCHC, and prothrombin, thromboplastin, and clotting times; and serum chemistry endpoints: calcium, chloride, phosphorus, potassium, sodium, albumin, blood urea nitrogen, glucose, creatinine, total protein, creatine phosphokinase, ALT, and AST. Additional endpoints can be added depending on predetermined target organs or other study objectives.

D. Necropsy

The most important information obtained from a long-term carcinogenicity study comes from the scheduled and unscheduled necropsies, when organ weights and tissue samples are collected. Complete necropsies should be conducted on all animals, whether they die on study or survive to their scheduled sacrifice. It is also important to establish criteria for determining if a test animal is sick or moribund and should be sacrificed before the end of the study. Even though it is desirable to keep an animal on study long enough to ascertain the effects of the drug, animals that die suddenly may lose tissues to cannibalism or autolysis.

A complete postmortem examination includes the organs and tissues listed in Table 1. These are examined for all animals, with males and females treated in a similar fashion. Any grossly visible lesions should be recorded, including location, size, shape, and number. For unscheduled sacrifices, it is important to try to determine the role of the lesion in the death of the animal. If a lesion contributed to the cause of death, either directly or indirectly, then it is observed in a fatal context, otherwise it was observed in an incidental context. The true cause of death can be difficult to determine, but it is generally considered sufficient if the lesion is assessed according to the following scale: (a) definitely fatal, (b) probably fatal, (c) probably incidental, or (d) definitely incidental. The context can then be possibly refined after histopathological examination and correlation with other study data. Lesions, such as skin tumors, which are observed before the death of the animal are classified as "mortality-independent." Tumors observed at a scheduled sacrifice will be, by definition, incidental.

Organ weights are usually recorded for selected organs. When this information is collected, the necropsy body weight should also be recorded for purposes of calculating relative values. It should also be

TABLE 1   Organs and Tissues Commonly Examined During a
Complete Necropsy

Gross lesions and tissue masses	Heart
Mandibular and mesenteric lymph node	Brain
Salivary gland	Thymus
Sternebrae, femur	Pancreas
Esophagus	Adrenals
Stomach	Pituitary
Small intestine	Thyroid
Cecum	Parathyroids
Colon and rectum	Spleen
Liver: left and right lobes	Kidneys
Gallbladder (mice)	Urinary bladder
Testes and epididymis	Spinal cord
Prostate and seminal vesicles	Eyes
Uterus	Mammary gland
Ovaries	Skin
Nasal cavity and turbinates	Thigh muscle
Trachea	Sciatic nerve
Lungs and main stem bronchi	Oral cavity
Preputial or clitoral gland (rats)	Zymbal glands

recorded whether the organ weighed was unilateral or bilateral (combined), and whether the organ as weighed contained a tumor or unusual mass.

E. Histopathology

The NCI–NTP protocols originally called for the routine examination of 32 sections of 25 organs or tissues from every animal on study. Subsequent experience increased the list to 43–44 sections of 31–33 organ-tissues. These are listed in Table 2. Additional sections are also examined based on necropsy findings of masses or other lesions or on study objectives. These guidelines result in the examination of 25,000–26,000 slides per carcinogenicity assay, approximately one-half man year of effort (51).

Various alternatives have been suggested to reduce the workload without loss of valuable information (52). These typically involve the use of an "inverse pyramid" type of approach. These approaches have a common (a) complete necropsy examinations are made of all animals,

TABLE 2   Organs and Tissues Commonly Examined Histopathologically

Gross lesions and tissue masses	Heart
Mandibular and mesenteric lymph node	Brain
Salivary gland	Thymus
Sternebrae, femur	Pancreas
Esophagus	Adrenals
Stomach	Pituitary
Small intestine	Thyroid
Cecum	Parathyroids
Colon and rectum	Spleen
Liver: left and right lobes	Kidneys
Gallbladder (mice)	Urinary bladder
Testes and epididymis	Spinal cord
Prostate and seminal vesicles	Eyes
Uterus	Mammary gland
Ovaries	Skin
Nasal cavity and turbinates	
Trachea	
Lungs and main stem bronchi	
Preputial or clitoral gland (rats)	

and (b) complete sets of tissues from all animals are collected and preserved. Histopathological evaluations are then made of either the complete list (see Table 2) or some predetermined subset of the list for all
control and high-dose animals. If there was significant mortality in the
high-dose group, then the next highest dose group would also receive the
complete examination. If target organs or tissues were identified in the
protocol of if drug-related neoplastic or nonneoplastic changes are seen
at the high dose, then all animals in the lower doses are also examined
for the particular tissue. The use of this type of strategy would result in
a savings of 20–60% in the histopathology evaluation cost.

The quality of histopathological slide preparation is of extreme
importance, and should be conducted by qualified professionals. Autolysis, poor histotechnique, inadequate tissue or sera samples, and concurrent disease can confound the results, and care should be taken to minimize these occurrences. Standardized techniques in the histopathology
laboratory should be used. Consistency in trimming is very important.
The direction in which the organ is cut and the localization (anatomical
site) should be the same for all samples. Like numbers of sections should

be obtained from the control and treated animals to avoid increased chances of observing a lesion in treated groups. There have been documented studies in the past during which multiple sections from treated animals were examined, whereas only single sections from the controls were.

Information that should be recorded for an observed lesion includes the organ or tissue it was observed in, whether it was neoplastic or nonneoplastic, and whether it was benign or malignant. The terminology used by pathologists for the classification of lesions is critical to the proper statistical assessment of the data. Ideally, there should be a uniform classification scheme used within the study. With computerized data collection systems in widespread use, this is especially critical. Lengthy descriptions of the lesion, overly detailed or subtly changing descriptions, ambiguity, and the use of synonyms can make the computerized tabulation of lesion data difficult. Because it is probably impossible to achieve complete uniformity, it is usually necessary to perform some rationalization (lumping or splitting of diagnosis) before tabulation and analysis. Any such actions should be well-documented in the raw data.

Because carcinogenesis is being increasingly recognized to be a multistage process, the handling of histopathology data can possibly be refined. The assessment of carcinogenicity might be improved by replacing the mere counting of tumors and preneoplastic lesions with a grading scale representing the proliferative process. A scale of say 1–5, with 1 representing the beginning stages of hyperplasia and 5 full carcinoma. A grading system could also help distinguish between spontaneous and chemically induced lesions and in ranking carcinogenic effects (53).

Probably the most controversial aspect of the histopathological evaluation is the issue of "blind" slide reading. Blind reading refers to the evaluation of slides in a random fashion without knowledge of which treatment group the slide came from. Blind reading helps assure that there is no statistical bias being introduced into the tests for treatment effect and that each observation is independent. Biostatisticians generally advocate this procedure, but toxicological pathologists are in almost universal agreement that this is not an appropriate procedure. In fact, the American College of Veterinary Pathologists (54), the Society of Toxicologic Pathologists (55) and others (56) have issued official positions that blind reading is inappropriate for the routine evaluation of slides. They feel that the pathologist should have all information available on the status of the animal. Besides knowledge of the treatment, this includes clinical chemistries, clinical observations, necropsy data, and any other observations on the particular animal.

A possible compromise involves a two-step procedure. The initial reading of all slides would be made with all information available. For selected endpoints, a second, blind evaluation would be done, either by the same pathologist or by peer review. Although pathologists quite adamantly reject blind reading, most do agree with the two-step approach.

VII. FUTURE DIRECTIONS

Study design and published guidelines for long-term carcinogenicity studies will continue to evolve as knowledge increases and new questions arise. Pressure to reduce the number of laboratory animals and cut costs in general will also influence future designs.

Conducting combined chronic toxicity and carcinogenicity studies is an option that could result in substantial savings in cost and laboratory animals. The Organisation for Economic Cooperation and Development (OECD) has issued guidelines that include a protocol for such a study. The protocol has four dose groups, each containing the standard 50 animals of each sex, plus additional satellite groups of 15–20 animals at the control and high-dose levels for the toxicity phase (57).

The use of two species is an area that may possibly undergo change in the future. Studies in mice have been called redundant (58). Review of the large NCI–NTP database suggests that a protocol using male rats and female mice would have found 90% of the carcinogens. Increased knowledge of chemical structure–activity, metabolism, and pharmacokinetics may also decrease the need for additional species.

The use of transgenic animals has great potential in carcinogenicity screening (59). Specific genes or segments can be altered or removed to genetically engineer an animal to answer specific questions concerning chemical–DNA interactions.

Medium-term carcinogenicity assays, taking from 8 to 36 weeks, have also been developed. These tests include the rat liver foci, preweanling mouse liver, mouse lung, and mouse skin assays. These assays look for preneoplastic changes as predictors of tumor development. They are highly target-specific, and the results depend on the class of chemical compounds.

In conclusion, although we may expect to see changes in the long-term assay, it will probably remain for some time the main tool in the search for human carcinogens.

REFERENCES

1. McAuslane JAN, Lumley CE, Walker RS. The need for control animal pathology database: an international survey. Hum Exp Toxicol 10:205–213, 1991.
2. International Agency for Research on Cancer. IARC Monographs on the Evaluaton of Carcinogenic Risk to Humans – Preamble. IARC Internal Technical Report 87/001. Lyon: IARC, 1987.
3. Boorman GA, Maronpot RR, Eustis SL. Rodent carcinogenicity bioassay: past, present and future. Toxicol Pathol 22:105–111, 1994.
4. Sontag JM, Page NP, Sanfiotti U. Guidelines for Carcinogen Bioassays in Small Rodents. DHHS Publication NIH/76-801. Bethesda, MD: National Cancer Institute, 1976.
5. Food and Drug Administration. Toxicological Principles for the Safety Assessment of Direct Food Additives Used in Food. Springfield, VA: National Technical Information Service, 1982, revised 1993.
6. Environmental Protection Agency. Risk Assessment Guidelines of 1986, EPA/600/8-87/045. Washington, DC: Office of Health and Environmental Assess, Environmental Protection Agency, 1987.
7. Kempthorne O. The Design and Analysis of Experiments. New York: John Wiley & Sons, 1952.
8. Quenouille MH. The Design and Analysis of Experiments. New York: Hafner Publishing, 1953.
9. Cochran WG, Cox GM. Experimental Design. New York: John Wiley & Sons, 1957.
10. Winer BJ. Statistical Priniciples in Experimental Design. New York: McGraw-Hill, 1972.
11. Montgomery DC. Design and Analysis of Experiments. New York: John Wiley & Sons, 1991.
12. Haseman JK, Huff JE, Rao GN, Eustis SL. Sources of variability in rodent carcinogenicity studies. Fundam Appl Toxicol 12:793–804, 1989.
13. Greenman DL, Bryant P, Kodell RL, Sheldon W. Influence of cage shelf level on retinal atrophy in mice. Lab Anim Sci 32:353–356, 1982.
14. Haseman JK. Do cage effects influence tumor incidence? An examination of laboratory animal carcinogenicity studies utilizing Fischer 344 rats. J Appl Toxicol 8:267–273, 1988.
15. Young SS. Are there local room effects on hepatic tumors in male mice? An examination of the NTP Eugenol study. Fundam Appl Toxicol 8:1–4, 1987.

16. Young SS. Evaluation of data from long-term rodent studies [Letter to the Editor]. J Nat Cancer Inst 80:3–4, 1988.
17. Young SS. What is the proper experimental unit for long-term rodent studies? An examination of the NTP benzyl acetate study. Toxicology 54:233–239, 1989.
18. Lagakos S, Mosteller F. A case study of statistics in the regulatory process: the FD&C Red 40 experiments. J Nat Cancer Inst 66:197–212, 1981.
19. Haseman JK. Lack of cage effects on liver tumor incidence in B6C3F1 mice. Fundam Appl Toxicol 10:179–187, 1988.
20. Gad S, Weil CS. Statistics and Experimental Design for Toxicologists. Caldwell, NJ: Telford Press, 1988.
21. Bickis M, Krewski D. Statistical design and analysis of the long-term carcinogenicity bioassay. In: Clayson DB, Krewski D, Munro I, eds. Toxicological Risk Assessment, vol. I. Biological and Statistical Criteria. Boca Raton, FL: CRC Press, 1985.
22. Ostle B. Statistics in Research. Ames, IA: Iowa State Press, 1963.
23. SAS Institute. SAS/STAT User's Guide, Version 6, 4 ed, vol 2. Cary, NC: SAS Institute, 1990.
24. Mohr U. The Syrian golden hamster as a model in cancer research. Prog Exp Tumor Res 24:245–252, 1979.
25. Littlefield NA, Kodell RL. Influence of genetic population structure on the results of chronic toxicity studies. J Toxicol Environ Health 5:121–129, 1979.
26. Schellabarger CJ, Stone JP, Holtzman S. Rat differences in mammary tumor induction with estrogen and neutron irradiation. J Nat Cancer Inst 61:1505–1508, 1978.
27. Greenman DL, Delongchamp RR, Highman B. Variability of response to diethylstilbestrol: a comparison of inbred with hybrid mice. J Toxicol Environ Health 5:131–143, 1979.
28. Haseman JK, Hoel DG. Statistical design of toxicity assays: role of genetic structure of test animal population. J Toxicol Environ Health 5:89–101, 1979.
29. Festing MFW. Use of a multistrain assay could improve the NTP carcinogenesis bioassay. Enviorn Health Perspect 103:44–52, 1995.
30. Festing MFW. Properties of inbred strains and outbred stocks, with special reference to toxicity testing. J Toxicol Environ Health 5:53–68, 1979.
31. Festing MFW. Phenotypic variability of inbred and outbred mice. Nature 263:230–232, 1976.
32. Festing MFW. Genetic variation in outbred rats estimated from DNA fingerprints: implications for toxicological screening [abstr]. Hum Exp Toxicol 11:590–591, 1992.
33. Festing MFW. A case for using inbred strains of laboratory animals in evaluating the safety of drugs. Food Cosmet Toxicol 13:369–375, 1975.
34. Felton RP, Gaylor DW. Multistrain experiments for screening toxic substances. J Toxicol Environ Health 26:399–411, 1989.

35. Wolff GL, Gaylor DW, Blackwell BN. Bladder and liver tumorigenesis induced by 2-acetylaminofluorine in different F_1 mouse hybrids: variations within genotypes and effects of using more than one genotype on risk assessment: J Toxicol Environ Health 33:327–348, 1991.
36. Festing MFW, Lovell DP. Reducing the use of laboratory animals in toxicological research and testing by better experimental design. J R Stat Soc Ser B 58:127–140, 1996.
37. Haseman JK, Seilkop SK. An examination of the association between maximum tolerated dose and carcinogenicity in 326 long-term studies in rats and mice. Fundam Appl Toxicol 19:207–213, 1992.
38. Gold LS, Bernstein L, Magaw R, Slone TH. Interspecies extrapolation in carcinogenesis: prediction between rats and mice. Environ Health Perspect 81:211–219, 1989.
39. International Life Sciences Institute. The selection of doses in chronic toxicity/carcinogenicity studies. In: Grice HC, ed. Current Issues of Toxicology. New York: Springer-Verlag, 1984, pp 6–49.
40. Haseman JK. Issues in carcinogenicity testing: dose selection. Fundam Appl Toxicol 5:66–78, 1985.
41. Frederick GL. The necessary minimal duration of final long-term toxicological tests of drugs. Fundam Appl Toxicol 6:385–394, 1986.
42. Davies TS, Munro A. The case for an upper dose limit of 1000 mg/kg in rodent carcinogenicity tests. Cancer Lett 95:69–77, 1995.
43. Munro A, Davies TS. High dose levels are not necessary in rodent studies to detect human carcinogens. Cancer Lett 75:183–194, 1993.
44. Contrera JF. Emerging trends in non-clinical safety assessment for therapeutics. Toxicol Pathol 22:89–94, 1994.
45. Swenberg JA. Bioassay design and MTD setting: old methods and new approaches. Regul Toxicol Pharmacol 21:44–51, 1995.
46. Hottendorf GH, Pachter IJ. Review and evaluation of the NCINTP carcinogenesis bioassays. Toxicol Pathol 13:141–146, 1985.
47. Portier C, Hoel D. Design of animal carcinogenicity studies for goodness-of-fit of multistage models. Fundam Appl Toxicol 4:949–959, 1984.
48. Grice HC, Burek JD. Age associated (geriatric) pathology: its impact on long-term toxicity studies. In: Grice HC, ed. Current Issues in Toxicology. New York: Springer-Verlag, 1984, pp 57–107.
49. Della Porta G, Dragani TA. Long-term assays for carcinogenicity. Teratogenesis Carcinog Mutagen 10:137–145, 1990.
50. Environmental Protection Agency. Studies/Chronic: Data formats for Chronic/Oncogenicity Rodent Bioassays. EPA 540/09-90-092. Washington, DC: EPA, 1990.
51. McConnell, EE. Pathology requirements for rodent two-year studies. I. A review of current procedures. Toxicol Pathol 11:60–64, 1983.
52. McConnell EE. Pathology requirements for rodent two-years studies. II. Alternative procedures (with discussion). Toxicol Pathol 11:65–76, 1983.

53. Squire, RA, Carcinogenicity testing and safety assessment. Fundam Appl Toxicol 4:S326–S334, 1984.
54. Prasse K, Hildebrandt P, Dodd D, et al. [Letter to the Editor] Toxicol Pathol 14:274–275, 1986.
55. Iatropoulous MJ. In Current Issues in Toxicology. New York: Springer-Verlag, 1988.
56. Newberne PM, de la Iglesia FA. Philosophy of blind slide reading in toxicologic pathology. Toxicol Pathol 13:255, 1985.
57. Feron VJ, Kroes R. The long-term study in rodents for identifying carcinogens: some controveries and suggestions for improvements. J Appl Toxicol 6:307–311, 1986.
58. Schach von Wittenau M, Estes PC. The redundancy of mouse carcinogenicity bioassays. Fundam Appl Toxicol 3:631–639, 1983.
59. Tennant RW, Hansen L, Spaulding J. Gene manipulation and genetic toxicology. Mutagen 9:171–174, 1994.

8

Analysis of Long-Term Carcinogenicity Studies

HONGSHIK AHN

State University of New York at Stony Brook, Stony Brook, New York

RALPH L. KODELL

National Center for Toxicological Research, Food and Drug Administration, Jefferson, Arkansas

I. INTRODUCTION

Animal carcinogenicity experiments are employed to test the carcinogenic potential of drugs and other chemical substances used by humans. In such experiments, animals are divided into several groups by randomization. A typical carcinogenicity study involves a control and two to three dose groups of 50 or more animals, usually rats or mice. Typically, a chemical is administered at a constant daily dose rate (i.e., a fixed amount daily, a fixed amount daily per unit body weight, or a fixed concentration) for a major portion of the lifetime of the test animal (e.g., 2 years). Sometimes, scheduled interim sacrifices are performed during the experiment. At the end of the study, all surviving animals are sacrificed and subjected to necropsy. For each animal in a given dose group, the age at death and the presence or absence of specific tumor types are recorded. Groups of animals are compared for tumor development. A possible carcinogenic response is an acceleration of tumor development in exposed groups.

Many methods have been proposed for analyzing tumor incidence data from animal bioassays. For nonlethal tumors, Hoel and Walburg (1972), Peto (1974), Gart (1975), and Lagakos (1982) recommended that some form of Mantel–Haenszel test (Mantel and Haenszel, 1959) be applied to experimental survival data to test for differences in tumor prevalence. For rapidly lethal tumors, Peto et al. (1980) recommended a log-rank test for comparing the rate of death with tumor across different doses. However, most tumors are neither strictly nonlethal nor rapidly lethal. Peto (1974) and Peto et al. (1980) proposed a method for analyzing tumor data in which tumors are observed in both the fatal and incidental contexts.

The estimation of incidence rates for certain diseases can be affected by competing causes of death. Hence, many analyses require cause-of-death information (Peto, 1974; Kodell and Nelson, 1980; Peto et al., 1980; Kodell et al., 1982, 1986; Dinse and Lagakos, 1982, 1983; Turnbull and Mitchell, 1984; Kodell and Chen, 1987; Dinse, 1988a; Archer and Ryan, 1989). These methods are popular because they do not require large numbers of animals to be sacrificed at multiple timepoints to observe the prevalence of occult tumors. These methods assume that pathologists can determine if a tumor affected an animal's risk of death. In practice, however, pathologists often claim that accurate determinations of the cause of death are impossible, and classification errors can produce biases (Lagakos, 1982; Racine-Poon and Hoel, 1984; Lagakos and Louis, 1988). Without cause-of-death information or simplifying assumptions, interim sacrifices of groups of animals are necessary to determine tumor incidence rates and for occult tumors to be identifiable from bioassay data (McKnight and Crowley, 1984). However, most of the animal carcinogenicity studies are designed with a single, terminal sacrifice.

Various analyses have been developed for experiments in which serial interim sacrifices are performed (Clifford, 1977; Turnbull and Mitchell, 1978; Berlin et al., 1979; Mitchell and Turnbull, 1979; Dewanji and Kalbfleisch, 1986; Portier and Dinse, 1987; Dinse, 1988b; Malani and Van Ryzin, 1988; Williams and Portier, 1992a,b; Malani and Lu, 1993; Ahn and Kodell, 1995; Kodell and Ahn, 1996, 1997). Portier and Dinse (1987) introduced a semiparametric test for comparing the tumor incidence rates of two treatments. McKnight and Crowley (1984), Dewanji and Kalbfleisch (1986), Malani and Van Ryzin (1988), Williams and Portier (1992a), and Ahn and Kodell (1995) proposed nonparametric methods for estimation and pairwise testing of the tumor incidence function. Recently, several authors developed tests for dose-related trend in tumor incidence rate across several dose groups (Portier and Dinse, 1987; Bailer and Portier, 1988; Dinse, 1991, 1994; Kodell and Ahn, 1996). The most important carcinogenic response is an increase in age-specific rates of tumor incidence in exposed animals over some portion of the life span of the test species, leading to an increased lifetime probability of developing a tumor. Malani and Lu (1993) and Kodell and Ahn (1997) proposed age-adjusted tests of the tumor incidence rate for dose-related trend, based on data from bioassays with sacrifices. Dinse (1991, 1993, 1994), Lindsey and Ryan (1994), and Kodell et al. (1996) proposed statistical methods for analyzing tumor incidence rates based on data with a single terminal sacrifice. Most trend tests in common use involve age-adjusted tests.

Gart et al. (1986) presented an excellent review of the statistical methods for analyzing animal carcinogenicity data. In addition to the methods covered in Gart et al., several new methods developed during the last decade in this area will be discussed in this chapter. We will focus on estimation and testing of tumor response data arising from animal tumorigenicity experiments. A review of methods for identification and testing of the tumor incidence rate will be given. Several statistical tests to be considered are described in detail.

II. NOTATION

Consider an experiment with g treatment groups, a control and $g - 1$ dose groups. Let d_i be the dose level of the ith group. Suppose N animals are initially placed on experiment, and N_i animals are assigned randomly to the ith treatment group. Let N_i animals in the ith treatment group be followed over time for the development of tumors. We assume that all animals come from the same population and are born tumor-free on day zero of the experiment. Divide the time span into m intervals such that the jth interval is $I_j = (t_{j-1}, t_j]$, $j = 1, \ldots, m$, where $t_0 = 0$ and t_m denotes the time at which the terminal sacrifice is scheduled. Let X_T be a random variable for time to onset of tumor and X_D be the time to natural death. Throughout this chapter, all the tumors are assumed to be irreversible. Individuals are assumed to be in the tumor-free state at the onset of the experiment.

III. KNOWN CAUSE OF DEATH

A. Testing

In survival–sacrifice experiments, information about onset of specific diseases is confounded with information about the effect of the presence or absence of all diseases on mortality. To avoid biases caused by differences in intercurrent mortality and at the same time to make some use of data on time of death, Peto (1974) and Peto et al. (1980) recommended that pathologists assign the context of observation to each observed tumor. Tumors that do not alter an animal's risk of death and are observed only as the result of a death from an unrelated cause are classified as incidental, whereas tumors that affect mortality by either directly causing death or indirectly increasing the risk of death from other causes are classified as fatal. Accurate data on cause of death allow the tumor incidence function to be estimated without requiring sacrifices. The analysis of data on occult tumors using cause of death is performed separately for nonlethal (incidental) tumors and rapidly lethal tumors.

First, consider the animals that did not have the specific tumor before death and tumor-bearing animals that did not die of that tumor. Let n_{ij} be the number of animals in group i dying during interval I_j from causes unrelated to the presence of the tumor of interest, and y_{ij} be the number of these animals in which the tumor was observed in the incidental context, for $i = 1, \ldots, g$. For each interval I_j, the tumor prevalence data may be summarized in a $2 \times g$ table as in Table 1. All tumors found in sacrificed animals are classified as incidental.

The expected number of tumors in the ith group for the jth interval is $E_{ij} = y_{\cdot j} K_{ij}$, where $K_{ij} = n_{ij}/n_{\cdot j}$. Thus, the observed and expected numbers of tumors in the ith group over the entire experiment are $O_i = \Sigma^m_{j=1} y_{ij}$ and $E_i = \Sigma^m_{j=1} E_{ij}$, respectively, for $i = 1, \ldots, g$. Define

TABLE 1 Tumor Prevalence Data for Incidental Tumors in Interval I_j

	Dose group				
	1	2	$\cdots$	g	Total
No. with tumors	y_{1j}	y_{2j}	$\cdots$	y_{gj}	$y_{\cdot j}$
No. without tumors	$n_{1j} - y_{1j}$	$n_{2j} - y_{2j}$	$\cdots$	$n_{gj} - y_{gj}$	$n_{\cdot j} - y_{\cdot j}$
No. deaths	n_{1j}	n_{2j}	$\cdots$	n_{gj}	$n_{\cdot j}$

$$D_i = O_i - E_i = \sum_{j=1}^{m} (y_{ij} - E_{ij}) \tag{1}$$

and

$$V_{ri} = \sum_{j=1}^{m} \kappa_j K_{rj}(\delta_{ri} - K_{ij}) \tag{2}$$

where $\kappa_j = y_{\cdot j}(n_{\cdot j} - y_{\cdot j})/(n_{\cdot j} - 1)$ and δ_{ri} is defined as 1 if $r = i$ and 0 otherwise. Let $D_a = (D_1, \ldots, D_g)'$ and V_a be the $g \times g$ matrix with (r,i) entry V_{ri}.

Second, consider tumors that were the cause of death. The method used is very similar to that used for the incidental tumors, except that each tumor-death time defines an interval. Table 2 is a contingency table for interval I_j. Let m_{ij} be the number of animals in group i surviving at the beginning of the interval, and x_{ij} be the number of these animals dying of the tumor in that interval. A vector D_b of differences of observed and expected values using the foregoing data is calculated the same way as that for the incidental tumors, and the corresponding covariance matrix V_b is computed.

The analysis of data on occult tumors using contexts of observation is based on the vector $D = D_a + D_b$, with covariance matrix $V = V_a + V_b$. Then

$$X_H = D'V^-D \tag{3}$$

can serve as a test for heterogeneity among the g groups, where V^- is a generalized inverse of V. If there is no difference among the groups, then X_H is asymptotically distributed as χ^2 distribution with $g - 1$ degrees of freedom. Also, a trend test can be considered by using

$$X_R = \frac{(l'D)^2}{l'Vl} \tag{4}$$

TABLE 2 Tumor Causing Death in Interval I_j

	Dose group				
	1	2	$\cdots$	g	Total
No. with tumors	x_{1j}	x_{2j}	$\cdots$	x_{gj}	$x_{\cdot j}$
No. surviving	m_{1j}	m_{2j}	$\cdots$	m_{gj}	$m_{\cdot j}$

where $l = (d_1, \ldots, d_g)'$. A test for departure from a monotone dose-response relation can be based on

$$X_M = X_H - X_R \tag{5}$$

which has a χ^2 distribution with $g - 2$ degrees of freedom under the null hypothesis that the dose-response relation is linear.

An experiment was conducted at the National Center for Toxicological Research to study the effects of feeding 2-acetylaminofluorene (2-AAF) to female BALB/C mice (ED_{01} study; Littlefield et al., 1980). Data in Table 3 are from groups of animals that were dosed continuously at concentrations of 0, 35, 75, or 150 ppm 2-AAF until the terminal

TABLE 3 Counts for Deaths for the ED_{01} Data

	Interval (wk)	Dose (ppm)				Total
		0	35	75	150	
Incidental tumor data						
No. with tumors	0–52	0	1	0	0	1
No. without tumors		9	9	10	5	33
No. with tumors	53–78	0	0	1	1	2
No. without tumors		15	31	16	14	76
No. with tumors	79–92	0	0	1	4	5
No. without tumors		34	35	28	25	122
No. with tumors	93–104	6	18	28	23	75
No. without tumors		197	272	142	51	662
Fetal tumor data						
No. with tumors	0–52	0	0	0	0	0
No. alive		264	391	232	133	1020
No. with tumors	53–78	0	3	0	1	4
No. alive		255	381	222	128	986
No. with tumors	79–92	1	1	2	2	6
No. alive		240	347	205	113	905
No. with tumors	93–104	2	1	4	8	15
No. alive		205	291	174	82	752

Dose-metric for trend test: Concentration in ppm.
Peto heterogeneity test: Incidental: $\chi_3^2 = 70.6$ Fatal: $\chi_3^2 = 27.2$ Combined: $\chi_3^2 = 90.5$.
Peto trend test: Incidental: $z = 8.3$ Fatal: $z = 4.8$ combined: $z = 9.5$.
All p-values < 0.00001.
Source: Littlefield et al., 1980.

sacrifice at 24 months. The tumors of interest were hepatocellular adenomas or carcinomas of the liver. The NTP (National Toxicology Program) time intervals (Bailer and Portier, 1988) were used for both the incidental tumor analysis and the fatal tumor analysis, although the latter could have been done with the time of death of each fatal tumor defining a time interval. Both the heterogeneity test and trend test show significant differences for both the incidental and fatal tumors in this example.

The choice of time intervals for calculating the incidental tumor component of the test of Peto et al. (1980) is an important consideration. The use of the so-called ad hoc time intervals that are determined by the observed data is problematic (Kodell et al., 1994). It is better to define fixed time intervals in advance, such as the NTP intervals, to maintain the nominal test size. For tumors that can be detected during life, an analysis identical with the fatal tumor component of the Peto analysis is performed. Each time of detection defines a time interval for the test, and there is no incidental tumor component.

The cause-of-death test allows an assessment of the carcinogenic potential of a substance without requiring extreme lethality assumptions of multiple sacrifices (Archer and Ryan, 1989). The test is valid when deaths from nontumor causes are representative of the live population for the tumor of interest (Lagakos and Ryan, 1985). The cause-of-death method is also more cost-effective than methods requiring multiple interim sacrifices (McKnight and Crowley, 1984). However, pathologists often cannot accurately assess every context of observation. As a compromise, an analysis can allow cause of death to be specified with uncertainty (Racine-Poon and Hoel, 1984; Dinse, 1986; Kodell and Chen, 1987). Alternatively, an incomplete data analogue of the cause-of-death method can be used to partition each tumor-bearing animal into a fatal portion and an incidental portion, based on an assumed value of a tumor lethality function (Lagakos and Louis, 1988). With this approach, the cause-of-death test is applied to each of several partitions determined by a range of assumed tumor lethalities.

B. Estimation

Kodell and Nelson (1980) presented a stochastic model that uses survival and sacrifice data to describe the sequence of events comprised by histological appearance of a tumor followed by death from that tumor. They used the Weibull distribution within their schematic representation of the tumor–death model provided in Fig. 1. Here, the random variable X_T defined in Section II represents the transition time from the initial normal state to the tumor state. Let X_{DT} be the potential time to death from the tumor, and X_{DNT} be the potential time to death from a competing risk (transition time from the normal state or the tumor state to the death from competing risk). Kodell and Nelson assumed that X_T, $X_{DT} - X_T$ (transition time from the tumor state to the death from tumor), and X_{DNT} have independent Weibull distributions. Sacrificed animals are considered to be dead from a competing risk. Within this framework, the likelihood function is developed by considering both natural deaths and scheduled sacrifices. Although analytical solutions to the likelihood equations are not possible, the likelihood function can be maximized numerically.

Tolley et al. (1978) also chose a Weibull function to describe transition to the tumor state for human stomach cancer data, but chose a Gompertz function for transition to death from a competing risk. Kalbfleisch et al. (1983) discussed likelihood estimation for an arbitrary parametric model without the assumption of independent competing risks. However, the formulation of Kodell and Nelson (1980), which does not require estimation of the distribution of time to death from competing risks, is somewhat simpler.

Kodell et al. (1982) proposed nonparametric estimates for disease

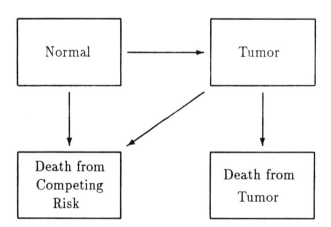

FIGURE 1   Illustration of illness and death, with possible transitions, in rodent bioassay. (From Kodell and Nelson, 1980.)

resistance and survival functions for the distribution of time to death caused by the disease. They relaxed the assumption of independence of the tumor onset time and the course of the disease from Kodell and Nelson (1980).

Consider three random variables X_T defined in Section II, and X_{DT} and X_{DNT} introduced earlier in this section. Define the tumor resistance function as

$$S_{X_T}(t) = \Pr(X_T \geq t \,|\, X_{DNT} \geq t)$$

and the survival function for the disease of interest as

$$S_{X_{DT}}(t) = \Pr(X_{DT} \geq t \,|\, X_{DNT} \geq t)$$

To obtain the maximum likelihood estimators $\hat{S}_{X_T}(t)$ and $\hat{S}_{X_{DT}}(t)$ of the foregoing functions, Kodell et al. assumed that the ratio $S_{X_T}(t)/S_{X_{DT}}(t)$ is monotonically nonincreasing. This assumption means that the proportion of disease-free animals in the population is monotonically nonincreasing. Let n_j be the number of animals alive just before t_j; c_j be the number of deaths at t_j caused by the tumor; and a_j and b_j be the number of deaths at t_j caused by a competing risk, for which the tumor of interest is present or absent, respectively. It should be assumed that tumor-bearing and tumor-free animals of the same age have identical hazard functions for death unrelated to tumor. The likelihood function under these assumptions is proportional to

$$\prod_{j=1}^{m} [S_{X_{DT}}(t_j - 0) - S_{X_{DT}}(t_j)]^{c_j}[S_{X_{DT}}(t_j) - S_{X_T}(t_j)]^{a_j}[S_{X_T}(t_j)]^{b_j}$$

By letting $p_j = S_{X_{DT}}(t_j)/S_{X_{DT}}(t_{j-1})$ and $r_j = S_{X_T}(t_j)/S_{X_{DT}}(t_j)$, the likelihood function may be written as

$$\prod_{j=1}^{m} p_j^{n_j - c_j}(1-p_j)^{c_j} \prod_{j=1}^{m} r_j^{b_j}(1-r_j)^{a_j} \tag{6}$$

Equation (6) can be maximized individually for the p_j's and the r_j's. The maximum likelihood estimator of p_j is $(n_j - c_j)/n_j$, $i = 1, \ldots, I$ and that of r_j is $b_j/(a_j + b_j)$, $j = 1, \ldots, J$, provided that the estimators of r_j's are monotonically nonincreasing. Consequently, the estimator of $S_{X_{DT}}(t)$ is the Kaplan–Meier product-limit estimator (Kaplan and Meier, 1958),

$$\hat{S}_{X_{DT}}(t) = \prod_{t_i \leq t} \frac{n_i - c_i}{n_i}$$

and that of $S_{X_T}(t)$ is the Hoel–Walburg estimator of prevalence of disease,

$$\hat{S}_{X_T}(t) = \prod_{t_i \le t} \left(\frac{n_i - c_i}{n_i} \right) \left(\frac{b_i}{a_i + b_i} \right)$$

provided that the disease of interest were strictly nonlethal. The variance of $\hat{S}_{X_{DT}}(t)$ is obtained by the Greenwood approximation

$$\text{var}[\hat{S}_{X_{DT}}(t)] \simeq [S_{X_{DT}}(t)]^2 \sum_{t_j \le t} \frac{1 - p_j}{n_j p_j}, \quad t_j \le t < t_{j+1}$$

and the variance of $\hat{S}_{X_T}(t)$ is obtained using a first-order Taylor series,

$$\text{var}[\hat{S}_{X_T}(t)] \simeq [S_{X_T}(t)]^2 \sum_{t_j \le t} \left[\frac{1 - p_j}{n_j p_j} + \frac{1 - r_j}{(a_j + b_j) r_j} \right],$$

$$t_j \le t < t_{j+1}$$

Table 4 shows the estimates of tumor onset function for the ED_{01} data, based on the method of Kodell et al.

Dinse and Lagakos (1982) weakened the restriction of monotonicity of $S_{X_T}(t)/S_{X_{DT}}(t)$ and proposed to estimate $S_{X_T}(t)$ and $S_{X_{DT}}(t)$, and approximated their variances. As in Kodell et al. (1982), Dinse and Lagakos obtained the Kaplan–Meier estimator for $S_{X_{DT}}$. To obtain an estimator for S_{X_T}, they used isotonic regression. The Kaplan–Meier estimator for $S_{X_{DT}}(t)$ is used as a starting point in this iterative approach. Given this estimator, the log-likelihood

$$\sum_{j=1}^{m} [b_j \log r_j + a_j \log(1 - r_j)]$$

TABLE 4 Nonparametric Estimates of Tumor Onset Function for the ED_{01} Data

Interval (wk)	0	35	75	150
0–52	0	0.010	0	0
53–78	0	0.018	0.044	0.079
79–92	0.004	0.021	0.053	0.160
93–104	0.043	0.075	0.192	0.394

Source: Kodell et al., 1982.

of the second half of Eq. (6) is maximized for r_j under the restriction that the resulting estimator must be monotonically decreasing. The foregoing estimator for $S_{X_T}(t)$ is inserted into the original likelihood function, which is maximized again for $S_{X_{DT}}$. This process is iterated until convergence. Although their method relaxed the monotonicity assumption of Kodell et al., there are computational difficulties. Instead of describing the algorithm explicitly, they described in detail a heuristic approximation to the nonparametric MLEs.

Turnbull and Mitchell (1984) proposed a simpler iterative procedure for finding the exact nonparametric MLEs in terms of the joint distribution of X_T and X_{DT}. They pointed out that the joint distribution cannot have any probability mass outside a finite set of disjoint vertical intervals in the (x, y) plane. They proposed a two-dimensional EM algorithm for the nonparametric MLE of the distributions of X_T and X_{DT}. The marginal distributions can be derived from the estimator of the joint distribution. Therefore, the survival functions $S_{X_T}(t)$ and $S_{X_{DT}}(t)$ can be obtained.

Kodell et al. (1986) proposed a method for adjusting tumor rates to reflect lifetime or near-lifetime tumor incidences that would be obtained if all dose groups experienced the same mortality from causes other than the tumor of interest. They assumed that death from other causes does not depend on the time of onset of the tumor of interest, and that death from other causes is nonprognostic for the future occurrence of the tumor and future death from the tumor. The probability that an animal dies of the tumor of interest at time t_j can be expressed as $S_{X_{DNT}}(t_j)[S_{X_{DT}}(t_j^-) - S_{X_{DT}}(t_j)]$, and the probability that an animal dies with the tumor, but of a competing risk can be expressed as $S_{X_T}(t_j^-) - S_{X_T}(t_j)[S_{X_{DNT}}(t_j^-) - S_{X_{DNT}}(t_j)]$. The probability that an animal dies with a tumor sometime during the experiment can be expressed as

$$R = \sum_{j=1}^{m} S_{X_{DNT}}(t_j)[S_{X_{DT}}(t_j^-) - S_{X_{DT}}(t_j)] + \sum_{j=1}^{m} [S_{X_{DT}}(t_j) - S_{X_T}(t_j)][S_{X_{DNT}}(t_j^-) - S_{X_{DNT}}(t_j)]$$

After reparameterization and substitution of sample quantities, we obtain

$$\hat{R} = \frac{\sum_{i=1}^{m} (c_i + a_j)}{N}$$

This adjusted lifetime tumor probability is useful for dose–response modeling in risk assessment.

IV. UNKNOWN CAUSE OF DEATH

In this section, cause-of-death information is assumed to be unavailable. Except for the tests in Section IV.A.4, the methods require multiple sacrifice times, including the terminal sacrifice.

A. Testing

1. Prevalence Test for Nonlethal Tumors

When cause-of-death information is unavailable, statistical tests for tumorigenicity must rely either on information from scheduled sacrifices, or on simplifying assumptions. Hoel and Walburg (1972) discussed nonparametric methods that apply when all tumors are assumed to be lethal or when all tumors are assumed to be nonlethal. If the tumor is rapidly lethal, the time to death following tumor onset is short, and it is reasonable to treat the time to death or sacrifice of an animal as an exact or right-censored observation of the time of interest. Accordingly, an analysis based on time to death with tumor is indicated. This analysis is completely analogous to the fatal tumor component of the test of Peto et al. (1980), described in Section III.A. If the tumor is nonlethal, tumors cannot cause death and do not alter the risk of death from other causes. In this case, the proportion of deaths at time t with tumor present provides an estimator of the prevalence of tumor at time t, and suitable analyses can be based on the prevalence function. For nonlethal tumors, information on the cause of death is no longer relevant and the time of death provides only a censored observation on the time until tumor onset. Nonlethal occult tumors are discovered at necropsy, either after terminal sacrifice or after an animal has died before terminal sacrifice because of illness unrelated to the presence of the tumor.

In this section, tests for the equality of prevalence rates for nonlethal occult tumors are presented. An assumption underlying the derivation of these prevalence tests is that, at least for the presence or absence of a nonlethal tumor, death is a random sampling mechanism. It is assumed that all tumors of a particular type observed in the carcinogenesis experiment under consideration are nonlethal.

The Hoel–Walburg test for nonlethal tumors (Hoel and Walburg, 1972) is completely analogous to the incidental tumor component of the test of Peto et al. (1980). For each interval I_j, the tumor prevalence data may be summarized in a $2 \times g$ table (see Table 1). The difference of the observed and expected number of tumors in the ith group over the entire experiment can be calculated as Eq. (1), and the corresponding variance can be calculated as Eq. (2). Let $D = (D_1, \ldots, D_g)'$ and V be the $g \times g$ matrix with (r,i) entry V_{ri}. The tumor prevalence of the animals killed at any interim or terminal sacrifice can be summarized in a similar table. Each time of such a sacrifice is treated as a separate interval. A test for heterogeneity among the g groups given in Eq. (3), and a trend test is given in Eq. (4). A test for departure from a monotone dose–response relation is given in Eq. (5).

Dinse and Lagakos (1983) and Finkelstein (1986) proposed model-based tests for tumors that are assumed to be nonlethal under logistic and proportional hazards models, respectively. Dinse and Lagakos considered the following logistic model for the tumor incidence rate $\lambda_i(t)$:

$$\frac{\exp(\mu + \tau t + \theta d_i)}{1 + \exp(\mu + \tau t + \theta d_i)} \tag{7}$$

They derived the likelihood ratio test of $\theta = 0$, which under the foregoing model is equivalent to a test of the null hypothesis of equality of the tumor incidence rates among groups. Recently, Sun and Kalbfleisch (1996) proposed a modification of the Hoel–Walburg test, which includes the tests of Dinse and Lagakos (1983) and Finkelstein (1986) as special cases.

Sun and Kalbfleisch (1996) considered the two-sample (control and treatment) case, assuming similar death rates for the two groups. Let z_i be the treatment indicator (0 or 1) of the ith animal, $i = 1, \ldots, n$, and define

$$h_i = \begin{cases} 0 & \text{if tumor absent} \\ 1 & \text{if tumor present} \end{cases}$$

Let $F(t) = \Pr(X_T \leq t)$ denote the probability that a tumor has occurred by time t, under the null hypothesis of the equality of tumor prevalence rates in the two groups. Let $s_1 < \ldots < s_{k_n}$ denote the distinct ordered times, and $\hat{F}(t)$ the maximum likelihood estimator of $F(t)$. Using isotonic regression, Sun and Kalbfleisch obtained

$$\hat{F}(s_j) = \frac{\sum\limits_{u \in S_r} \bar{n}_u}{\sum\limits_{u \in S_r} l_u}, j \in S_r$$

$r = 1, \ldots, K_n$, where $\bar{n}_j$ denotes the number of tumors detected at time s_j, l_j the number of animals who died or were sacrificed at time s_j, K_n the number of the blocks of the isotonic estimator, and $\{S_1, \ldots, S_{K_n}\}$, a partition of $\{1, \ldots, k_n\}$, the blocks of the isotonic estimator of $F(t)$.

For the null hypothesis, consider

$$U = \sum_{i=1}^{N} w_i z_i (h_i - h_i^*)$$

where w_i is some weight and $h_i^* = \hat{F}(s_j)$ if $t_i = s_j$. Provided $w_i z_i$ are independent with the same means and variances, under the null hypothesis,

$$U / \left[\hat{\sigma}^2 \sum_{i=1}^{N} (h_i - h_i^*)^2 \right]^{1/2}$$

converges in distribution to the standard normal as $N \to \infty$, where $\hat{\sigma}^2 = \sum_{i=1}^{n}(w_i z_i - \sum_{i=1}^{n} w_i z_i / N)^2 / N$. If $w_i = 1$, $i = 1, \ldots, N$, then U becomes the Hoel–Walburg log-rank type of statistic. In Dinse and Lagakos (1983), weights are prespecified, and in Finkelstein (1986), $w_i = -\log[1 - \hat{F}(t_i)]/\hat{F}(t_i)$.

2. Pairwise Testing

If there are no material differences between dose groups relative to death of a competing risk, no adjustment for longevity is needed, and unadjusted tumor rates can be compared. In this case, the Fisher's exact test (Fisher, 1935; Gart et al., 1986, pp. 80–81) often is used for testing for the equality of tumor rates in a control and a treated group. From Table 5, the probability, $\Pr(y_2)$, of obtaining y_1 animals with tumor out of N_1 control animals and y_2 animals with tumor out of N_2 treated animals is

TABLE 5   Number of Animals

	No. without tumor	No. with tumor	Total
Control	$N_1 - y_1$	y_1	N_1
Treated	$N_2 - y_2$	y_2	N_2
Total	$N - y$	y	N

$$\Pr(y_2) = \frac{\binom{N_1}{y_1}\binom{N_2}{y_2}}{\binom{N}{y}}$$

The exact P-value for a possible increase in tumor incidence in the dose group is then

$$\sum_{k=y_2}^{y} \Pr(k)$$

A long-term feeding study was carried out at the National Center for Toxicological Research to investigate the effects of gentian violet on the F_{1a} generation of Fischer 344 rats (Littlefield et al., 1989). Data on thyroid follicular cell adenoma or carcinoma from the control group and the group fed 600 ppm gentian violet continuously for 24 months are given in Table 6. Fisher's exact test shows a significant difference of tumor rates between the two groups.

McKnight and Crowley (1984) proposed a method of testing for differences in tumor incidence rates using data from planned sacrifices. They proved that if no assumptions about tumor lethality are made and cause-of-death data are unavailable, then sacrifice information is necessary to identify the tumor incidence rate. Let z be the treatment indicator defined in Section IV.A.1. The tumor incidence function (rate of tumor onset among live tumor-free animals) in group z is defined as

$$\lambda_z^T(t) = \lim_{\epsilon \downarrow 0} \Pr(X_T \in [t,t + \epsilon) \,|\, X_D \geq t, X_T > t, z)/\epsilon \qquad (8)$$

TABLE 6   Number of Animals with and Without Tumor in Each Dose Group for Gentian Violet Data

Dose (ppm)	No. without tumor	No. with tumor	Total
0	157	2	159
600	68	9	77
Total	225	11	236

Fisher's exact test: $p = 0.0009$ (one-sided test).

the death rate for tumor-free animals is

$$\lambda_z^{DNT}(t) = \lim_{\epsilon \downarrow 0} \Pr(X_D \in [t, t + \epsilon), X_T > t \,|\, X_D \geq t, z)/\epsilon \qquad (9)$$

the death rate for tumor-bearing animals is

$$\lambda_z^{DT}(t) = \lim_{\epsilon \downarrow 0} \Pr(X_D \in [t, t + \epsilon), X_T \leq t \,|\, X_D \geq t, z)/\epsilon \qquad (10)$$

and the overall death rate is

$$\begin{aligned} \lambda_z^{D}(t) &= \lambda_z^{DNT}(t) + \lambda_z^{DT}(t) \\ &= \lim_{\epsilon \downarrow 0} \Pr(X_D \in [t, t + \epsilon) \,|\, X_D \geq t, z)/\epsilon \end{aligned} \qquad (11)$$

The likelihood can be expressed in terms of $\lambda_z^{T}(t)$, $\lambda_z^{DNT}(t)$, and $\lambda_z^{DT}(t)$. McKnight and Crowley derived an approximate normal pairwise test for the equality of two groups.

Portier and Dinse (1987) proposed a parametric model for the tumor incidence function. They developed a likelihood ratio test for comparing the control and a treatment group. This procedure needs a terminal sacrifice and at least one interim sacrifice. The likelihood is expressed in terms of $\lambda_z^{T}(t)$ in Eq. (8) and the following discrete versions of $\lambda_z^{DNT}(t)$ and $\lambda_z^{D}(t)$:

$$\lambda_{z_j}^{DNT} = \Pr(X_D = t_j, X_T > t_j \,|\, X_D \geq t_j, z)$$

and

$$\lambda_{z_j}^{D} = \Pr(X_D = t_j \,|\, X_D \geq t_j, z)$$

Define

$$S_z(t) = \exp\left[-\int_0^t \lambda_z^{T}(u)\,du \right]$$

Then in group z at t_j, the following formulas contribute to the likelihood: A sacrificed animal without tumor contributes

$$S_z(t_j) \prod_{k=1}^{j} (1 - \lambda_{z_k}^{DNT})$$

a sacrificed animal with tumor contributes

$$\prod_{k=1}^{j} (1 - \lambda_{z_k}^{D}) - S_z(t_j) \prod_{k=1}^{j} (1 - \lambda_{z_k}^{DNT}) \qquad (12)$$

a dead animal without tumor contributes

$$\lambda_{z_j}^{DNT} S_z(t_j) \prod_{k=1}^{j-1} (1 - \lambda_{z_k}^{DNT})$$

and a dead animal with tumor contributes

$$\lambda_{z_j}^{D} \prod_{k=1}^{j-1} (1 - \lambda_{z_k}^{D}) - \lambda_{z_j}^{DNT} S_z(t_j) \prod_{k=1}^{j-1} (1 - \lambda_{z_k}^{DNT}) \tag{13}$$

The likelihood ratio statistic for testing for the equal incidence rates can be formulated using an appropriate parameterization for $\lambda_z^T(t)$.

Dewanji and Kalbfleisch (1986) considered a discrete time process and used the EM algorithm to obtain the nonparametric maximum likelihood estimator of the discrete tumor incidence function. They provided sufficient conditions for the nonparametric model for tumor incidence to be estimable and identifiable. They also developed a log-rank type score test for comparing the tumor incidence rate of two groups from a bioassay with sacrifices. They initially assumed that animals were sacrificed at every time point and later suggested that the same methods could be applied if the natural deaths were grouped into intervals determined by the sacrifice times.

Malani and Van Ryzin (1988) proposed a nonparametric MLE of the tumor incidence rate and a pairwise test for the difference of two treatments. They defined the discrete version of the tumor incidence rate given in Eq. (8) for group i and interval I_j as

$$\begin{aligned}
\lambda_i^T(t_j) &= \Pr(X_T = t_j | X_D \geq t_j, X_T \geq t_j) \\
&\quad 1 - \{[1 - p_i^A(t_j)][1 - \lambda_i^D(t_j)] \\
&\quad + [1 - p_i^D(t_j)]\lambda_i^D(t_j)\} / [1 - p_i^A(t_{j-1})]
\end{aligned} \tag{14}$$

where $p_i^A(t_j) = \Pr(X_T \leq t_j | X_D > t_j)$ is the tumor prevalence rate among live animals, $p_i^D(t_j) = \Pr(X_T \leq t_j | X_D = t_j)$ is the tumor prevalence rate among dying animals and $\lambda_i^D(t_j) = \Pr(X_D \leq t_j | X_D = t_j)$ is the discrete hazard rate for X_D. Let $N_i^1(t_j)$ and $N_i^2(t_j)$ denote the number of natural deaths with and without tumors, respectively, and let $N_i^3(t_j)$ and $N_i^4(t_j)$ denote the number of sacrifices with and without tumors, respectively. The log-likelihood function is defined as

$$\begin{aligned}
l = \sum_{j=1}^{m} &\{N_i^1(t_j) \log p_i^D(t_j) + N_i^2(t_j) \log[1 - p_i^D(t_j)] \\
&+ N_i^3(t_j) \log p_i^A(t_j) + N_i^4(t_j) \log[1 - p_i^A(t_j)] \\
&+ N_i(t_j) \log \lambda_i^D(t_j) + [A_i(t_j) - N_i(t_j)] \log[1 - \lambda_i^D(t_j)]\}
\end{aligned}$$

$$+ \sum_{j=2}^{m} \{S_i(t_j) \log \lambda_i^S(t_{j-1}) + A_i(t_j) \log[1 - \lambda_i^S(t_{j-1})]\}$$
$$+ \text{constant}$$

where $N_i(t_j) = N_i^1(t_j) + N_i^2(t_j)$; $S_i(t_j) = N_i^3(t_j) + N_i^4(t_j)$; $A_i(t_j)$ denotes the numbers of animals alive at the start of interval I_j; and $\lambda_i^S(t_j)$ is the hazard function for the time to sacrifice (Table 7). Maximum likelihood estimators of $\lambda_i^T(t_j)$ are obtained by substituting the parameter estimators of $p_i^A(t_j)$; $p_i^D(t_j)$; and $\lambda_i^D(t_j)$ in Eq. (14).

By using the delta method, Malani and Van Ryzin obtained the asymptotic variances and covariances of the tumor incidence rate. The variance of the cumulative tumor incidence rate $A_i^T(t_j) = \sum_{k=1}^{j} \lambda_i^T(t_k)$ is

$$\sigma_i^2(t_j) = \text{var}[\hat{\Lambda}_i^T(t_j)] = \sum_{k=1}^{j} \text{var}[\hat{\lambda}_i^T(t_k)]$$
$$+ 2 \sum_{k=2}^{j} \text{cov}[\hat{\lambda}_i^T(t_{k-1}), \hat{\lambda}l_i^T(t_k)], j = 2, \ldots, m$$

Malani and Van Ryzin showed that

$$Z_{MV} = \frac{\hat{\Lambda}_{i_1}^T(t_m) - \hat{\lambda}_{i_2}^T(t_m)}{\sqrt{\hat{\sigma}_{i_1}^2(t_m) + \hat{\sigma}_{i_2}^2(t_m)}}$$

can serve as an approximate normal test under $\lambda_{i_1}^T(t_j) = \lambda_{i_2}^T(t_j)$, $j = 1$, $\ldots, m$, where i_1 and i_2 are different treatment groups.

Williams and Portier (1992a) proposed analytic solutions for the MLE of the hazard rates. Their tumor incidence rate estimator and the estimator of the overall death rate turned out to be identical to Malani and Van Ryzin's $\hat{\lambda}_i^T(t_j)$ and $\hat{\lambda}_i^D(t_j)$. They derived an approximate normal statistic for the equality of tumor incidence rates in two groups. The variances and covariances are estimated from the observed information matrix.

Malani and Van Ryzin's test suffers from a loss of power when the

TABLE 7   Counts of Key Events in Interval I_j

	With tumors	Without tumors	Total
Natural deaths	$N_i^1(t_j)$	$N_i^2(t_j)$	$N_i(t_j)$
Sacrifices	$N_i^3(t_j)$	$N_i^4(t_j)$	$S_i(t_j)$
Total	$N_i^1(t_j) + N_i^3(t_j)$	$N_i^2(t_j) + N_i^4(t_j)$	$N_i(t_j) + S_i(t_j)$

estimated tumor incidence rate is negative, as often happens. It may occur when small numbers of natural deaths or sacrifices are observed in some intervals. Malani and Lu (1993) suggested using an EM algorithm to estimate the tumor incidence rate to guarantee a nonnegative tumor incidence rate, but they did not provide a detailed instruction. Ahn and Kodell (1995) proposed a numerical method to maximize the likelihood function iteratively, under a sufficient condition for a positive tumor incidence rate. The resulting estimator reduces standard error and gives the test of two heterogeneous groups more power. A linear contrast of more than two groups can be tested using Ahn and Kodell's procedure. The statistic

$$Z_{AK} = \frac{a_1 \hat{\Lambda}_{i_1}^T(t_m) + \ldots + a_r \hat{\Lambda}_{i_r}^T(t_m)}{\sqrt{a_1^2 \hat{\sigma}_{i_1}^2(t_m) + \ldots + a_r^2 \hat{\sigma}_{i_r}^2(t_m)}}$$

converges in distribution to the standard normal in distribution under $\lambda_{i_1}^T(t_j) = \ldots = \lambda_{i_r}^T(t_j)$, $j = 1, \ldots, m$, when $\Sigma_{k=1}^r a_k = 0$. Here, the asymptotic variance

$$\sigma_i^2(t_j) = \sum_{k=1}^{j} \text{var}[\hat{\lambda}_i^T(t_k)] + 2 \sum_{k=1}^{j-1} \sum_{k'=k+1}^{j} \text{cov}[\hat{\lambda}_i^T(t_k), \hat{\lambda}_i^T(t_{k'})],$$

$$j = 2, \ldots, m$$

of $\Lambda_i^T(t_j)$ is recalculated under the constraint.

A study was carried out at the National Center for Toxicological Research to assess the modulatory effect of caloric restriction on the occurrence of spontaneous neoplasms and mortality in Fischer 344 rats (Thurman et al., 1994). The study involved up to six scheduled sacrifices. Frequency data on pituitary adenoma or carcinoma in males are given in Table 8, for comparison of tumor rates in ad libitum-fed animals with those in calorically restricted animals. The Ahn-Kodell test shows a significant difference of the tumor incidence rates in two groups, but the Malani-Van Ryzin test fails to detect this difference. The main reason for this is that the Ahn-Kodell test is able to correct the negative tumor incidence rate estimate problem in this example.

3. Trend Tests

Cochran (1954) and Armitage (1955) introduced a trend test (Cochran-Armitage test) for detecting a linear trend across dose groups in the overall proportions of animals with the tumor. This test needs an assumption of equal risk of getting the tumor among the dose groups over

TABLE 8　Frequency Data on Pituitary Adenoma/Carcinoma in Males (Fischer 344 Rats) from a Caloric Restriction Study

	Interval (days)	Dead/ moribund with tumor	Dead/ moribund w/o tumor	Sacrificed with tumor	Sacrificed w/o tumor
Ad lib	0–368	0	0	3	9
Restricted		0	2	0	12
Ad lib	369–555	4	5	6	4
Restricted		3	4	2	10
Ad lib	556–754	57	16	9	2
Restricted		7	19	3	9
Ad lib	755–919	31	15	9	0
Restricted		25	40	7	5

Ahn–Kodell two-group test: $z = 5.342, p < 0.0001$ (one-sided test).
Malani–Van Ryzin test: $z = 0.069, p = 0.285$.

the duration of the study. By pooling all the time intervals, Table 1 can be modified to Table 9. The expected number of tumors in the ith group is $E_i = y.K_i$, where $K_i = N_i/N$. Defining D_i as in Eq. (1), the test statistic for possible monotonic trend with dose is based on

$$X = \sum_{i=1}^{g} d_i D_i$$

and the variance is estimated by

$$V = \{y.(N - y.)/[N(N - 1)]\} \sum_{i=1}^{g} N_i(d_i - \bar{d})^2$$

where $\bar{d} = (\sum_{i=1}^{g} N_i d_i/N$. The Cochran–Armitage test is

TABLE 9　Tumor Data for the Intervals Combined in Each Group

	Dose group				
	1	2	$\cdots$	g	Total
No. with tumors	y_1	y_2	$\cdots$	y_g	$y.$
No. without tumors	$N_1 - y_1$	$N_2 - y_2$	$\cdots$	$N_g - y_g$	$N - y.$
No. deaths	N_1	N_2	$\cdots$	N_g	N

$$Z_{CA} = \frac{X}{\sqrt{V}}$$

where Z_{CA} is asymptotically distributed as a standard normal variate under the null hypothesis of equal tumor incidence rates among the groups. Two-tailed tests may be based on Z_{CA}^2, which is an approximate χ^2 with 1 degree of freedom.

If the mortality patterns are similar across dose groups, then the Cochran–Armitage test will be appropriate, but it may not be valid if the mortality rates differ across dose groups. Bailer and Portier (1988) proposed the Poly-3 trend test, which made an adjustment of the Cochran–Armitage test by modifying the value of N to reflect decreased survival. Define the number at risk as the sum of N_i weights:

$$r_i = \sum_{k=1}^{N_i} \omega_{ik},$$

where ω_{ik} is the weight for the kth animal in the ith dose group. Note that this test becomes the Cochran–Armitage test if the weights, ω_{ik}, are all equal to 1. Bailer and Portier defined the weights as $\omega_{ik} = 1$ if the kth animal in the ith dose group dies with the tumor, and $\omega_{ik} = (t_i/t_{\max})^3$ if not, where $t_{\max}$ is the maximum survival time. This weighting gives proportionally less weight to a tumor-free animal that dies at time t_i. The third power comes from the observation that tumor incidence often seems to be a low-order polynomial in time (Portier et al., 1986). Bailer and Portier suggested a Poly-k test if the shape of the tumor incidence function is expected to follow time to some power k. Gart et al. (1979) suggested the truncated trend test which defines the weights as $\omega_{ik} = 1$ if the age at death for the kth animal in the ith group exceeds the time of the first death with tumor present and $\omega_{ik} = 0$ if not.

Kodell and Ahn (1996) extended the test of Ahn and Kodell (1995) to a dose-related trend test. It relaxed the sufficient condition for non-negativity of the tumor incidence to provide a general, improved numerical method for obtaining constrained MLE. Define weights $a_i = f(d_i) - \Sigma_{i=1}^{g} f(d_i)/g$, where $f(d)$ is any appropriate dose metric. A test for dose-related trend is obtained as:

$$Z = \frac{a_1 \hat{\Lambda}_1^T(t_m) + \ldots + a_g \hat{\Lambda}_g^T(t_m)}{\sqrt{a_1^2 \hat{\sigma}_1^2(t_m) + \ldots + a_g^2 \hat{\sigma}_g^2(t_m)}}$$

Under the nonnegativity constraint of the tumor incidence rate, the asymptotic variance

$$\sigma_i^2(t_j) = \sum_{k=1}^{j} \text{var}[\hat{\lambda}_i^T(t_k)] + 2 \sum_{k=2}^{j} \text{cov } [\hat{\lambda}_i^T(t_{k-1}),\hat{\lambda}_i^T(t_k)]$$

$$+ 2 \sum_{k=2}^{j-1} \text{cov } [\hat{\lambda}_i^T(t_{k-1}),\hat{\lambda}_i^T(t_{k+1})]$$

of $\Lambda_i^T(t_j)$ can be obtained.

Malani and Lu (1993) proposed an age-specific test of the tumor incidence rate for dose-related trend. Define the risk as

$$R_i(t_j) = A_i(t_j)[1 - \hat{p}_i^A(t_{j-1})]$$

The number of animals developing tumors in interval I_j can be expressed as $y_i(t_j) - R_i(t_j)\hat{\lambda}_i^T(t_j)$. Malani and Lu's approximate normal test is given by $Z_{ML} = \Delta/V$, where

$$\Delta = \sum_{j=1}^{m} \sum_{i=1}^{g} y_i(t_j)[d_i - \bar{d}(t_j)]$$

$$\bar{d}(t_j) = \frac{\sum_{i=1}^{g} R_i(t_j)d_i}{\sum_{i=1}^{g} R_i(t_j)}$$

$$V^2 = \sum_{j=1}^{m} \sum_{i=1}^{g} \text{vâr}[\hat{\lambda}_i^T(t_j)]R_i^2(t_j)[d_i - \bar{d}(t_j)]^2$$

$$+ 2 \sum_{j=1}^{m-1} \sum_{i=1}^{g} \text{côv}[\hat{\lambda}_i^T(t_j),\hat{\lambda}_i^T(t_{j+1})]R_i(t_j)R_i(t_{j+1})[d_i - \bar{d}(t_j)]$$

$$[d_i - \bar{d}(t_{j+1})]$$

They did not restrict the tumor incidence rate to be nonnegative, instead basing their test on the closed-form unrestricted MLE. In the two-group situation, the numerators of the Dewanji–Kalbfleisch and Malani–Lu test statistics have the same formulation, although the data values that appear in the numerator are imputed differently. The variances of both test statistics are based on Fisher information, but the respective information matrices arise from differently formulated likelihood functions.

Kodell and Ahn (1997) modified the age-adjusted trend test of Malani and Lu by maximizing their likelihood function subject to a nonnegativity constraint on the tumor incidence rate. Their test statistic is formulated as many of the other trend test statistics,

$$Z_{KA} = \frac{d'(O - E)}{\sqrt{d'Vd}} \tag{15}$$

where d is a vector of length g containing an appropriate dose metric, $O = (O_1, \ldots, O_g)'$ is a vector of observed frequencies of tumors, $E = (E_1, \ldots, E_g)'$ is a vector of expected frequencies, and V is a $g \times g$ estimator of the variance of O with (i,k) entry V_{ik}. Further, $O_i = \Sigma_{j=1}^{m} y_i(t_j)$, $E_i = \Sigma_{j=1}^{m} R_i(t_j)[y.(t_j)/R.(t_j)]$, $R_i(t_j) = A_i(t_j)[1 - \hat{p}_i^A(t_{j-1})]$, $y_i(t_j) = R_i(t_j)\, \hat{\lambda}_i^T(t_j)$, $R.(t_j) = \Sigma_{i=1}^{g} R_i(t_j)$, and $y.(t_j) = \Sigma_{i=1}^{g} y_i(t_j)$. Here, $R_i(t_j)$ is the imputed number of animals alive and tumor-free at the beginning of interval I_j, and $y_i(t_j)$ is the imputed observed number of the $R_i(t_j)$ animals that develop a tumor in I_j. The statistic Z_{KA} is approximate standard normal under $\lambda_1(t_j) = \ldots = \lambda_g(t_j)$, $j = 1, \ldots, m$. The elements of V are given by

$$
\begin{aligned}
V_{ii} = \sum_{j=1}^{m} &\{ ([R_i(t_j)/R.(t_j)][1 - R_i(t_j)/R.(t_j)] \\
&- [A_i^2(t_j)/R.^2(t_j)]\text{vâr}[\hat{p}_i^A(t_{j-1})]) \\
&\times (y.(t_j)[R.(t_j) - y.(t_j)]/[R.(t_j) - 1]) \\
&+ [y.(t_j)/R.(t_j)]^2 A_i^2(t_j)\text{vâr}[\hat{p}_i^A(t_{j-1})]\} \\
V_{ik} = -\sum_{j=1}^{m} &\{ [R_i(t_j)R_k(t_j)/R.^2(t_j)]y.(t_j)[R.(t_j) \\
&- y.(t_j)]/[R.(t_j) - 1]\}, \quad k \neq i
\end{aligned}
$$

Kodell and Ahn showed that their test controls the type I error rate better than the Malani and Lu test. The two tests performed comparably relative to power according to Kodell and Ahn (1997).

A survival–sacrifice experiment was conducted at the National Center for Toxicological Research to study the carcinogenic effects of benzidine dihydrochloride in two strains of mice. For the F_2 females, frequencies of animals with and without liver tumors in each sacrifice interval for four dose groups are given in Table 10. Both the Kodell–Ahn and Malani–Lu age-adjusted trend tests show highly significant dose-related trend in this example. The Malani–Lu trend test gives a smaller p-value than the Kodell–Ahn trend test. This result agrees with the simulation results reported in Kodell and Ahn (1997).

4. Data with Single Terminal Sacrifice

Both interim sacrifice data and cause-of-death data add expense to rodent bioassays, so that neither type of information is always available in the standard 2-year rodent study. In the absence of both interim sacrifices and cause-of-death information, the tumor incidence rate is not identifiable from bioassay data, unless simplifying assumptions are

TABLE 10   Counts for Fitting the Discrete Model to Data from
Benzidine Dihydrochloride Equipment (F2-strain Female Mice)

Dose (ppm)	Interval (days)	Dead/ moribund with tumor	Dead/ moribund w/o tumor	Sacrificed with tumor	Sacrificed w/o tumor
60	0–40	0	2	0	70
120		0	7	2	44
200		1	2	4	43
400		0	3	8	14
60	40–60	0	1	10	38
120		6	4	15	26
200		17	1	23	12
400		17	4	13	1
60	60–80	7	4	15	20
120		16	2	20	1
200		11	2	3	0
400		9	1	1	0

Dose-metric: Concentration in ppm.
Kodell–Ahn age-adjusted trend test: $z = 8.5, p < 10^{-7}$.
Malani–Lu age-adjusted trend test: $z = 11.1, p < 10^{-7}$.
Source: Ann and Kodell, 1995.

made. We will discuss a few recently developed methods of analyzing data without interim sacrifices.

   For data with no interim sacrifices, Dinse (1991) and Lindsey and Ryan (1994) proposed parametric statistical tests for dose-related trend. Dinse's test is based on the assumption of a constant difference between the death rates of animals with and without tumors, whereas Lindsey and Ryan's test assumes a constant ratio for those death rates.

   The constant risk difference analysis assumes

$$\lambda_i^{DT}(t) - \lambda_i^{DNT}(t) = \Delta$$

and the constant risk ratio analysis assumes

$$\lambda_i^{DT}(t)/\lambda_i^{DNT}(t) = \rho$$

where Δ and ρ are constants, and $\lambda_i^{DNT}(t)$ and $\lambda_i^{DT}(t)$ are defined in Eqs. (9) and (10), respectively. Dinse assumes linear-logistic models of the form of Eq. (7) for $\lambda_i^{T}(t)$ and $\lambda_i^{DNT}(t)$. A likelihood ratio test is used to compare the full model to the reduced model in which the dose coefficient for $\lambda_i^T(t)$ is constrained to be zero. Dinse (1991, 1993) showed that the constant risk difference model performs well over a wide range of tumor lethalities, but the constant risk ratio does not perform as well.

Kodell et al. (1996) proposed a nonparametric age-adjusted trend test for a single terminal sacrifice. They assume the constant proportionality of tumor prevalence for live and dead animals:

$$p_i^A(t_j) = \frac{p_i^D(t_j)p_i^A(t_m)}{p_i^D(t_m)}, \qquad j = 1, \ldots, m$$

This constraint can be rewritten as

$$\frac{\lambda_i^D(t_j)/[1 - \lambda_i^D(t_j)]}{\lambda_i^{D|T}(t_j)/[1 - \lambda_i^{D|T}(t_j)]} = C, \qquad j = 1, \ldots, m$$

where $\lambda_i^{D|T}(t_j) = \Pr(X_D = t_j | X_D \geq t_j, X_T \leq t_j)$ is the discrete death rate for animals with tumors (Malani and van Ryzin, 1988) and C is a constant. This means that the ratio of the odds of death for any animal, irrespective of tumor status, to the odds of death for an animal that has a tumor, is constant over time. The variances and covariances can be calculated under the constraint. The test in Eq. (15) can be used to test the dose-related trend.

To illustrate this method, the data are collapsed in the first example (ED_{01}; see Table 3), ignoring cause-of-death data. Table 11 shows the

TABLE 11 Single-Sacrifice Tumor Data (ED_{01})

| | | \multicolumn{8}{c|}{Dose (ppm)} | | | | | | | |
| | Interval (wk) | \multicolumn{2}{c|}{0} | \multicolumn{2}{c|}{35} | \multicolumn{2}{c|}{75} | \multicolumn{2}{c|}{150} |
		d/m	sac	d/m	sac	d/m	sac	d/m	sac
No. with tumors	0–52	0		1		0		0	
No. w/o tumor		9		9		10		5	
No. with tumors	53–78	0		3		1		2	
No. w/o tumor		15		31		16		14	
No. with tumors	79–92	1		1		3		6	
No. w/o tumor		34		55		28		25	
No. with tumors	93–104	3	5	2	17	12	20	16	15
No. w/o tumor		75	122	81	191	41	101	19	32

Kodell–Ahn–Pearce–Turturro age-adjusted trend test: $z = 8.9, p < 10^{-7}$.

combined data. Kodell et al.'s age-adjusted trend test shows highly significant dose-related trend in this example. The z-value obtained by this method is close to the z-value obtained by the Peto trend test in Section III.A.

B. Estimation

Turnbull and Mitchell (1978) and Mitchell and Turnbull (1979) developed a model that was parameterized in terms of illness-state prevalences and lethalities, for multiorgan tumorigenicity data from survival experiments with interim sacrifices. Berlin et al. (1979) considered general Markov processes in modeling very complex disease mechanisms that incorporate serial sacrifice. They performed a test for dependence of diseases. They also discussed problems of identifiability of models. There are difficulties in these methods of estimating many model parameters, because the typical bioassay experiment is usually only of a limited size.

Portier (1986) parametrically modeled tumor incidence as a function of time and dose and placed nonparametric stochastic restrictions on the death rates. In this work, an approximate maximum likelihood method is proposed for parametric estimation of the distribution of occult tumor onset times in the presence of competing risks. Dinse (1986) proposed nonparametric prevalence and mortality estimates, but the prevalence function is assumed to be constant over time intervals for stabilization purposes.

The tumor incidence rate estimation of Portier and Dinse (1987) in Section IV.A.2 has computational difficulties. The maximization of the likelihood involves a constrained nonlinear optimization because the MLEs of $\lambda_z(t)$, $\lambda_{z_j}^{DNT}$ and $\lambda_{z_j}^{D}$ should lie in the interval [0, 1] when they are substituted into Eqs. (12) and (13). Dinse (1988a) proposed a computationally simpler method of estimation by using the onset-specific death rate for tumor-bearing animals.

$$\alpha_{z_j} = \Pr(X_D = t_j \mid X_D \geq t_j)$$

instead of $\lambda_{z_j}^{D}$. Dinse derived the relation between $\lambda_{z_j}^{D}$ and α_{z_j} as

$$\lambda_{z_j}^{D} = \alpha_{z_j} - (\alpha_{z_j} - \lambda_{z_j}^{DNT})S_z(t_j) \prod_{k=1}^{j-1} \left[\frac{(1 - \lambda_{z_k}^{DNT})}{(1 - \lambda_{z_k}^{D})} \right]$$

The MLE of $\lambda_z^T(t)$ can be calculated by making a modification to the EM algorithm.

To estimate the tumor incidence rate, Dinse (1988b) proposed parametric models for a set of functions that can be estimated directly from data. This approach is based on the hazard functions [see Eqs. (8), (9), and (11)]. These estimators are transformed to obtain estimators for the tumor incidence rate, the conditional death rates, and the relative risk.

For the tumor incidence rate estimate in Williams and Portier (1992a), they imposed a boundary condition (1992b) for a nonnegative tumor incidence rate for up to three sacrifices. For study designs with more than two interim sacrifices, they suggested alternative estimates of the tumor incidence rate and discrete death rates developed heuristically by pooling data together from adjacent intervals.

As we mentioned in Section IV.A, Dinse and Lagakos (1983) and Dinse (1987, 1991, 1993) proposed parametric estimation of the tumor onset distribution, and McKnight and Crowley (1984), Dewanji and Kalbfleisch (1986), Malani and Van Ryzin (1988), Ahn and Kodell (1995), Kodell and Ahn (1996, 1997), and Kodell et al. (1996) proposed nonparametric tumor onset estimation.

V. DISCUSSION

Besides the approaches we have covered in the previous sections, Meng and Dempster (1987), Finkelstein and Schoenfeld (1989), Lu and Malani (1995), and Chen (1996) developed methods of simultaneous testing of multiple tumor types. Multiple testing of individual tumor types requires an adjustment of significance levels of individual tests to control experiment-wise type I error. Heyse and Rom (1988), Farrar and Crump (1988), and Westfall and Young (1989) used permutation and bootstrap resampling methods to adjust individual *p*-values for multiplicity of testing. An approach commonly used by regulatory agencies is to employ different significance levels for rare and common tumors (e.g., Haseman, 1983). Kodell and George (1993) reviewed various methods of carcinogenicity tests involving multiple tumor sites.

It seems desirable to investigate the following issues in the analysis of animal carcinogenicity data in future studies: (a) In the analyses of some carcinogenicity data, it would be reasonable to make adjustments between body weight and tumor occurrence. (b) To reduce the cost of experiments, effects of shortening study duration on power of statistical tests could be investigated. (c) Power and sample size calculations could be performed to see how reasonable the standard size of 50 animals per sex per group is. (d) Overall false-negative error might be investigated. (e) It would be worthwhile to develop formal statistical procedures to incorporate the information from historical control data into the analysis of carcinogenicity study data. (f) An in-depth study of the accuracy of cause-of-death assignment would be useful. (g) Numerical comparisons of power among different procedures under various conditions could be performed.

REFERENCES

Ahn H, Kodell RL. Estimation and testing of tumor incidence rates in experiments lacking cause-of-death data. Biometr J 37:745–763, 1995.

Archer LE, Ryan LM. On the role of cause-of-death data in the analysis of rodent tumorigenicity experiments. Appl Stat 38:81–93, 1989.

Armitage P. Tests for linear trends in proportions and frequencies. Biometrics 11:375–386, 1955.

Bailer AJ, Portier CJ. Effects of treatment-induced mortality and tumor-induced mortality on tests for carcinogenicity in small samples. Biometrics 44:417–431, 1988.

Berlin B, Brodsky J, Clifford P. Testing disease dependence in survival experiments with serial sacrifice. J Am Stat Assoc 74:5–14, 1979.

Chen JJ. Global tests for analysis of multiple tumor data from animal carcinogenicity experiments. Stat Med 15:1217–1225, 1996.

Clifford P. Nonidentifiability in stochastic models of illness and death. Proc Nat Acad Sci USA 74:1338–1340, 1977.

Cochran WG. Some methods for strengthening the common χ^2 tests. Biometrics 10:417–451, 1954.

Dewanji A, Kalbfleisch JD. Nonparametric methods for survival/sacrifice experiments. Biometrics 42:325–341, 1986.

Dinse GE. Nonparametric prevalence and mortality estimators for animal experiments with incomplete cause-of-death data. J Am Stat Assoc 81:328–336, 1986.

Dinse GE. Estimating tumor incidence rates in animal carcinogenicity experiments. Biometrics 44:405–415, 1988a.

Dinse GE. Simple parametric analysis of animal tumorigenicity data. J Am Stat Assoc 83:638–649, 1988b.

Dinse GE. Constant risk differences in the analysis of animal tumorigenicity data. Biometrics 47:681–700, 1991.

Dinse GE. Evaluating constraints that allow survival-adjusted incidence analyses in single-sacrifice studies. Biometrics 49:399–407, 1993.

Dinse GE. A comparison of tumour incidence analyses applicable in single-sacrifice animal experiments. Stat Med 13:689–708, 1994.

Dinse GE, Lagakos SW. Nonparametric estimation of lifetime and disease onset distributions from incomplete observations. Biometrics 38:921–932, 1982.

Dinse GE, Lagakos SW. Regression analysis of tumor prevalence data. Appl Stat 32:236–248, 1983.

Farrar DB, Crump KS. Exact statistical tests for any carcinogenic effect in animal bioassays. Fundam Appl Toxicol 11:652–663, 1988.

Finkelstein DM. A proportional hazards model for interval-censored failure time data. Biometrics 42:845–854, 1986.

Finkelstein DM, Schoenfeld DA. Analysis of multiple tumor data from a rodent carcinogenicity experiments. Biometrics 45:219–230, 1989.

Fisher RA. The logic of inductive inference. J R Stat Soc 98:39–54, 1935.

Gart JJ [Letter to the Editor]. Br J Cancer 31:696–697, 1975.

Gart JJ, Chu KC, Tarone RE. Statistical issues in interpretation of chronic bioassay tests for carcinogenicity. J Nat Cancer Inst 62:957–974, 1979.

Gart JJ, Krewski D, Lee PN, Tarone RE, Wahrendorf J. The design and analysis of long-term animal experiments. In: Statistical Methods in Cancer Research, vol 3. IARC Scientific Publication 79. Lyon: International Agency for Research on Cancer, 1986.

Haseman JK. A reexamination of false-positive rates for carcinogenesis studies. Fundam Appl Toxicol 3:334–339, 1983.

Hayse JF, Rom D. Adjusting for multiplicity of statistical tests in the analysis of carcinogenicity studies. Biometr J 8:883–896, 1988.

Hoel DG, Walburg HE. Statistical analysis of survival experiments. J Nat Cancer Inst 49:361–372, 1972.

Kalbfleisch JD, Krewski DR, Van Ryzin J. Dose-response models for time-to-response toxicity data (with discussion). Can J Stat 11:25–49, 1983.

Kaplan EL, Meier P. Nonparametric estimation from incomplete observations. J Am Stat Assoc 53:457–481, 1958.

Kodell RL, Ahn H. Nonparametric trend test for the cumulative tumor incidence rate. Commun Stat Theory Methods 25:1677–1692, 1996.

Kodell RL, Ahn H. Age-adjusted trend test for the tumor incidence rate. Biometrics 1997 (in press).

Kodell RL, Ahn H, Pearce BA, Turturro A. Age-adjusted trend test for the tumor incidence rate for single-sacrifice experiments. Drug Inf J 31:471–487, 1996.

Kodell RL, Chen JJ. Handling cause of death in equivocal cases using the EM algorithm (with discussion). Commun Stat Theory Methods 16:2565–2585, 1987.

Kodell RL, Chen JJ, Moore GE. Comparing distributions of time to onset of disease in animal tumorigenicity experiments. Commun Stat Theory Methods 23:959–980, 1994.

Kodell RL, Gaylor DW, Chen JJ. Standardized tumor rates for chronic bioassays. Biometrics 42:867–873, 1986.

Kodell RL, George EO. Carcinogenicity tests involving multiple tumor sites. In: Patil GP, Rao CR, eds. Multivariate Environmental Statistics. Amsterdam: Elsevier Science, 1993.

Kodell RL, Nelson CJ. An illness-death model for the study of the carcinogenic process using survival/sacrifice data. Biometrics 36:267–277, 1980.

Kodell RL, Shaw GW, Johnson AM. Nonparametric joint estimators for disease resistance and survival functions in survival/sacrifice experiments. Biometrics 38:43–58, 1982.

Lagakos SW. An evaluation of some two-sample tests used to analyze animal carcinogenicity experiments. Util Math 21B:239–260, 1982.

Lagakos SW, Louis TA. Use of tumour lethality to interpret tumorigenicity experiments lacking cause-of-death data. Appl Stat 37:169–179, 1988.

Lindsey JC, Ryan LM. A comparison of continuous- and discrete-time three-state models for rodent tumorigenicity experiments. Environ Health Perspect 102(suppl 1):9–17, 1994.

Littlefield NA, Farmer JH, Gaylor DW, Sheldon WG. Effects of dose and time in a long-term, low-dose carcinogenic study. J Environ Pathol Toxicol 3: 17–34, 1980.

Littlefield NA, Gaylor DW, Blackwell B-N, Allen RR. Chronic toxicity/carcinogenicity studies of gentian violet in Fischer 344 rats: two-generation exposure. Food Chem Toxicol 27:239–247, 1989.

Lu Y, Malani HM. Analysis of animal carcinogenicity experiments with multiple tumor types. Biometrics 51:73–86, 1995.

Malani HM, Lu Y. Animal carcinogenicity experiments with and without serial sacrifice. Comm Stat Theory Methods 22:1557–1584, 1993.

Malani HM, Van Ryzin J. Comparison of two treatments in animal carcinogenicity experiments. J Am Stat Assoc 83:1171–1177, 1988.

Mantel N, Haenszel W. Statistical aspects of the analysis of data from retrospective studies of disease. J Nat Cancer Inst 22:719–748, 1959.

McKnight B, Crowley J. Tests for differences in tumor incidence based on animal carcinogenesis experiments. J Am Stat Assoc 79:639–648, 1984.

Meng CYK, Dempster AP. A bayesian approach to the multiplicity problem for significance testing with binomial data. Biometrics 43:301–311, 1987.

Mitchell TJ, Turnbull BW. Log-linear models in the analysis of disease prevalence data from survival/sacrifice experiments. Biometrics 35:221–234, 1979.

Peto R. Guidelines on the analysis of tumour rates and death rates in Experimental animals. Br J Cancer 29:101–105, 1974.

Peto R, Pike MC, Day NE, Gray RG, Lee PN, Parish S, Peto J, Richards S, Wahrendorf J. Guidelines for simple, sensitive significance tests for carcinogenic effects in long-term animal experiments. Annex to: Long-Term and Short-Term Screening Assays for Carcinogens: A Critical Appraisal. IARC Monogr Suppl 2. Lyon: International Agency for Research on Cancer, 1980, pp 311–426.

Portier CJ. Estimating the tumour onset distribution in animal carcinogenesis experiments. Biometrika 73:371–378, 1986.

Portier CJ, Dinse GE. Semiparametric analysis of tumor incidence rates in survival/sacrifice experiments. Biometrics 43:107–114, 1987.

Portier CJ, Hedges J, Hoel DG. Age-specific models of mortality and tumor onset for historical control animals in the National Toxicology Program's carcinogenicity experiments. Cancer Res 46:4372–4378, 1986.

Racine-Poon A, Hoel DG. Nonparametric estimation of the survival function when cause of death is uncertain. Biometrics 40:1151–1158, 1984.

Sun J, Kalbfleisch JD. Nonparametric tests of tumor prevalence data. Biometrics 52:726–731, 1996.

Thurman JD, Bucci TJ, Hart RW, Turturro A. Survival, body weight, and spontaneous neoplasms in ad libitum-fed and food-restricted Fischer-344 rats. Toxicol Pathol 22:1–9, 1994.

Tolley HD, Burdick D, Manton KG, Stallard E. A compartment model approach to the estimation of tumor incidence and growth: investigation of a model of cancer latency. Biometrics 34:377–389, 1978.

Turnbull BW, Mitchell TJ. Exploratory analysis of disease prevalence data from survival/sacrifice experiments. Biometrics 34:555–570, 1978.

Turnbull BW, Mitchell TJ. Nonparametric estimation of the distribution of time to onset for specific diseases in survival/sacrifice experiments. Biometrics 40:41–50, 1984.

Westfall PH, Young SS. *p*-Value adjustments for multiple tests in multivariate binomial models. J Am Stat Assoc 84:780–786, 1989.

Williams PL, Portier CJ. Analytic expressions for maximum likelihood estimators in a nonparametric model of tumor incidence and death. Commun Stat Theory Methods 21:711–732, 1992a.

Williams PL, Portier CJ. Explicit solutions for constrained maximum likelihood estimators in survival/sacrifice experiments. Biometrika 79:717–729, 1992b.

9

Design of Developmental and Reproductive Toxicology Studies

R. John Weaver and Marshall N. Brunden*
Pharmacia & Upjohn, Inc., Kalamazoo, Michigan

I. INTRODUCTION

During the late 1950s and early 1960s, normally rare but extremely severe limb malformations were observed in an unusually high incidence in babies in a number of countries. Thousands of such births occurred before it was determined that thalidomide, a sedative given to pregnant mothers for hyperemesis gravidarum, was responsible for the defects (1). Less dramatically, but no less important, the infertility rate in couples aged 15–24 years increased threefold between 1965 and 1982 (2). The cause of this increase remains unknown, but is thought to be due to increased exposures to various exogenous chemicals. These examples illustrate both the importance of and the difficulty in identifying compounds that can affect reproduction and fetal development.

Animal studies are an important part of assessing chemicals and drugs for potential reproductive toxicity. Reproductive toxicity can be expressed in a broad range of manifestations, including adult male and/ or female reproductive function and mating behavior, embryonic and fetal development, major organ formation and development, neurological and behavioral development, and pre- and postweaning development

---

*Retired.

and growth. As such, numerous study designs and protocols are used to assess the effects of exposure.

A general overview of studies in developmental and reproductive toxicology (sometimes abbreviated DART) is presented, followed by discussions of specific study protocols. These include the three study design, dominant lethal assay, behavioral teratology, and a protocol that combines the three study design with aspects of behavioral teratology.

II. GENERAL EXPERIMENTAL CONCEPTS

A. Introduction

Most of the concepts of experimental design discussed in Chapter 7, on the design of carcinogenicity studies, are equally important in developmental and reproductive toxicity studies. These include specification of the experimental unit, identification of sources of experimental variation and their control, randomization, replication, and choice of experimental design. We briefly discuss these in the context of DART studies and refer the reader to Section II in Chapter 7 for further details.

B. The Experimental Unit

The concept of the experimental unit has probably been discussed more in the context of DART studies than for any other type of animal study (3,4). As stated in Chapter 7, the experimental unit is defined as the unit to which the treatment is applied in a single replication of the experiment. Somewhat unique to DART studies is the idea that the effect of treatment can be expressed and measured not only in the entity actually treated but also in other attributes of that entity. For example, in many studies the treatment is given to the pregnant animal, and, along with maternal observations, measurements on the individual fetuses or offspring are made. In this situation, the entire litter must be considered as an attribute of the experimental unit in the design and as the unit of statistical analysis.

Another example is a study design to assess male fertility that utilizes treated males, each mated to a pair of females. The male's fertility is expressed by the pair of females, and they must be considered together as the experimental unit in the statistical analysis.

C. Animals: Choice of Species and Strain

As with carcinogenicity studies, because there is no one animal species that exactly mimics the human in reproductive physiology other criteria, such as practicality, are used in choosing the animal model. For many of the same reasons discussed in Chapter 7, the two rodent species are commonly used for DART studies. Rats and mice are small and highly fertile, and have relatively short gestation periods. Other advantages include their genetic homogeneity, nonseasonal breeding, low incidence of spontaneous birth defects, and large litters. Because they have been widely used, there is substantial historical information on reproductive endpoints in these species. Some disadvantages include stress sensitivity, malformation clusters, the small size of the fetuses, and possible cannibalization of offspring. The commonly used strains include Sprague-Dawley outbred albino, Fisher 344 inbred albino, Wistar outbred albino and Long-Evans white and black hooded rats, and the CD-1 (Swiss) outbred albino, non-Swiss outbred albino, and Swiss-Webster outbred albino mice. Hybrid strains are generally avoided.

Rabbits are also often used in DART studies, in part because of their high fertility, especially in the males. Another reason may be historical, since rabbits were the only commonly used test animal to respond to thalidomide in testing subsequent to the drug's ban in the early 1960s. Rabbit strains frequently used are the New Zealand white albino and the Dutch belted black and white. Other, less used species are the dog, cat, pig, and monkey. A major disadvantage with these higher species is that they are seasonal breeders.

It is usually desirable to use the same species/strains of animals used in the other toxicological studies on the compound being investigated. During the acclimation periods, the estrus cycles of the females should be monitored, with any abnormal females excluded from the study. In rats, the failure to have two estrus cycles in a 10-day monitoring period is a criterion that might be employed. Monitoring of female mice is more difficult, because they must be in close proximity to males to become cyclic.

D. Choice of Dose Levels

Selection of dose levels is one of the most important issues in the design of the study. If available, information from earlier subchronic toxicity studies and pharmacokinetic studies is helpful in setting dose levels. Similarity in structure and/or activity to previously studied compounds may also be useful. Small dose-finding studies are also routinely conducted.

The high dose should elicit some maternal toxicity, but care should be taken that the dose chosen is not too high. Doses that result in substantial maternal toxicity are to be avoided, as it is difficult to distinguish actual drug effects on development of the fetus from nutritional deficiency due to the ill health of the mother. A common objective in choosing the high dose is to select a dose expected to result in a 10% reduction in mean body weight.

The route and frequency of administration depend on the intended route in humans and the specific objectives of the study. Frequently used routes are food, water, and gavage. Dermal exposure can be troublesome during the breeding phase, because some oral ingestion is likely to occur during the cohabitation. The stage of the reproductive cycle that is of interest will help determine the dosing scheme, as will become clear in the next section.

III. OVERVIEW OF REPRODUCTIVE PHYSIOLOGY

A. Reproductive and Developmental Toxicity

We begin by defining reproductive toxicity and developmental toxicity, then discussing some general concepts of reproductive physiology in mammals. This is followed by a discussion of some of the specific protocol types currently in use.

The purpose of reproductive toxicology is to identify the effect of a xenobiotic on mammalian reproduction. The definition is therefore very broad, encompassing virtually any adverse effect on male or female reproduction. Kimmel et al. (5) defines reproductive toxicology as "the occurrence of adverse effects on the reproductive system that may result from exposure to agents from exogenous sources. The toxicity may be expressed as alterations to the reproductive organs, the related endocrine system, or pregnancy outcomes. The manifestation of such toxicity may include adverse effects on sexual maturation, gamete production and transport, cycle normality, sexual behavior, fertility, gestation, parturition, lactation, pregnancy outcomes, premature reproductive senescence, or modifications in other functions that are dependent on the integrity of the reproductive system."

Developmental toxicology, also known as teratology, is a subset of reproductive toxicology that looks at the causes, mechanisms, and manifestations of abnormal development, of either a structural or a functional nature. The word *teratology* comes from the Greek *terat,* meaning "monster." One medical dictionary (6) defines teratology as: "that division of embryology and pathology which deals with abnormal development and congenital malformations." The entity that produces these physical defects in the developing embryo is called a teratogen. Teratology as a discipline is in its relative infancy, beginning in this century and really coming into its own after the thalidomide disaster.

B. Male Reproductive Physiology

There are two concerns in testing for male reproductive toxicity: 1) the ability of the male to produce sperm capable of fertilizing the female ovum and 2) that the sperm produced has normal genetic components. Toxicity may manifest itself in preventing fertilization or, more insidiously, damage the genetic material in the germ cell, resulting in fertilization but causing fetal death or malformation.

The development of mature, fertile sperm in mammals is called spermatogenesis. It beings with the spermatogonia, which as it progresses through stages of maturity is known sequentially as a primary spermatocyte, a secondary spermatocyte, a spermatid, and finally a spermatozoa. In human males this spermatogenic cycle takes approximately 64 days. In animals, the sequence is variable. Even within species, it varies somewhat—in rats, ranging from 48 days in Long-Evans rats to 53 days in Wistar rats. In the rabbit, the cycle is approximately 43 days and in mice 60 days. There is an additional period of approximately 12 days of maturation in the epididymis, when the sperm gains motility and the potential to fertilize. New cohorts of spermatogonia are released in waves, about every 12 days in rats and 16 days in humans, so there are about four or five waves in the various stages of maturity at a given point in time. These waves, sometimes referred to as cycles of the germinal epithelium, may be selectively susceptible to the effects of a xenobiotic.

While damage to mature and developing sperm is a major concern, the male reproductive cycle involves more than just the testis and epididymis. It is a complicated, interorgan system involving hormones released by the hypothalamus and anterior pituitary, and the actions of the efferent ducts, ductus deferens, and accessory sex glands. Effects on any of these sites can compromise the reproductive ability of the male. Toxicant-related activity may involve effects on the sex organ function. The males must be monitored for changes in mating patterns, decrease in libido, inability to achieve erection, etc. As such, it is evident that numerous protocols can be used, each designed to assess different aspects of the male reproductive cycle from early fetal life to sexual maturity.

C. Female Reproductive Physiology

The female reproductive process is a complex, hormone-mediated system that is yet to be fully understood. It involves the hypothalamus and pituitary, ovaries, fallopian tubes, and uterus.

The ovary contains a collection of follicles in a dormant state. These follicles originated from primordial germ cells formed during embryonic development. After puberty a follicle, or in multiparous animals, groups of these follicles begin to develop at the beginning of each menstrual cycle. At ovulation, each follicle ruptures and releases an ovum, which begins to travel down the fallopian tube. The ruptured follicle collapses into a glandlike structure. If fertilization does not occur, the structure undergoes luteolysis into a mass of tissue called the corpus albicans and the ovum deteriorates. If fertilization of the ovum occurs, the collapsed follicle, now called the corpus luteum, begins to secrete progesterone. The successfully fertilized ovum continues down the fallopian tube into the uterus, which, under the influence of progesterone from the corpus luteum, has prepared itself for implantation. The embryo implants into the uterine wall and continues development through parturition. The timing of these events and hormones involved varies from species to species.

The timing of exposure to the xenobiotic is critical in reproductive toxicity. Identical exposures can cause miscarriage or malformation or have no effect at all depending on when the exposure occurs in the reproductive cycle. Conversely, the effects of the exposure, either direct or latent, can also be observed any time during the complete life cycle, i.e. from conception in one generation through conception in the next generation. The expression of the toxicity may occur long after the exposure.

For convenience, the International Conference on Harmonization (ICH) divides the life cycle into the following stages:

1. Premating to conception
2. Conception to implantation
3. Implantation to closure of the hard palate
4. Closure of the hard palate to end of pregnancy

5. Birth to weaning
6. Weaning to sexual maturity

It is evident that no single study design will cover all the complexity of the reproductive life cycle. A combination of study protocols designed to cover all these stages of development is usually employed in the safety assessment of a drug.

IV. COMMON STUDY PROTOCOLS

A. Introduction

Because of the complexity of the reproductive process, many basic study designs are used, along with numerous variations and permutations of these designs. Some of the more common types of studies and their protocols have been described extensively by Ecobichon (7), Hoar (8), and Hutchins (9).

In vivo reproductive toxicity testing can involve single or multigeneration studies with males, females, or both sexes exposed to the chemical entity. Standardized testing protocols in rodents include single-, two-, or three-generation tests. In discussing the various studies, Collins (10) defines a single generation: "The test compound is administered prior to and throughout gestation within a single generation. The parental animals may be mated once or several times in order to detect possible cumulative effects of the compound." His definition of a multigeneration study is "an expansion of the test undertaken in the single-generation study. The parents are exposed continuously to the compound prior to mating, during gestation, and during lactation. Offspring from the mating are also continuously exposed to the compound, and are weaned, allowed to mature, and mated among themselves (sibling matings are avoided). The procedure is followed for each succeeding generation until the desired number of generations is obtained." Multigeneration studies are less commonly required for drugs than for pesticides and food additives, but may be appropriate when the drug is expected to be given chronically and/or bioaccumulation is expected.

B. Common Endpoints

There is an overlapping of the objectives of developmental toxicity and reproductive toxicity trials, and many of the endpoints observed are common to both. Data collected can be broadly categorized as either parental or litter data. It is important to collect general toxicity data on the maternal animals, because pregnancy causes many physiological changes that may alter the susceptibility to drugs, and data of this type are not available from the usual acute and chronic toxicology studies. It is also useful in determining to what extent maternal toxicity has influenced the observations made on the embryos/fetuses. Parental data include clinical observations, body weight, food and water consumption, mortality, organ weights, and, on occasion, hematology, blood chemistries, and urinalysis.

Other parental data are related to fertility and reproductive performance. Usually both the parental males and females are examined for fertility and reproductive organ histopathology. Mating behavior is sometimes observed. Data on numbers of abortions, early births, and gestation lengths are also collected. Kimmel et al. (5) provide a complete list of endpoints categorized as couple-mediated, male-specific, or female-specific. A number of indices commonly used in presenting the results of studies are listed in Table 1. Generally the numbers obtained are multiplied by 100 to express the index as a percentage. The statistical analysis and interpretation of indices can be complicated by the fact that the denominator and/or the numerator may be affected by the treatment.

TABLE 1   Commonly Used Reproduction and Fertility Indices

Index	Numerator (number of)	Denominator (number of)
Mating	Confirmed copulations	Estrus cycles
Male fertility	Males that impregnated a female	Males housed with a fertile female
Female fertility	Confirmed pregnancies	Females housed with a fertile male
Female fecundity	Confirmed pregnancies	Confirmed copulations
Parturition	Females giving birth	Confirmed pregnant
Gestation	Litters with live pups	Confirmed pregnant
Live birth	Viable pups born	Pups born
Day 1 Survival	Viable on day 1	Pups born
Preimplantation loss	Corpora lutea—implantations	Corpora lutea
Postimplantation loss	Implantations—live fetuses	Implantations

Data based on the litter numbers of corpora lutea, implantation sites, resorptions (early and late), fetal deaths, and live fetuses; sex ratios; crown-rump lengths; fetal weights; and malformations and variations. Malformations are the most serious finding, defined as permanent morphological changes that are detrimental to postnatal survival and normal growth or development. Variations are less serious findings, such as delays in structural development. Generally all fetuses are examined for gross or external abnormalities, and then randomly divided into two equal-sized groups by litter, with half examined viscerally and half skeletally. Observations on litters delivered include number of live births and dead pups, vitality and viability of pups, and pup body weights.

C. The Three Study Designs for Pharmaceutical Testing

1. Introduction

Pharmaceuticals are generally tested using the three study design described in this section. These studies provide a good general screen for developmental and reproductive toxicity. They address a) fertility and early embryonic development, b) embryo-fetal development, and c) prenatal and post natal development, including maternal function. Guidelines for this testing regimen were prepared under the direction of the ICH and evolved in part from guidelines published by the Food and Drug Administration in 1966 in response to the thalidomide disaster (11). Guidelines on the ICH three study design were published in the Federal Register (12), where the reader is referred for more details.

2. Fertility and Early Embryonic Development Study

The purpose of this study is to test for effects of treatment on the period from premating through implantation of the embryo. It assesses the effect of the compound on maturation of the gametes, mating behavior, fertility, preimplantation development of the embryo, and implantation.

Treatment generally begins 4 weeks prior to mating for males and 14–15 days prior to mating for females. If there is histologic evidence of effects on the male sex organs from previous studies, then treatment may begin up to 10 weeks prior to mating in males. Treatment continues through mating in males and at least through implantation in the females. Males are sacrificed after mating, and females at any point after midpregnancy. This treatment regimen covers up to the entire spermatogenesis cycle in males and several estrus cycles in females. Data collected include parental data, and numbers of corpora lutea, implantation sites, live and dead embryos. Organs are generally preserved for possible histological evaluation.

3. Embryo-Fetal Development Study

This testing pertains specifically to the screening of the capability of drugs to produce toxicity during the period of primary organogenesis. Organogenesis is the critical period of differentiation of organs in the embryos, when the embryo is most susceptible to xenobiotic exposure. It is relatively short, beginning in humans at implantation at about week 1 and ending by week 8 of pregnancy. Individual organ systems have highly specific time periods within the overall period when they are most vulnerable to exposure, which in rodents may be as short as 24 hours.

These studies typically use rats and rabbits. The typical design consists of a control and three to five dose groups of the drug in question. Usually 20 to 30 females are used per group, depending on the species. Because pregnancy rates are normally expected to be 80–90%, this will allow for an adequate number of litters. Average litter sizes are 12 in mice, 14 in rats, and 8–12 in rabbits. The experiments begin with untreated females being bred with untreated males. Treatment during the study is usually restricted to the females during the period of primary organogenesis, although some protocols utilize exposure from implantation to sacrifice and others for the entire gestational period. Extended treatment periods are indicated if the drug is known to be slowly absorbed, resulting in delayed attainment of peak or steady-state levels. In rats and mice, the period of primary organogenesis is over approximately days 6–17 of gestation, while in rabbits it is days 6–20. Pregnancy is timed by detection of a vaginal plug or the vaginal smear method, and the day that pregnancy is detected is usually designated as gestation day 0. Approximately 24 hours prior to expected delivery the dams/does are killed and caesarean sections performed. The uterus is opened and examined for the presence of early and late deaths, and corpora lutea are counted. The fetuses are removed, weighed, sexed, and examined for gross malformations. The reason for this early termination of the pregnancy is that rats often will cannibalize abnormal or malformed offspring, increasing the probability that these events will be missed. Some variations of the design, particularly those using original Japanese guidelines, allow some of the females (usually 25–33%) to deliver normally and then follow the pups through lactation.

A number of maternal and fetal outcomes are recorded in these studies. Examples of maternal outcomes for each treatment group are number of dams inseminated, number of dams pregnant, percent conceived, initial body weight, maternal body weight changes at several times during gestation, body weight at sacrifice, weight of the uterus and contents at sacrifice, maternal organ weight, food consumption measurements, and mortality counts.

Examples of fetal outcomes are number of implantations, number of early and late resorptions, number of fetal deaths (occurring later in gestation), fetal weights, sex ratios and number and type of malformations observed externally, viscerally, and skeletally.

4. Prenatal and Postnatal Development Study

In humans, it may take years before the effects of exposure are observed in the offspring, a prime example being vaginal cancer in females caused by exposure to diethylstilbesterol in the womb some 20 years earlier. The objective of this testing is to assess the effect of xenobiotics during late pregnancy and throughout the life of the offspring. Treatment begins in the female after implantation and continues through lactation. This protocol provides an ongoing assessment during fetal and neonatal life, looking for adverse effects of a drug on delivery, lactation, neonatal survival, and the continued health of the offspring.

Similar to the convention for time of mating, the day of birth is usually designated as postnatal or lactational day 0. In some protocols, one male and one female per litter are randomly chosen at the time of weaning to continue on study. Other protocols follow more offspring during maturation. Maternal data as described previously are usually collected, as are data on the growth and development of the offspring. The latter include mortality, body weights, and behavioral observations.

D. Behavioral Teratology

The integration of experimental psychology and teratology forms the basis of behavioral teratology. It is the study of possible neurobehavioral changes that may result from exposure of germ cells, embryos, fetuses, and postnatal subjects to xenobiotics. Its emergence as a scientific discipline began in the early 1960s, and in 1975 Japan and Great Britain took regulatory action requiring developmental neurotoxicity testing of medicinal products.

These studies involve the measurement of various psychological endpoints in the offspring. The teratological aspects are brought in by exploration of the relationship between developmental stage at the time of treatment with drug and the nature of the behavioral effects produced in the progeny.

The drugs may be administered at various times. The critical periods are embryo predifferentiations, embryo development, and fetal development. The drugs may be thought to produce biochemical alterations in the developing central nervous system, possibly in the absence of gross structural malformations. Behavioral testing is often included as a part of segment I studies.

Endpoints of interest may be motor activity measures such as open field and inclined plane activity, seizure susceptibility, hyperactivity, and neuropathology produced by the agent such as brain size, brain damage (dead cells), and brain lesions.

E. Reproductive Assessment by Continuous Breeding

Another fairly common design, reproductive assessment by continuous breeding (RACB), has been in use for about 15 years. It is a two-generation design that was developed by the National Toxicology Program, and has been described in detail by Chapin and Sloane (13).

A complete RACB consists of four tasks, although all four are not necessary in all situations. Task 1 is the dose-range-finding study. It is recommended that groups consist of five to eight animals, given 1 week of exposure followed by 3 weeks of cohabitation and exposure, leading to the birth of the pups. Data collected include body weights, food consumption, and litter data.

Task 2 is the main part of the study. A control group of 40 animals and three or four treated groups consisting of 20 animals per group comprise the design. Exposure begins 1 week prior to cohabitation, and continues as animals are housed together for 14 weeks. Litters are generally produced about every 3 to 4 weeks, yielding four or five litters per breeding pair. After 14 weeks, the breeding pair is separated, and the female is allowed to deliver her last litter, which is nursed and weaned at postnatal day 21. Data collected include body weights, food consumption, and litter data.

Task 3 is a crossover mating test. It usually utilizes control and high-dose animals only. Three testing groups of 20 pairs each are formed, consisting of control males × treated females, treated males × control females, and control males × control females. The animals used are obtained from task 2, and pairs are cohabited for a week without exposure, with the females allowed to carry and deliver their litters. This task aids in identifying gender-specific effects on fertility and reproduction.

Task 4 is the evaluation of the second generation. Pups begin exposure at the same level as their parents, beginning at weaning on postnatal day 21. At 74–80 days of age, they are assigned breeding partners within treatment groups, being careful to avoid sibling matings. Females carry and deliver their litters.

F. Male Fertility and Reproductive Toxicity: Study Protocols

1. Introduction

Male fertility and reproductive performance can be assessed as part of a larger study that also investigates female reproduction (such as a segment I study) or as a separate standalone study. In this section, we discuss some study protocols specifically designed to assess effects to the male reproductive system. As noted previously, the complete spermatogenesis cycle takes approximately 40 to 60 days, depending on the species used. To ensure covering the entire cycle, treatment typically has extended a week or so longer, for example, from 70 to 75 days in rats. Recent guidelines (14), however, suggest a much shorter premating treatment period in males, from 2 to 4 weeks. This is based on observations that selective toxic effects are rare, with most appearing in the postmeiotic stages. Use of the shorter treatment period must be justified, based on the results of earlier repeated dose toxicity studies of at least 4 weeks' duration. If previous studies show evidence of effects on the reproductive organs, then longer treatment periods should be considered.

2. Sperm Assessment

The easiest and most direct assessment of reproductive toxicity in males is the examination of the sperm. Male animals are treated, and sperm is collected from the vas deferens or the cauda epididymis. Sperm count, motility, and morphology (alterations in the head or tail) are common observations. Assessments of functional status may also be made including pH and viscosity. Reproductive organs should be weighed and preserved for later histopathological evaluation. In many cases, the most sensitive method of detection of toxicity is the histopathological examination of the testes and epididymis. These assessments can often be made as part of the repeated dose toxicity study, thereby allowing later studies to examine more specific exposures and effects.

3. Serial and Extended Mating Studies

In these designs, males are treated, then mated with untreated females over a period of time. Depending on the objective of the study and the proposed use of the investigational drug, treatment may range from a single dose to daily dosing over the duration of the study. During each breeding period, males are housed with from one to four females. As discussed previously, the male is considered the experimental unit, and housing with multiple females does not increase the overall sample size. In each successive breeding period, new virgin females are used, for a total of up to 50 females used for each male. Data collected include fertility indices and fetal data such as numbers of live, dead, and malformed fetuses. The timing of the effects will yield evidence as to what portion of the spermatogenic cycle was affected.

4. Dominant Lethal Assay

The dominant lethal assay is a common variation of the serial mating study in which the male animals are treated at subtoxic levels and are mated with untreated virgin females, with new females each week, throughout a complete spermatogenic cycle. The doses selected are estimated to cause chromosomal damage that results in fetal lethality. The dams are euthanized at midgestation, with the numbers of corpora lutea and live, dead and resorbed conceptuses counted. The timing of the appearance of the lethal effects indicates the stage or stages of the spermatogenic cycle that were affected.

G. A Hypothetical Example of a Combined Study Design with Aspects of Behavioral Teratology

The purpose of this study is to determine potential adverse effects of a drug at all stages of the reproductive life cycle in both males and females. It examines effects on the F_0 parental generation, fetal development, the peri- and postnatal development of the offspring, and the reproductive performance of the offspring. A relatively detailed outline of the entire experiment is given below. The relationship of this experimental sequence to the three study design and facets of behavioral teratology should become clear.

The study design employed is completely randomized with a single-factor treatment layout. Randomization is used throughout the study to control for potential bias. Animals are transferred in a random fashion from shipping cartons to cages, followed by the random assignment of treatment levels to the cages. Further randomizations are used during the study for estrus cycle monitoring assignments, the culling of litters, offspring selection for developmental observation, behavioral testing, all mating assignments, and the assignment of males for sperm analysis.

The design consists of 24 male rats and 48 female rats per treatment group. Half of the females arrive unbred and half timed-mated. Animals are housed singly in cages except during mating periods, when the breeding pairs cohabitate. Male rats begin treatment 70 days prior to cohabitation, and the unbred females begin 14 days prior to cohabitation. They are then randomly assigned on a 1 : 1 basis for a 14-day cohabitation period. With evidence of mating, the males and females are returned to their individual cages. The body weights of the male and unbred female F_0 animals are recorded on arrival and twice weekly, beginning with the day of the first dose. F_0 food consumption is monitored in the males and females on a weekly basis during the treatment period, until the cohabitation begins. Food consumption is not monitored during cohabitation.

The F_0 timed-mated females compose the teratology portion of the protocol. They are treated on gestation days 6 through 15. Body weights and food consumption for pregnant females are recorded on gestation days 0, 6, 9, 12, 15, 17, and 20. Dams are observed, weighed, and sacrificed on gestation day 20. The entire uterus and contents are removed and weighed intact. Nongravid uteri are stained for implantation sites. A gross necropsy is performed on each dam for major organ examination. Unusual tissue masses are fixed for histopathological examination. Liver weights are also taken.

Live and dead fetuses are recorded and early and late resorptions counted. The number of corpora lutea are recorded for each ovary. Fetuses are numbered sequentially from the ovarian end of the left horn to cervix to the ovarian end of the right horn. This is done to uniquely identify all fetuses, and to identify cases in which there is a concentration gradient of the test article in the uterine blood vessels. Approximately one-half of the fetuses receive a fresh visceral examination, the remaining ones are given skeletal examinations. Findings are tabulated as gross, visceral, and skeletal malformations.

Half of the males are randomly selected for sperm analysis and sacrificed after the cohabitation period. They receive a gross necropsy and the liver, testes, epididymides, and seminal vesicles are weighed. After sperm analysis, the reproductive organs are fixed for possible histopathological examination. Dosing of the remaining F_0 males continues until the females scheduled to deliver have cast their offspring, at which time the males are sacrificed and given a gross necropsy. Target organs may be weighed and the reproductive organs from any male that did not impregnate a female fixed.

Blood samples to be used for toxicokinetics are collected from the lateral tail vein to provide plasma samples for determination of drug levels. Five F_0 males and five F_0 unbred females per group and five bred F_0 females per treated group are bled. Samples are collected 0, 1, 4, 8, 12, 16, and 24 hours after the dose on day 24 for F_0 males, dose day 12 for unbred F_0 females, and gestation days 6 and 17 for F_0 timed-pregnant females.

The 24 dams per group that were cohabited and bred are allowed to deliver their litters. Any difficulties at the time of parturition and the length of gestation are recorded. In addition, each litter is processed and the following data collected:

Number of live newborn
Number of dead newborn
Number of abnormal newborn
Weight and sex of each newborn
Number of cannibalized newborn

All dead pups are given a gross examination. Pups born dead or that die on postpartum days 0–21 are given a visceral examination. This includes detection of hydrocephaly and heart dissection. Lungs of dead pups found on day 0 will be examined for air-filled alveoli to distinguish between stillborns and deaths that occurred after birth. Live pups are sexed and weighed on postpartum days 0, 1, 4, 7, 14, and 21. The F_0 females that delivered are weighed and sacrificed on postpartum day 21. Females that failed to deliver are sacrificed on the 24th day following insemination or when determined to be not pregnant. Dams with total litter loss are sacrificed within 48 hours of parturition. All dams are given gross necropsies consisting of examination of the major organs in the abdominal and thoracic cavities. Target organs of each dam may also be weighed, and unusual tissue masses are fixed for histopathological examination. Implantation scars are counted and recorded.

On postpartum day 4, the F_1 litter size is reduced to eight pups. This is accomplished by randomly selecting pups by sex, while trying to maintain the most even sex distribution. This will usually result in four males and four females retained in a litter, but occasionally sex ratios of 3 : 5, 2 : 6, etc., are necessary. In litters with fewer than eight pups, extra pups from the same dose group are randomly fostered into the litter to maintain a size of eight. The pups are returned to their cages and monitored for developmental milestones, behavioral testing, and F_1 fertility evaluation. Body weights of F_1 offspring are recorded weekly after weaning and until sacrifice. Postnatal development milestones of eye opening, pinna detachment, vaginal patency, balanopreputial separation, auditory startle response, negative geotaxis, and M-maze are monitored and the results recorded.

In order to obtain at least 20 F_1 males and 20 F_1 females per group, a minimum of one male and one female pup per litter are randomly selected for the assessment of reproductive performance. The selected pups are housed individually until they are at least 70 days old. They are then randomly paired on a 1 : 1 basis, avoiding sibling matings. Vaginal smears are examined for presence of sperm each morning after pairing, continuing until the 15th day of cohabitation. The date of pairing, length of gestation, and fertility indexes are determined. The F_1 dams are allowed to deliver. Measures similar to those recorded for the F_0 dams and F_1 pups are recorded for the F_1 dams and F_2 pups. F_1 sires are sacrificed when it has been established that fertility has not been adversely affected. A gross necropsy is also conducted on the F_1 males.

F_1 females that fail to deliver or have a total litter loss are handled in the same fashion as those in the F_0 generation. Any abnormal findings during the gross necropsy or results from microscopic examinations made on lesions or tissues saved for histopathology from the dams, sires, and pups are recorded.

V. CONCLUSION

The preceding discussions emphasize the great complexity of the reproductive life cycle, with the resulting myriad of study designs used in assessing reproductive and developmental toxicity. The combination of studies employed in testing a drug should encompass exposure at all stages of the reproductive life cycle. When effects are detected, further studies, with more specific objectives and defined exposures, should be employed to more fully characterize the stage(s) of the reproductive life cycle affected. In all individual situations, there should be flexibility in the strategy employed, utilizing all previous knowledge gained on the compound and its anticipated exposure to humans in designing the study protocols.

REFERENCES

1. Mcbride WG. Thalidomide and congenital abnormalities. Lancet ii:1138, 1961.
2. Mosher WD, Pratt WF. Fecundity and infertility in the United States, 1965–1982. Publication PHS 85-1250. NCHS Advance Data 104. Washington, DC: US Public Health Service, 1985.
3. Staples RE, Haseman JK. Selection of appropriate experimental units in teratology. Teratology 9:259–260, 1974.
4. Palmer AK. Statistical sampling and choice of sampling units. Teratology 10:301–302, 1974.
5. Kimmel GL, Clegg ED, Crisp TM. Reproductive toxicity testing: A risk assessment perspective. In: Witorsch RJ, ed. Reproductive Toxicology, 2nd ed. New York: Raven Press, 1995.
6. Dorland's Illustrated Medical Dictionary, 28th ed. Philadelphia: WB Saunders, 1994.
7. Ecobichon DJ. The Basis of Toxicity Testing. Boca Raton, FL: CRC Press, 1992.
8. Hoar RM. Reproduction/teratology. Fundam Appl Toxicol 4:S335–S340, 1984.
9. Hutchins DE. Behavioral teratology: A new frontier in neurobehavioral research. In: Johnson EM, Kochhar DM, eds. Teratology and Reproductive Toxicology. Berlin: Springer-Verlag, 1983.
10. Collins TF. Multigeneration reproduction studies. In: Wilson JG, Fraser FC, eds. Research Procedures and Data Analysis, Handbook of Teratology, Vol 4. New York: Plenum Press, 1978.
11. Food and Drug Administration. Guidelines for Reproduction Studies for Safety Evaluation of Drugs for Human Use. Washington, DC: US Food and Drug Administration, 1966.
12. Food and Drug Administration, Guideline on Detection of Toxicity to Reproduction for Medicinal Products. Federal Register: September 22, 1994.
13. Chapin RE, Sloane RA. Reproductive assessment by continuous breeding: Evolving study design and summaries of ninety studies. Environmental Health Perspectives 105(suppl 1):199–395, 1997.
14. International Conference on Harmonization S5B. Guideline for Industry: Detection of Toxicity to Reproduction for Medicinal Products. Addendum on Toxicity to Male Fertility, April 1996.

10

Analysis of Reproductive and Developmental Studies

JAMES J. CHEN

National Center for Toxicological Research, Food and Drug Administration, Jefferson, Arkansas

I. INTRODUCTION

Reproductive and developmental toxicity experiments are conducted in laboratory animals for the evaluation of potential adverse effects of chemical compounds on fertility, reproduction, and fetal development. Regulatory agencies in the United States routinely require such experiments for approval of drugs, pesticides, or food additives. A test compound is administered to either parent before conception, during prenatal development, or postnatally. A typical reproductive or developmental study involves one control and two to four dose groups of 20–30 (pregnant) animals, usually rats, mice, or rabbits. The highest dose is chosen to produce minimal maternal toxicity, ranging from marginal body weight reduction to not more than 10% mortality (Environmental Protection Agency [EPA], 1991). The pregnant dams normally are humanely killed just before term, and the uterine contents are then examined to study reproductive and developmental toxicity of the test compound. The experimental outcomes for each female typically include numbers of corpora lutea, implantation sites, dead or resorbed implants, individual malformation of viable fetuses, normal fetuses, fetal weight, fetal lengths, and such.

Soper and Clark (1991) provided an excellent overview of stages in reproductive development as follows. During the reproductive process, ovarian follicles release eggs that are fertilized by sperm to form embryos. These embryos subsequently implant into the wall of the uterus. The discharged ovarian follicles differentiate into corpora lutea, which secrete hormones necessary to sustain pregnancy. The embryos undergo organogenesis to form fetuses. Each step in this process is a potential target for toxic effects of a test compound. Depending on when treatment begins, a test compound may affect the number of corpora lutea, the number of embryos implanting into the wall of uterus on gestational days, and the number of live fetuses surviving to term. For surviving fetuses, growth reduction, such as weight loss, may occur or may exhibit one or more types of structural malformations. Figure 1 is a sketch of the outcomes from a dam in a developmental and reproductive toxicity experiment.

A. Developmental Toxicity Endpoints

The most commonly used protocol for assessing reproductive and developmental toxicity is the segment II design, which involves an administration of a test substance to pregnant dams during a period of organogenesis (after implantation). In a segment II study, the two primary toxicity outcomes of interest are the number of resorptions (early deaths) and deaths, and the number of malformations in viable fetuses. The number of deaths and resorptions combined (equivalently, the number of viables) provides a measure of embryotoxic lethality (prenatal death). However, the proportion of the number of deaths and resorptions among the implants to the total number of implants provides a better measure of embryotoxic lethality because it adjusts for the variability in the number of implants from dam to dam. Likewise, the proportion of the number of fetuses with anomaly (malformation) of a specific type to the number of live fetuses in a litter provides a better measure of developmental effects than the number of anomalies. Finally, the proportion of the total number of deaths, resorptions, and malformations combined to the total number of implants measures the total developmental toxic effects of a test substance. Other developmental toxicity measures are discussed by the EPA (1991).

In addition to the proportion of deaths or resorptions and the

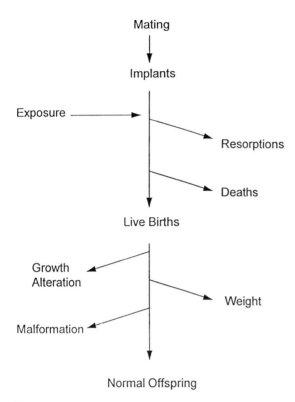

FIGURE 1   Schematic representation of the outcomes from a dam in a developmental toxicity experiment.

proportion of malformations, the number of implantations and the number of corpora lutea are both counted, and have been the primary toxicity endpoints in some reproductive studies. For example, if a compound is administered before implantation, such as the segment I design or dominant lethal assay, then both the numbers of implantations and corpora lutea provide a measure of the effects of a test substance on the reproduction system. Other reproductive toxicity endpoints involving count data will be discussed later.

Fetal weight reduction, which measured in a continuous variable scale, generally is a more sensitive developmental toxicity endpoint than the prenatal deaths or resorptions and malformations; in some cases, fetal weight reduction may be the only indicator of developmental toxicity (Kimmel and Gaylor, 1988). Reduced fetal growth may represent a mechanism that is different from a dose effect, resulting in malformations and fetal deaths. The associations among the number of implants, number of viables, and fetal weight have been reported previously by several authors (Barr et al., 1969; Jensh et al., 1970; Cornwall et al., 1984). Ryan et al. (1991) investigated the correlations between fetal weight and malformation using the data from ten developmental toxicity studies conducted for the National Toxicology Program (NTP). They found a tendency for malformed fetuses to have a lower weight at term than nonmalformed fetuses. Chen and Gaylor (1992) examined a large-scale study of 2,4,5-trichlorophenoxyacetic (2,4,5-T) acid exposure, and found a negative correlation between the number of live fetuses and fetal weight, and between cleft palate incidence and fetal weight. Statistically, a quantitative response (continuous) variable is more sensitive to treatment effects than a quantal response variable such as presence or absence of a particular malformation type.

B. Multiple Developmental Outcomes

The standard approach for assessment of developmental risks of a compound has been based on the analysis of each developmental endpoint separately. It has been suggested that the developmental toxicity outcomes (i.e., death or resorption, malformation, growth retardation, or other) may represent different degrees of responses to a toxic insult and occur in a dose-related manner (Kimmel and Gaylor, 1988). These developmental outcomes are likely to be correlated. Therefore, a joint analysis of multiple developmental outcomes can have some advantages: it can increase the power of detecting effects if the multiple outcomes are manifestations of some common biological effects, and it allows investigations of associations among the multiple outcomes if they are the results of different biological mechanisms.

   Recently, several authors have proposed multivariate models for simultaneous analysis of multiple endpoints. Statistical procedures for the analysis of multiple malformation types have been proposed (Lefkopoulou et al., 1989; Lefkopoulou and Ryan, 1993; Chen and Ahn, 1997). Statistical models for the analysis of death or resorption and malformation jointly have been proposed (Chen et al., 1991; Chen and Li, 1992, 1994; Ryan, 1992; Zhu et al., 1994; Krewski and Zhu, 1994). Statistical modelings of the relations among malformation, fetal weight or number of viables have been considered (Rai and Van Ryzin, 1985; Catalano and Ryan, 1992; Chen, 1993b; Fitzmaurice and Laird, 1995).

C. Litter Effect

In developmental and reproductive toxicity experiments, chemicals are administered to the dam, but the observations are made on individual fetuses. The treatment affects the fetuses only indirectly by the dam. Rosenkranz and Uhl (1991) discussed two extreme points of view in the evaluation of fetal data. One extreme view is that if "a foetus belongs to a certain litter does not influence the analysis, then assigning the individual foetuses to specific litters is irrelevant." This leads to performing the analysis at an individual fetus level, without adjusting for possible correlations among the littermates. The other extreme view is to ignore the differences of individual fetuses within a litter and perform the analysis based on the litter means. Because an individual dam is treated, the fetal responses from the same dam are expected to be more alike than responses from different dams (this phenomenon is referred to as *litter effect*). The litter-based analysis is generally considered to be more appropriate than the fetal-based analysis (Healy, 1972; Haseman and Hogan, 1975). However, the litter-based approach may not be a satisfactory analysis; for example, it does not account for differences in litter sizes. Two approaches, parametric and quasi-likelihood, to account for the litter effect are considered in this chapter.

D. Scope of the Chapter

The reproductive and developmental toxicity endpoints described in the foregoing can generally be divided into three categories: (a) dichotomous (e.g., presence or absence of a particular malformation) or proportion, (b) count (e.g., number of implants), and (c) continuous (e.g., fetal body weight). The purpose of this chapter is to review common statistical methods for the analysis of the three types of fetal data, and methods for the analysis of multiple malformation types and a joint analysis of deaths or resorptions and malformations.

    Statistical analysis of developmental toxicity endpoints have focused either on the qualitative testing for an adverse effect (e.g., Williams, 1975; Gladen, 1979) or the quantitative estimation by dose–response modeling (e.g., Chen and Kodell, 1989; Ryan, 1992) for risk estimation. This chapter mainly focuses on the procedures for testing developmental and reproductive effects.

II. GENERAL MODELS AND HYPOTHESES

A. Quasi-Likelihood and Generalized Estimating Equations

Let Y be a random variable for a response with mean $E(Y) = \mu$ and variance $Var(Y) = \sigma^2 v(\mu)$, where σ^2 may be unknown, and $v(\mu)$ is a known function of μ. Assume that the mean parameter μ is related to a set of covariates $z = (z_1, \ldots, z_p)$ (e.g., dose, sex, and such), by a link function

$$h(\mu|z) = z\beta$$

where $\beta = (\beta_0, \ldots, \beta_p)$ is a vector of parameters. Wedderburn (1974) defined the log quasi-likelihood Q for an observation y by

$$Q(y;\mu) = \int_y^\mu \frac{y - t}{\sigma^2 v(t)} dt + (\text{function of } y)$$

or equivalently, the quasi-score function is

$$U = \frac{\partial Q(y;\mu)}{\partial \mu} = \frac{y - \mu}{\sigma^2 v(\mu)}$$

The score function has the following properties in common with a log-likelihood derivative:

$$E(U) = 0$$

$$Var(U) = [\sigma^2 v(\mu)]^{-1}$$

and

$$-E\left(\frac{\partial U}{\partial \mu}\right) = [\sigma^2 v(\mu)]^{-1}$$

Let y denote the $N \times 1$ vector of responses, and $E(y) = \mu$ and $Cov(y) = \sigma^2 V(\mu)$, where $V(\mu)$ is a diagonal matrix containing $v(\mu)$'s. The quasi-likelihood estimating equations for β are

$$\frac{\partial Q(y;\mu)}{\partial \beta}\Big|_\beta = U(\hat{\beta}) = \hat{D}'\hat{V}^{-1}(y - \hat{\mu}) = 0, \tag{1}$$

where $D = [d_{ij}]$ is an $N \times p$ matrix such that $d_{ij} = \partial\mu_i/\partial\beta_j$, and $\hat{V} = \text{diag}\{v(\hat{\mu}_1), \ldots, v(\hat{\mu}_N)\}$. The regression parameters β can be estimated by the Newton–Raphson method (see McCullagh and Nelder, 1989, Chap. 9). The dispersion parameter σ^2 is estimated by the moment method in each iteration of the Newton–Raphson algorithm.

Under appropriate regularity conditions, the quasi-likelihood estimate $\hat{\beta}$ or β is approximately unbiased and asymptotically normal with the covariance matrix $\text{Cov}(\hat{\beta}) = (D' V^{-1} D)^{-1}\hat{\sigma}^2$ (see Davidian and Carroll, 1987; Smyth, 1989; Moore and Tsiatis, 1991). Equation (1) is known as the (generalized) estimating equations. Liang and Zeger (1986) showed that the robust variance estimate $M_0^{-1} M_1 M_0^{-1}$ is a consistent estimate of the covariance matrix of $\hat{\beta}$, even when $\text{Var}(Y)$ is misspecified, where $M_0 = \hat{D}' \hat{V}^{-1} \hat{D}$ and $M_1 = \hat{D}' \hat{V}^{-1}(y - \hat{\mu})(y - \hat{\mu})' \hat{V}^{-1}\hat{D}$. The matrix $M_0^{-1} \hat{\sigma}^2$ is known as the model-based variance estimate and the matrix $M_0^{-1} M_1 M_0^{-1}$ is the robust variance estimate. If the distribution of Y is completely specified by its mean and variance, then the estimate $\hat{\beta}$ in Eq. (1) is the maximum likelihood estimate.

The quasi-likelihood and generalized estimating equations approaches depend on only the assumptions of the form of the first two moments. The estimated coefficients $\hat{\beta}$ are consistent even if the variance function is misspecified. The estimates based on either the quasi-likelihood or generalized estimating equations method are more robust and easier to compute than the maximum likelihood estimates based on a parametric model. Detailed discussions and applications of the quasi-likelihood and generalized estimating equations are given by Liang and Zeger (1986) and Zeger and Liang (1986). Zeger and associates (1988) proposed methods of estimating the regression parameters β and the covariance matrix for some applications.

In this chapter, the quasi-likelihood approach will be applied to analyzing proportions, such as the incidence of malformation, and counts, such as the number of implants. The general estimating equations approach will be applied to analyzing fetal weight, and joint analysis of the incidences of death or resorption and malformation, and the multiple malformation types.

B. Testing for Developmental Effects

Consider an experiment with g treatment groups, a control and $g - 1$ dose groups. Assume that the ith group contains m_i female animals. Let y_{ijk} be the response of an implant or a fetus out of n_{ij} examined for a particular developmental toxicity outcome, $1 \leq i \leq g$, $1 \leq j \leq m_i$, and $1 \leq k \leq n_{ij}$. Note that y_{ijk} may be an indicator variable representing the presence or absence of a particular malformation type or a continuous variable representing a fetal weight. Depending on the toxicity endpoint of interest, n_{ij} may represent the number of viables, number of implants, or number of corpora lutea.

Let μ_i represent the mean of the ith group for a developmental endpoint of interest (e.g., fetal weight, probability of a malformation, or other). The following three hypotheses are tested to evaluate the treatment effects:

1. Test for homogeneity among means:

$H_{a0} : \mu_1 = \cdots = \mu_g$

$H_{a1} : \mu_i \neq \mu_j$, for some $i \neq j$ (not all the μ_i's are equal).

2. Pairwise comparisons with the control:

$H_{b0} : \mu_1 = \mu_i$, $(i = 2, \cdots, g)$

$H_{b1} : \mu_1 < \mu_i$ (or $\mu_1 > \mu_i$)

3. Test for dose–response trend:

$H_{c0} : \mu_1 = \cdots = \mu_g$

$H_{c1} : \mu_1 < \cdots < \mu_g$ (or $\mu_1 > \cdots > \mu_g$)

The hypothesis H_a is two-sided, and the hypotheses H_b and H_c are one-sided. The hypothesis H_a is to determine if there are differences among the experimental groups. The hypothesis H_b is to determine whether the compound induces an effect above (or below) the background effect observed in controls, and H_c is to determine if there is an increasing trend in response to increasing dose.

In the parametric model, the likelihood ratio χ^2 test is applied to the hypothesis testing. Let L_1 represent the maximum value of log-likelihood with the constraints $\mu_1 = \cdots = \mu_g$, and let L_m represent the maximum value subject to no constraints on μ's. Under the null hypothesis, the likelihood ratio statistic $2(L_m - L_1)$ has a χ^2 distribution with ($g - 1$) degrees of freedom. The likelihood ratio test can also be used to compare control and dose groups.

An alternative test for the treatment differences is to compute the Wald test directly from a fitted model. The Wald test is based on the fact that the MLE has an asymptotic normal distribution. In the generalized linear model framework, the link function for the ith mean can be modeled as

$$h(\mu_i) = \beta_1 + \beta_i, i = 2, \ldots, g$$

The link function h describes a relation between the treatment and response. For binary (proportion) data, h is a logit function; for continuous data, h is an identity function; for count data, h is a logarithm function. Let $\hat{\beta}_i$ be the maximum likelihood estimate (or quasi-likelihood estimate) of β_i, $i = 1, \ldots, g$. The null hypothesis of the homogeneity, $\mu_1 = \cdots = \mu_g$, is equivalent to the hypothesis, $\beta_2 = \cdots = \beta_g = 0$. The Wald test statistic is

$$X_w = \hat{\beta}'_0 \Sigma_{\hat{\beta}_0}^{-1} \hat{\beta}_0$$

where $\hat{\beta}_0 = (\hat{\beta}_2, \ldots, \hat{\beta}_g)$, and $\Sigma_{\hat{\beta}_0} = [\hat{\sigma}_{ij}]$ is the covariance matrix of $\hat{\beta}_0$. Under the null hypothesis, X_w has an approximate χ^2 distribution with $g - 1$ degrees of freedom. Similarly, the null hypothesis $\mu_1 = \mu_i$ is equivalent to the hypothesis $\beta_i = 0$, $i = 2, \ldots, g$. The Wald test statistic $\beta_i^2/\hat{\sigma}_{ii}$ has a χ^2 with 1 degree of freedom.

The score test is also often used to test for treatment effects. Define the score statistic $U_{g \times 1}(\beta) = U_{g \times 1}(\beta_1, \beta_0) = \partial L/\partial \beta$ with the variance matrix $I_\beta = -E(\partial^2 L/\partial \beta^2)$. Denote $U_{g \times 1}(\beta) = [U_{\beta_1}(\beta_1, \beta_0), U_{\beta_0}(\beta_1, \beta_0)]$, where $U_{\beta_1}(\beta_1, \beta_0)$ and $U_{\beta_0}(\beta_1, \beta_0)$ are 1 and $(g - 1)$ score vectors for β_1 and β_0, respectively. Let I^{β_0} be lower right-hand $(g - 1) \times (g - 1)$ submatrix of the inverse matrix I_β^{-1} corresponding to the score vector $U_{\beta_0}(\beta_1, \beta_0)$. Under the null hypothesis, the score test statistic.

$$X_s = U_{\beta_0}(\hat{\beta}_1, O)' \, I^{\beta_0} U_{\beta_0}(\hat{\beta}_1, O)$$

has an approximate χ^2 distribution with $g - 1$ degrees of freedom.

A dose effect on the mean μ_i can be modeled by a link function,

$$h(\mu_i) = \beta_0 + \beta_1 d_i$$

The inverse function h^{-1} is a dose response function that describes a relation between μ_i and d_i. The hypothesis of a dose-related trend (H_c) can be expressed as

$$H_{c'0}: \beta_1 = 0$$

$$H_{c'1}: \beta_1 < 0 \ (\text{or } \beta_1 > 0).$$

The likelihood ratio, Wald test, or score statistic can be applied to testing for $H_{c'0}: \beta_1 = 0$. Under the null hypothesis, the test statistic has a χ^2 distribution with 1 degree of freedom.

C. Litter-Based Analysis

Conventional methods of litter-based analysis (e.g., Healy, 1971) are based on the analysis of litter means $y_{ij.} = \Sigma_k y_{ijk}/n_{ij}$. The classic analysis of variance F test is used to test for homogeneity among the treatment groups. For comparisons between control and a dose group, a vector of constant L such that $L_i'\mu = (\mu_1 - \mu_i)$ can be used in conjunction with the analysis of variance. Alternatively, a Student's t-test can be applied directly to compare two groups. Similarly, the linear regression coefficient is used to test for a dose-related trend. Note, that the litter means may be transformed by an angular or Freeman–Tukey transformation (1950) if $y_{ij.}$ is a proportion variable, and transformed by a square root transformation if $y_{ij.}$ is a count variable. An alternative approach to analyzing the litter proportion or count data is the nonparametric Kruskal–Wallis or Wilcoxon rank test. Nonparametric tests will not be considered in this chapter.

III. ANALYSIS OF BINOMIAL PROPORTIONS

The statistical method for the analysis of proportions from reproductive and developmental toxicity studies has been considered by many authors (e.g., Williams, 1975, 1987; Kupper and Haseman, 1978; Haseman and Kupper, 1979; Gladen, 1979; Paul, 1982; Rai and Van Ryzin, 1985; Pack, 1986; Kupper, et al., 1986; Chen and Kodell, 1989; Rao and Scott, 1992; Ryan, 1992, 1993; Carr and Portier, 1993; Chen, 1993a; Fung et al., 1994; Liang and Hanfelt, 1994; Donner et al., 1994; Bieler and Williams, 1995; Bowman and George, 1995; Paul and Islam, 1995; Bowan et al., 1995, and others).

Let y_{ijk} denote the presence or absence of a response. Assume that the mean and variance of y_{ijk} are

$$E(y_{ijk}) = \mu_i, \quad \text{and} \quad \text{Var}(y_{ijk}) = \mu_i(1 - \mu_i)$$

and the correlation is

$$\text{Corr}(y_{ijk}, y_{ijk'}) = \phi_i$$

where $k, k' = 1, \ldots, n_{ij}$, and $k \neq k'$. The parameter μ_i is the probability of a developmental effect of the ith group, and ϕ_i is the intralitter correlation coefficient. The binary responses $y_{ij1}, \ldots, y_{ijn_{ij}}$ within each litter are modeled by a multivariate (correlated) binary distribution. A simple multivariate binary model is the multivariate equicorrelated probit model proposed by Ochi and Prentice (1984). This model is a multivariate tolerance distribution with an underlying multivariate normal with an equicorrelation matrix. Other multivariate distribution, such as a multivariate Student's t-test and log-normal, and a correlation matrix, such as tridiagonal and autocorrelated structures, can also be used to generate a multivariate binary model. Bowman and George (1995) proposed a multivariate exchangeable binary model by assuming the binary responses within each litter are exchangeable. Specifically, if $\{k_1, \ldots, k_l\}$ is a subset of $\{1, \ldots, n_{ij}\}$, then

$$Pr(y_{ij1} = 1, \ldots, y_{ijl} = 1) = Pr(y_{ij_{k_1}} = 1, \ldots, y_{ij_{k_l}} = 1)$$

for all $l = 1, \ldots, n_{ij}$. A multivariate probit model based on an equicorrelation structure is an exchangeable model.

Let $y_{ij} = (y_{ij1} + \ldots + y_{ijn_{ij}})$, then the mean and variance of y_{ij} are

$$E(y_{ij} \mid n_{ij}) = n_{ij}\mu_i$$

and

$$Var(y_{ij} \mid n_{ij}) = n_{ij}\mu_i(1 - \mu_i)[\phi_i(n_{ij} - 1) + 1]$$

The intralitter correlation coefficient generally is positive ($\phi_i > 0$). Thus, the variance $n_{ij}\mu_i(1 - \mu_i)[\phi_i(n_{ij} - 1) + 1]$ is greater than the nominal binomial variance $n_{ij}\mu_i(1 - \mu_i)$. The distribution of y_{ij} is known as an extrabinomial variate. Note that if $\phi_i = 0$, then all y_{ijk}'s are independent binary random variables and y_{ij} is a binomial,

$$P(y_{ij}) = \binom{n_{ij}}{y_{ij}} \mu_{ij}^{y_{ij}} (1 - \mu_{ij})^{n_{ij} - y_{ij}}$$

In a binomial or extrabinomial model, the mean function is often modeled by a logit function,

$$\text{logit}(\mu_i \mid z_{ij}) = \beta' z_{ij}$$

The logistic function for the dose-related trend is given by

$$\mu_i = \frac{\exp(\beta_0 + \beta_1 d_i)}{1 + \exp(\beta_0 + \beta_1 d_i)}$$

The logit function can include any additional explanatory variables (e.g., fetal weight or litter size).

Many authors have proposed extrabinomial models based on an exchangeable correlation structure. Kupper and Haseman (1978) derived a correlated binomial model that assumed an equal second-order (pairwise) correlation and all the correlations higher than the order of 2 were 0. Other "generalized" binomial distributions have also been proposed (Altham, 1978; Ochi and Prentice, 1984; Paul, 1987; Bowman and George, 1995). A fundamental relation between a binomial and generalized binomial was given by Bahadur (1961), who showed that the probability density function of a generalized binomial can be expressed as the product of a binomial density and a correction factor,

$$
\begin{aligned}
P(y_{ij}) = C(n_{ij},\mu_i)[1 &+ \sum_{k_1 < k_2} E(W_{ik_1} W_{ik_2}) w_{ik_1} w_{ik_2} \\
&+ \sum_{k_1 < k_2 < k_3} E(W_{ik_1} W_{ik_2} W_{ik_3}) w_{ik_1} w_{ik_2} w_{ik_3} \\
&+ E(W_{ij1} \cdots W_{ijn_{ij}}) w_{ij1} \cdots w_{ijn_{ij}}]
\end{aligned}
$$

where $C(n_{ij}, \mu_i)$ is the density of the binomial distribution with parameters n_{ij} and μ_i, and $W_{ijk} = (y_{ijk} - \mu_i)/[\mu_i(1 - \mu_i)]^{1/2}$.

The correlated binomial and multivariate probit models have not been widely used in practice because their maximum likelihood estimates are difficult to compute. A traditional approach to modeling the extrabinomial variation data is the beta-binomial model.

A. Beta-Binomial Model

The beta-binomial distribution was proposed by Williams (1975) to modeling the litter effect. The beta-binomial model assumes that responses within the same litter occur according to a binomial distribution and the probability of responses is assumed to vary among litters according to a beta distribution:

$$
P(y_{ij}) = \binom{n_{ij}}{y_{ij}} \frac{B(a_i + y_{ij}, b_i + n_{ij} - y_{ij})}{B(a_i,b_i)}
$$

where $B(a_i,b_i) = \Gamma(a_i)\Gamma(b_i)/\Gamma(a_i + b_i)$, where $\Gamma(\cdot)$ is the gamma function, $a_i > 0$, and $b_i > 0$.

The beta-binomial model implicitly assumes an underlying variance–covariance structure for the intracluster correlation induced by the random effects for the distribution of litter-to-litter variation. It can be viewed as an exchangeable model with an infinite cluster (litter) size.

Under the reparameterization $\mu_i = a_i/(a_i + b_i)$ and $\phi_i = (a_i + b_i + 1)^{-1}$, the parameters μ_i and ϕ_i are, respectively, the mean and the intralitter correlation parameters in the ith group. That is, the mean of y_{ij} is $E(y_{ij}) = n_{ij}\mu_i$, and the intralitter correlation is $\text{Corr}(y_{ijk}, y_{ijk'}) = \phi_i$. The variance of y_{ij} is $\text{Var}(y_{ij}) = [\phi_i(n_{ij} - 1) + 1][n_{ij}\mu_i(1 - \mu_i)]$. When $\phi_i = 0$, then y_{ij} becomes a binomial variable.

The parameters can be estimated by the maximum likelihood method. Ignoring the terms involving only the observations, the log-likelihood function of a beta-binomial is given by

$$
L \propto \sum_{i=0}^{g} \sum_{j=0}^{m_i} \left[\sum_{k=0}^{y_{ij}-1} \log\left(\mu_i + k\frac{\phi_i}{1 - \phi_i}\right) + \sum_{k=0}^{n_{ij}-y_{ij}-1} \right.
$$

$$
\log\left(1 - \mu_i + k\frac{\phi_i}{1 - \phi_i}\right) + \sum_{k=0}^{n_{ij}-1}
$$

$$
\left. \log\left(1 + k\frac{\phi_i}{1 - \phi_i}\right)\right]
$$

The maximum likelihood estimates (MLE) are obtained by solving the equation $\partial L/\partial \mu_i = 0$ (or $\partial L/\partial \beta_l = 0$) and $\partial L/\partial \phi_i = 0$, $i = 1, 2, \ldots g$. The MLEs cannot be represented in a closed form; the Newton–Raphson method is used to solve the system of nonlinear equations. The likelihood ratio test is often used to test for the significance of parameters. A general discussion about the beta-binomial likelihood ratio tests was described by Crowder (1978). An alternative test is to compute the Wald statistic directly from a fitted model. However, the likelihood ratio test is preferable.

An advantage of the use of the likelihood-based beta-binomial model is that the litter effect (i.e., $\phi_i = 0$ vs. $\phi_i > 0$) can be tested directly by either the likelihood ratio or Wald test. However, one problem with the beta-binomial model is the bias and instability of the maximum likelihood estimates of the coefficients as noted by Kupper et al. (1986), Williams (1982, 1987, 1988), and Liang and Hanfelt (1994). Williams (1982) proposed a quasi-likelihood approach as an alternative to the beta-binomial model.

B. Quasi-Likelihood Model

Several authors have proposed using the quasi-likelihood procedure to analyze developmental toxicity data (Williams, 1987, 1988; Lefkopoulou et al., 1989; Ryan, 1993; Chen and Li, 1994). In the quasi-likelihood approach, only assumptions on the mean and variance are required:

$$E(y_{ij} \mid n_{ij}) = n_{ij}\mu_i$$

and

$$\text{Var}(y_{ij} \mid n_{ij}) = n_{ij}\mu_i(1 - \mu_i)[\phi_i(n_{ij} - 1) + 1]$$

The coefficients of the β's can be obtained by solving the quasi-likelihood estimating (score) equations:

$$S(\beta_l) = \sum_{i=1}^{g} \sum_{j=1}^{m_i} z_{ijl} \frac{y_{ij} - n_{ij}\mu_i}{[1 + (n_{ij} - 1)\phi_i]} = 0, l = 1, \dots, p$$

The intralitter correlation coefficients are calculated by equating with the mean of Pearson χ^2 statistics; that is

$$\phi_i = \frac{1}{n_i - p} \sum_{j=1}^{m_i} \frac{(y_{ij} - n_{ij}\mu_i)^2}{n_{ij}\mu_i(1 - \mu_i)[\phi_i^{-1} + (n_{ij} - 1)]}$$

where $n_i = \sum_j^{m_i} n_{ij}$. The parameters β's and ϕ's are estimated by solving $S(\beta_k) = 0$ and ϕ_i alternately until convergence. In the quasi-likelihood estimation, the intralitter correlations typically are either modeled as constant across groups, or they are not modeled at all. If the intralitter correlation parameters are constant then

$$\phi = \frac{1}{N - p} \sum_{i=1}^{g} \sum_{j=1}^{m_i} \frac{(y_{ij} - n_{ij}\mu_i)^2}{n_{ij}\mu_i(1 - \mu_i)[\phi_i^{-1} + (n_{ij} - 1)]}$$

where $N = \sum_i^g \sum_j^{m_i} n_{ij}$. The Wald test is often used to test for the significance of parameters. Recently, several authors have proposed the quasi-likelihood score tests.

Paul and Islam (1995) recently proposed a $C(\alpha)$ or score statistic for testing homogeneity. The score statistic under the null hypothesis is given by

$$X_s \sum_{i=1}^{g} \frac{\{\sum_j (x_{ij} - n_{ij}\bar{\mu})[1 + (n_{ij} - 1)\phi_i]^{-1}\}^2}{\bar{\mu}(1 - \bar{\mu})\sum_j n_{ij}[1 + (n_{ij} - 1)\phi_i]^{-1}}$$

where $\bar{\mu}$ is the estimate of μ computed under the null hypothesis of homogeneity ($\mu_1 = \cdots = \mu_g$). Under the null hypothesis, X_s has an approximate χ^2 distribution with $g - 1$ degrees of freedom.

Chen (1993a) and Ryan (1993) proposed a score statistic for a dose-related trend test

$$Z_s = \frac{\sum_{i=1}^{g} (y_i - n_i\bar{\mu})d_i}{[\sum_{i=1}^{g} (d_i - \bar{d})^2 n_i\bar{\mu}(1 - \bar{\mu})]^{1/2}}$$

where $\bar{\mu}$ is the estimate of μ computed under the null hypothesis of no dose–response trend ($\beta = 0$), and $\bar{d} = (\sum_i \sum_j n_{ij}d_i)/(\sum_i \sum_j n_{ij})$. Under the null hypothesis, the statistic Z_s has an asymptotic normal distribution. Note that under the binomial model, the score test becomes the Cochran–Armitage trend test (Cochran, 1954; Armitage, 1955). This test has been the most powerful unbiased test against certain alternatives (Cox, 1958; Tarone and Gart, 1980).

The score test has an advantage over the Wald test because it is simple to compute. Unlike the Wald test statistic, the score test does not require a fit of the full model, which may sometimes fail to converge in estimating the coefficients of the link function. Brooks (1984) proposed an approximate likelihood ratio test for the quasi-likelihood analysis.

C. Related Results

Chen et al. (1994) and Paul and Islam (1995) conducted simulation studies comparing score test of homogeneity among the quasi-likelihood (Wedderburn, 1974), extended quasi-likelihood (Nelder and Pregibon, 1987), pseudo-likelihood (Carroll and Ruppert, 1982), beta-binomial likelihood, and Rao and Scott (1992) approaches. Paul and Islam (1995) recommended the quasi-likelihood score test. The Chen et al. (1994) simulation result showed that when the intralitter correlations were large or were heterogeneous among dose groups, the Wald test performed better than the score test. Moreover, the extended quasi-likelihood approach was the least favorable when μ was close to 0 or 1. In the same simulation, Chen et al. (1994) compared the model-based and robust variance estimators among the quasi-likelihood, extended quasi-likelihood, and pseudo-likelihood. They found that the model-based quasi-likelihood approach performed the best in maintaining the nominal level and the robust variance estimator performed poorly when the sample size was small.

Chen (1993a) and Fung et al. (1994) conducted simulation studies comparing several trend test procedures. They showed that all tests properly controlled the type I error rate and in the meantime maintained the power of detecting the dose effect even under the binomial model. In another simulation, Carr and Portier (1993) found that the Wald test based on the quasi-likelihood method was often more powerful than the likelihood ratio test based on the beta-binomial model when the intralitter correlations were heterogeneous.

The parameter for the extrabinomial variation in the variance function is expressed in terms of the intralitter correlation ϕ_i. A simpler model is to parameterize the extravariation in terms of the variance function directly; the variance of y_{ij} has the form

$$\text{Var}(y_{ij}) = \kappa n_{ij}\mu_i(1 - \mu_i)$$

Note that κ is no longer dependent on n_{ij}. Under the binomial model or when all n_{ij}'s are equal, this model is equivalent to the intralitter correlation structure model; that is, $\kappa = [1 + (n - 1)\phi]$. This model has been discussed by many authors (Lefkopoulou et al., 1989; McCullagh and Nelder, 1989). More recently, Liang and McCullagh (1994) has recommended that both models be adopted in seeking appropriate variance expression. This model provides the simplest approach to model the extrabinomial data, and it is computationally attractive.

Finally, it has been observed that the intralitter correlation may vary with dose. Kupper et al. (1986) concluded that when intralitter correlations were dose-dependent, the use of a common intralitter correlation in the beta-binomial model fitting might lead to bias in the estimation of dose–response coefficients. They suggested fitting a different intralitter correlations model to avoid the bias. However, Williams (1988) noted that the estimates obtained from the saturated correlation model, in which a different correlation parameter was fitted to each dose group, might not be reliable. Liang and Hanfelt (1994), who found that the bias and coverage probability for coefficients could still be substantial even when the saturated correlation model was fitted, recommended using the quasi-likelihood method with the constant correlation model when the number of litters was small or modest. It is generally true that fitting a separate intralitter correlation model tends to reduce the rejection rate (power) when the intracluster correlations have dispersion. A saturated correlation model that uses either the beta-binomial or quasi-likelihood does not perform well in terms of coverage probability, and may have convergence difficulty when sample sizes are small or modest. Bowman et al. (1995) proposed a logistic dose–response model to fit the intralitter correlations. This model provided an alternative to the constant correlation and saturated correlation models.

D. Example: Hydroxyurea Data

A study, conducted at the National Center for Toxicological Research, on developmental effects resulting from exposure to hydroxyurea in mice was used for illustration. The experiment consisted of four treatment groups, 0, 150, 200, and 250 ppm. Table 1 shows the frequency table of females according to the numbers of implants (n_{ij}), deaths/resorptions (y_{ij}), and malformations (x_{ij}). The probabilities of death/resorption (μ) and malformation (ξ) were considered in the example, but only the analysis for death/resorption was described in detail. Table 2 contains the means and standard errors from litter-based analysis, fetus-based analysis (binomial model), and the beta-binomial model. Note that fetus-based analysis is based on the likelihood-based binomial model. In the beta-binomial model, the mean parameters and intralitter correlation parameters were estimated by fitting a separate beta-binomial distribution to each group.

The mean estimates from the three procedures were close, but the standard errors based on the binomial model were much smaller than those based on the litter-based analysis and beta-binomial model, except

TABLE 1   The Trinomial Observations of (y) Dead/Resorbed Fetuses, (x) Malformations, and (n) Implantation Sites, Per Litter Following Exposure to Hydroxyurea, BAHC

Control	(y)	0	0	0	0	2	0	1	1	0	0	1	0	0	0	0	0	1
	(x)	0	0	0	0	0	0	0	0	0	0	0	0	0	0	0	0	0
	(n)	10	10	12	13	11	9	9	12	11	8	11	13	12	6	8	11	9
150 ppm	(y)	1	0	0	5	1	0	2	2	1	0	2	1	0				
	(x)	0	0	0	0	0	2	0	2	0	0	4	0	0				
	(n)	14	11	11	8	12	8	11	10	12	14	13	7	9				
200 ppm	(y)	2	0	12	9	12	5	3	3									
	(x)	0	0	1	0	0	5	1	0									
	(n)	14	11	16	11	13	13	13	11									
250 ppm	(y)	7	8	6	10	7	3	4	9	7	4	11	5	10	10	6	8	6
	(x)	1	3	1	0	2	1	0	0	1	1	0	4	0	0	0	1	3
	(n)	9	11	11	11	11	11	9	10	8	5	12	12	12	11	11	13	12
	(y)	8	11	2	11	2												
	(x)	0	0	4	0	1												
	(n)	9	12	10	12	9												

TABLE 2 The Maximum Likelihood Estimates with Standard Error Under the Binomial Model and beta-Binomal Model

Endpoint	Model	Parameter	0	100	200	250
Deaths/resorption	Litter-based	μ	0.034 (0.014)	0.119 (0.047)	0.440 (0.122)	0.671 (0.052)
	Binomial	μ	0.034 (0.014)	0.107 (0.026)	0.451 (0.054)	0.671 (0.031)
	beta-Binomial	μ	0.034 (0.014)	0.115 (0.039)	0.440 (0.107)	0.669 (0.049)
		ϕ	0.002 (0.040)	0.103 (0.085)	0.332 (0.125)	0.158 (0.060)
Malformation	Litter-based	ξ	0.0	0.066 (0.036)	0.122 (0.078)	0.284 (0.076)
	Binomial	ξ	0.0	0.064 (0.022)	0.125 (0.044)	0.303 (0.053)
	beta-Binomial	ξ	0.0	0.062 (0.039)	0.131 (0.077)	0.300 (0.064)
		θ	0.0	0.271 (0.194)	0.294 (0.200)	0.120 (0.119)

for the 0 ppm group. The estimated intralitter correlations for the four groups were 0.002, 0.103, 0.332, and 0.128. All three dosed groups showed evidences of overbinomial variations. The maximum values of the log-likelihood for dose 0, 150, 200, and 250 ppm, respectively, were -26.13, -45.76, -57.27, and -137.71 under the beta-binomial model, and were -26.13, -47.67, -70.21, and -146.33 under the binomial model. The likelihood ratio χ^2 tests for extrabinomial variation from the litter effect for the 200 and 250 ppm groups were significant.

The three hypotheses: homogeneity, pairwise comparisons with control, and trend tests were conducted using the litter-based analysis, beta-binomial, and quasi-likelihood approaches. In the analysis, the beta-binomial model assumed separate intralitter correlations in each group, and the quasi-likelihood approach assumed a constant intralitter correlation model. Table 3 contains the summary of the analyses.

In the litter-based analysis, the proportions were transformed by an angular transformation for normalization and variance stabilization. The analysis of variance F test for homogeneity was 38.86 with 3 and 56 degrees of freedom. For comparisons between the control and each dose group, the t_{56} values were 1.637 (0 versus 150 ppm), 5.070 (0 versus 200 ppm), and 9.962 (0 versus 250 ppm). In the linear regression analysis for test of trend, the t_{58} value was 10.32.

In the beta-binomial model, the maximum value of the log-likelihood was $L_{\max} = (-26.13) + (-45.76) + (-57.27) + (-137.71) = -266.87$. The maximized log-likelihood under the homogeneity constraint was 298.11. The likelihood ratio χ_3^2 statistic for homogeneity was $2(298.11 - 266.87) = 62.48$. For paired comparisons between control and dosed groups, the likelihood ratio statistics were computed separately in each comparison. The z values (converted from the χ^2 values) are 2.244 (0 versus 150 ppm), 4.274 (0 versus 200 ppm), and 6.178 (0 versus 250 ppm). The Wald test statistics were computed by fitting the full model. The χ_3^2 statistic for homogeneity was 91.92. The z values for pairwise comparisons between control and the three dose groups were 2.272, 5.141, and 8.531. The trend test statistics were computed by fitting the logistic dose–response function, the likelihood ratio test had a z value of 7.020 and the Wald test had a value of 7.819.

In the quasi-likelihood analysis, the score χ_3^2 statistic for homogeneity was 38.64. The score statistics were computed separately for each paired comparison between control and dose group. The z values were 1.632, 3.530, and 5.263. The z values for the trend statistic was 5.563. The Wald statistics were computed by fitting the full model. The χ_3^2

TABLE 3 The Test Statistics for the Parametric Litter-Based, beta-Binomial, and Quasi-Likelihood Approaches Computed Under the Three Null Hypotheses

Endpoint	Procedures	Homogeneity	$\mu_1 = \mu_2$	$\mu_1 = \mu_3$	$\mu_1 = \mu_4$	Trend
			Control vs. dose			
Deaths/resorption	Litter-based analysis[a]	38.86	1.637	5.070	9.962	10.32
	beta-Binomial[b,c]	62.48	2.245	4.275	6.179	7.020
	beta-Binomial[b,d]	91.92	2.272	5.141	8.531	7.819
	Quasi-likelihood[b,e]	38.64	1.632	3.530	5.263	5.563
	Quasi-likelihood[b,d]	56.07	1.621	4.127	5.727	6.163
Malformation	Litter-based analysis[a]	5.43	0.938	1.356	3.873	3.908
	beta-Binomial[b,c]	14.42	1.346	1.854	3.199	3.780
	beta-Binomial[b,d]	27.79	1.584	1.705	4.731	2.970
	Quasi-likelihood[b,e]	15.41	2.023	2.252	3.316	2.989
	Quasi-likelihood[b,d]	10.52	1.775	1.354	2.362	4.192

[a]The column under homogeneity represents an F value, other columns represent t scores.
[b]The column under homogeneity represents a χ^2 value, other columns represent z scores.
[c]Likelihood ratio test.
[d]Wald test.
[e]Score test.

statistic for homogeneity test was 56.07. The z values for the paired comparisons were 1.621, 4.127, and 5.727. The Wald test for the dose-related trend was 6.163.

IV. ANALYSIS OF TRINOMIAL RESPONSES

Two frequently used developmental toxicity endpoints are the proportion of deaths/resorptions and the proportion of malformations. Additionally, the proportion of deaths/resorptions/malformations measures the total reproductive and developmental effects of a test substance. The standard approach has been based on the analysis of the three endpoints independently.

Let y_{ij} and x_{ij}, respectively, represent the number of deaths/resorptions, and the number of malformation (in live fetuses) among the n_{ij}, then $(x_{ij} + y_{ij})$ is the number of affected fetuses and $(n_{ij} - x_{ij} - y_{ij})$ is the number of normal fetuses. Assume that y_{ij} has the beta-binomial

$$P(y_{ij}) = \binom{n_{ij}}{y_{ij}} \frac{B(a_i + y_{ij}, w_i + n_{ij} - y_{ij})}{B(a_i, w_i)}$$

and conditional on y_{ij} (equivalently, on $n_{ij} - y_{ij}$), x_{ij} has the beta-binomial

$$P(x_{ij} \mid y_{ij}) = \binom{n_{ij} - y_{ij}}{x_{ij}} \frac{B(b_i + y_{ij}, c_i + n_{ij} - y_{ij} - x_{ij})}{B(b_i, c_i)}$$

where $a_i > 0$, $b_i > 0$, $c_i > 0$, and $w_i > 0$. The joint distribution of (x_{ij}, y_{ij}) is the product of the marginal distribution y_{ij} and conditional distribution, $x_{ij} \mid y_{ij}$

$$P(x_{ij}, y_{ij}) = P(y_{ij}) P(x_{ij} \mid y_{ij}).$$

This model is referred to as a doubly beta-binomial model (Chen et al., 1991). Because the distribution of $(x_{ij} + y_{ij})$ is completely determined by the joint distribution $P(x_{ij}, y_{ij})$, it is not appropriate to model the number of affected by a beta-binomial distribution independently. This section described a Dirichlet-trinomial model proposed by Chen et al. (1991) for the analysis of the three endpoints simultaneously.

A. The Dirichlet Trinomial Model

The Dirichlet trinomial model assumes that fetuses within a litter behave independently and the distribution for the numbers of adverse responses

(x_{ij},y_{ij}) follows a trinomial distribution the probability parameters of which vary from litter to litter according to a three-parameter Dirichlet distribution, then the unconditional distribution of (x_{ij},y_{ij}) is a Dirichlet-trinomial,

$$P(x_{ij},y_{ij}) = \binom{n_{ij}}{y_{ij},x_{ij}} \frac{\Gamma(a_i + b_i + c_i)\Gamma(a_i + x_{ij})\Gamma(b_i + y_{ij})\Gamma(c_i + n_{ij} - x_{ij} - y_{ij})}{\Gamma(a_i + b_i + c_i + n_{ij})\Gamma(a_i)\Gamma(b_i)\Gamma(c_i)}$$

The distribution of (x_{ij},y_{ij}) can be expressed as a product of the distribution of the marginal distribution y_{ij} and conditional distribution $x_{ij} \mid y_{ij}$

$$P(x_{ij},y_{ij})$$
$$= \binom{n_{ij}}{y_{ij}} \frac{B(a_i + y_{ij}, w_i + n_{ij} - y_{ij})}{B(a_i,w_i)} \binom{n_{ij} - y_{ij}}{x_{ij}} \frac{B(b_i + y_{ij}, c_i + n_{ij} - y_{ij} - x_{ij})}{B(b_i, c_i)}$$

Therefore, the Dirichlet trinomial model is a special case of the doubly beta-binomial model with the constraint $w_i = b_i + c_i$. In the Dirichlet trinomial model, the responses between fetuses in the same litter (of the same treatment group) have the constant correlation $\phi_i = (a_i + b_i + c_i + 1)^{-1}$. The litter effect is explained by only one parameter. The doubly beta-binomial model contains two intralitter correlations: $(a_i + w_i + 1)^{-1}$ and $(b_i + c_i + 1)^{-1}$. A discussion on the assumptions of these two models was given by Chen et al. (1991) and Chen and Li (1992).

The marginal distribution y_{ij} of the Dirichlet trinomial (y_{ij},x_{ij}) is a beta-binomial with mean and variance

$$E(y_{ij}) = n_{ij}\mu_i \qquad \text{and}$$
$$\text{Var}(y_{ij}) = n_{ij}\mu_i(1 - \mu_i)[\phi_i(n_{ij} - 1) + 1]$$

where $\mu_i = a_i/(a_i + b_i + c_i)$. The conditional distribution $x_{ij} \mid y_{ij}$ is a beta-binomial with mean and variance

$$E(x_{ij} \mid y_{ij}) = (n_{ij} - y_{ij})\xi_i$$

and

$$\text{Var}(x_{ij} \mid y_{ij}) = (n_{ij} - y_{ij})\xi_i(1 - \xi_i)[\phi_i(n_{ij} - y_{ij} - 1) + 1]$$

where $\xi_i = b_i/(b_i + c_i)$. The marginal distribution $(x_{ij} + y_{ij})$ is a beta-binomial with mean and variance

$$E(x_{ij} + y_{ij}) = n_{ij}\eta_i \qquad \text{and}$$
$$\text{Var}(x_{ij} + y_{ij}) = n_{ij}\eta_i(1 - \eta_i)[\phi_i(n_{ij} - 1) + 1]$$

where $\eta_i = (a_i + b_i)/(a_i + b_i + c_i)$. Any two of the three distributions can be used to model the Dirichlet trinomial.

The parameters μ_i, ξ_i, and η_i are the probability for death/resorption, malformation, and death/resorption/malformation (combined toxic effect), respectively. The relation of the three probabilities is

$$\eta_i = \mu_i + (1 - \mu_i)\xi_i$$

The parameters can be estimated by the maximum likelihood method. Ignoring the terms involving only the observations, the log-likelihood function in terms of μ_i and ξ_i is given by

$$
L \propto \sum_{i=0}^{g} \sum_{j=0}^{m_i} \left[\sum_{k=0}^{y_{ij}-1} \log\left(\mu_i + k\frac{\phi_i}{1-\phi_i}\right) \right.
$$
$$
+ \sum_{k=0}^{x_{ij}-1} \log\left\{ (1-\mu_i)\xi_i + k\frac{\phi_i}{1-\phi_i}\right\}
$$
$$
+ \sum_{k=0}^{n_{ij}-y_{ij}-1} \log\left\{ (1-\mu_i)(1-\xi_i) + k\frac{\phi_i}{1-\phi_i}\right\}
$$
$$
\left. + \sum_{k=0}^{n-1} \log\left(1 + k\frac{\phi_i}{1-\phi_i}\right) \right]
$$

The log- likelihood function can also be expressed in terms of μ_i and η_i,

$$
L \propto \sum_{i=0}^{g} \sum_{j=0}^{m_i} \left[\sum_{k=0}^{y_{ij}-1} \log\left(\mu_i + k\frac{\phi_i}{1-\phi_i}\right) \right.
$$
$$
+ \sum_{k=0}^{n_{ij}-x_{ij}-z_{ij}-1} \log\left\{ \eta_i + k\frac{\phi_i}{1-\phi_i}\right\}
$$
$$
+ \sum_{k=0}^{y_{ij}-1} \log\left\{ (1-\mu_i-\xi_i) + k\frac{\phi_i}{1-\phi_i}\right\}
$$
$$
\left. + \sum_{k=0}^{n-1} \log\left(1 + k\frac{\phi_i}{1-\phi_i}\right) \right]
$$

The likelihood ratio test or Wald test can be applied to test for the treatment effects. Additionally, the goodness-of-fit for the Dirichlet trinomial model against the doubly beta-binomial model can be tested using the likelihood ratio test.

B. Quasi-Likelihood Model

Assume that the mean and variance of the proportion of deaths/resorptions y_{ij}/n_{ij} are

$$E\left(\frac{y_{ij}}{n_{ij}}\right) = \mu_i \qquad \text{and}$$

$$Var\left(\frac{y_{ij}}{n_{ij}}\right) = \frac{\mu_i(1 - \mu_i)}{n_{ij}}[\phi_i(n_{ij} - 1) + 1]$$

Further assume that $n_{ij} > y_{ij}$. Conditional on y_{ij}, the mean for the proportion of malformations $x_{ij}/(n_{ij} - y_{ij}) \mid y_{ij}$ is

$$E\left(\frac{x_{ij}}{n_{ij} - y_{ij}} \mid y_{ij}\right) = \xi_i$$

and the conditional variance is

$$Var\left(\frac{x_{ij}}{n_{ij} - y_{ij}} \mid y_{ij}\right) = \frac{\xi_i(1 - \xi_i)}{n_{ij} - y_{ij}}\left[\frac{\phi_i(n_{ij} - y_{ij} - 1)}{1 - \mu_i + \mu_i\phi_i} + 1\right]$$

The conditional variance can be expressed as

$$Var\left(\frac{x_{ij}}{n_{ij} - y_{ij}} \mid y_{ij}\right) = \frac{\xi_i(1 - \xi_i)}{h_{ij}}\left[\frac{\phi_i(h_{ij} - 1)}{1 - \mu_i + \mu_i\phi_i} + 1\right],$$

where $h_{ij}^{-1} = h_{ij}^{-1} = (n_{ij} - y_{ij})^{-1}$. The expectation of $(n_{ij} - y_{ij})^{-1}$ is

$$E\left(\frac{1}{n_{ij} - y_{ij}}\right) = \frac{1}{n_{ij}}E\left[1 + \frac{y_{ij}}{n_{ij}} + \cdots\right] \simeq \frac{1 + \mu_i}{n_{ij}}$$

Therefore, the first-order approximation for the unconditional variance is by replacing h_{ij} with $n'_{ij} = n_{ij}/(1 + \mu_i) > 1$. That is

$$Var\left(\frac{x_{ij}}{n_{ij} - y_{ij}}\right) = \frac{\xi_i(1 - \xi_i)}{n'_{ij}}\left[\frac{\phi_i(n'_{ij} - 1)}{1 - \mu_i + \mu_i\phi_i} + 1\right]$$

Note that when $n_{ij} = 1$ and $\mu_i > 0$, $n_{ij}/(1 + \mu_i) < 1$. In these cases, n'_{ij} will be set to 1. That is, when the litter size is one, the Bernoulli variance for x_{ij} is assumed. Moreover, let the correlation coefficient between y_{ij}/n_{ij} and $x_{ij}/(n_{ij} - y_{ij})$ be

$$Corr\left(\frac{y_{ij}}{n_{ij}}, \frac{x_{ij}}{n_{ij} - y_{ij}}\right) = \rho_i$$

The mean and the variance functions given in the quasi-likelihood model were based on the same relation between the mean and variance under the parametric model. The correlation between death/resorption and malformation is zero under the parametric model. But, the quasi-likelihood model allows for a nonzero correlation coefficients between the two endpoints. The correlation is set to be zero if an independence between the proportion of deaths/resorptions and the proportion of malformations is assumed.

The parameters in the quasi-likelihood model consist of the mean parameters, which include the coefficients in the mean functions, the intralitter correlation ϕ, and the correlation coefficients between the two proportions ρ. The mean parameters are estimated by solving the quasi-score equations. If we assume a homogeneous intralitter correlation across all groups, the intralitter correlation is estimated by

$$
\phi = \frac{1}{M + M' - 4} \sum_{i=1}^{g} \sum_{j=1}^{m_i} \frac{(y_{ij}/n_{ij} - \mu_i)^2}{\mu_i(1 - \mu_i)[\phi^{-1} + (n_{ij} - 1)]/n_{ij}},
$$

$$
+ \sum_{i=1}^{g} \sum_{j=1}^{m_i} \frac{[x_{ij}/(n_{ij} - y_{ij}) - \xi_i]^2}{\xi_i(1 - \xi_i)[\phi_i^{-1} + (1 - \mu_i + \mu_i\phi)^{-1}(n'_{ij} - 1)]/n'_{ij}},
$$

where $N = \Sigma_i^g \Sigma_j^{m_i} n_{ij}$ and M' is the total number of litters with at least one living fetuses. The parameters for the correlation coefficients can be estimated from the cross product of the standardized residuals,

$$
\rho = \frac{1}{M'} \sum_{i=1}^{g} \sum_{j=1}^{m_i} \frac{\left(\frac{y_{ij}}{n_{ij}} - \mu_i\right)\left(\frac{x_{ij}}{n_{ij} - y_{ij}} - \xi_i\right)}{\sqrt{\left[\frac{\mu_i(1 - \mu_i)}{n_{ij}}\{\phi(n_{ij} - 1) + 1\}\right]\left[\frac{\xi_i(1 - \xi_i)}{n'_{ij}}\left(\frac{\phi(n'_{ij} - 1)}{1 - \mu_i + \mu_i\phi_i} + 1\right)\right]}}
$$

C. Example: Hydroxyurea Data

The hydroxyurea data considered in the preceding section were used for illustration. The product–moment correlation coefficients between the proportion of malformation and proportion of death/resorption were 0, 0.013, 0.041, and -0.105. The data showed no evidence of association between the two proportions. In the analysis, the two proportions were modeled using the parametric doubly beta-binomial and Dirichlet trinomial models, and the quasi-likelihood approach under both doubly beta-binomial and Dirichlet trinomial models. In the quasi-likelihood analysis, the correlation coefficient between the two proportions were assumed to be zero.

The maximum likelihood estimates (MLEs) of the parameters were obtained by fitting separate Dirichlet trinomial distributions to the four treatment groups. The parameter estimates (with standard deviations) are

$$\mu_1 = 0.034(0.031), \mu_2 = 0.126(0.044),$$
$$\mu_3 = 0.428(0.100), \mu_4 = 0.664(0.045)$$

$$\xi_1 = 0.0(0.), \xi_2 = 0.054(0.030),$$
$$\xi_3 = 0.152(0.085), \xi_4 = 0.312(0.072)$$

$$\phi_1 = 0.002(0.069), \phi_2 = 0.155(0.082),$$
$$\phi_3 = 0.293(0.101), \phi_4 = 0.118(0.045)$$

By using the equality $\eta_i = \mu_i(1 - \xi_i)$, the MLEs for the η's were

$$\eta_1 = 0.034(0.031), \eta_2 = 0.173(0.051),$$
$$\eta_3 = 0.515(0.100), \eta_4 = 0.769(0.040)$$

These estimates can also be obtained by directly maximizing the log-likelihood for μ's and η given in Section IV.A.

Under the Dirichlet trinomial model, the MLEs for μ's, ξ's, η's, and ϕ's are unique. Under the beta-binomial model, the MLEs for μ's and ϕ_μ's, and ξ's and ϕ_ξ's were given in Table 2. The MLEs for η's and ϕ_η using a third beta-binomial model were

$$\eta_1 = 0.343(0.014), \eta_2 = 0.172(0.053),$$
$$\eta_3 = 0.490(0.111), \eta_4 = 0.770(0.040)$$

$$\phi_1 = 0.002(0.040), \phi_2 = 0.176(0.097),$$
$$\phi_3 = 0.357(0.125), \phi_4 = 0.114(0.057)$$

The estimates of η's did not appear to satisfy the probability constraint $\eta_i = \mu_i + (1 - \mu_i)\xi_i$, which the Dirichlet trinomial model ensures. In the beta-binomial model, each toxicity endpoint in a treatment group has its own estimates of the probabilities of response and the intralitter correlations. In each group, six parameters are estimated under the beta-binomial, but only three parameters are estimated under the Dirichlet trinomial.

The Dirichlet trinomial model is a doubly beta-binomial model, with the linear constraint $w_i = b_i + c_i$. The likelihood ratio can be used to test whether there is a significant lack of fit on this constraint. The maxima of the log-likelihood for death/resorption and malformation under the doubly beta-binomial were -26.13, -70.74, -74.38, and -183.54 for 0, 150, 200, and 250 ppm, respectively; the sum of the log-likelihood values was -354.79. The maxima of the log-likelihoods for the four groups under the Dirichlet trinomial model were -26.13, -71.06, -74.60, and -184.53; the sum of the log-likelihood values was -356.32. The likelihood ratio χ_1^2 statistics for the Dirichlet trinomial model against the doubly beta-binomial model were 0, 0.64, 0.24, and 1.98 for the four groups. Thus, the Dirichlet trinomial model fitted the data as well as the doubly beta-binomial for all four groups.

Logistic dose–response models for death/resorption and malformation were further fitted under both doubly beta-binomial and Dirichlet trinomial models. The logistic dose–response models for μ_i and ξ_i are

$$\mu_i = \frac{\exp(\beta_0 + \beta_1 d_i)}{1 + \exp(\beta_0 + \beta_1 d_i)}$$

and

$$\xi_i = \frac{\exp(\alpha_0 + \alpha_1 d_i)}{1 + \exp(\alpha_0 + \alpha_1 d_i)}$$

The parametric analysis assumed different intralitter correlations for different groups, and the quasi-likelihood analysis assumed a constant intralitter correlation for all groups.

In the parametric analysis, the maximum value of log-likelihood was -357.97 under the doubly beta-binomial model, and was -359.25 under the Dirichlet trinomial model. (The Dirichlet trinomial model fitted the data as well as the doubly beta-binomial.) The likelihood ratio test of whether the logistic dose–response function differs from the full-saturated model was not significant under either the doubly beta-binomial or the Dirichlet trinomial model.

The estimates of (β_0, β_1) and (α_0, α_1) and their estimated standard errors were

1. Parametric analysis under doubly beta-binomial model

$\beta_0 = -3.70(0.478), \beta_1 = 0.017(0.0022)$
$\alpha_0 = -6.39(1.256), \alpha_1 = 0.022(0.0054)$

2. Parametric analysis under Dirichlet trinomial model

$\beta_0 = -3.77(0.476), \beta_1 = 0.017(0.0022)$
$\alpha_0 = -6.25(1.226), \alpha_1 = 0.022(0.0056)$

3. Quasi-likelihood analysis under doubly beta-binomial model

$\beta_0 = -4.42(0.754), \beta_1 = 0.020(0.0035)$
$\alpha_0 = -5.70(1.329), \alpha_1 = 0.019(0.0058)$

4. Quasi-likelihood analysis under Dirichlet trinomial model

$\beta_0 = -4.42(0.704), \beta_1 = 0.020(0.0032)$
$\alpha_0 = -5.78(1.315), \alpha_1 = 0.019(0.0058)$

In testing for dose-related trend, the Wald test statistic gave a χ_2^2 value of 76.84 under the Dirichlet trinomial model and of 77.94 under the double beta-binomial model. In the quasi-likelihood analysis, the χ_2^2 were 44.67 and 50.04 under the Dirichlet trinomial and double beta-binomial variation, respectively.

In this example, the correlation coefficient between the proportion of death/resorption and proportion of malformations were assumed to be zero. An example in which the two proportions had a nonzero correlation coefficient was presented by Chen and Li (1994).

V. ANALYSIS OF COUNTS

Statistical procedures for the evaluation of reproductive and developmental toxicity effects generally focus on the analysis of proportion data. Methods for the analysis of count data have seldom been discussed. One reason for the lack of attention is that the commonly used segment II design, in which a test substance is administered after implantation, considers the proportion, rather than the number of deaths/resorptions per litter, because the proportion is a better measure of developmental effects. However, in some reproductive experiments, the primary endpoints of interest can be the count variable. In ovarian toxicity studies, female animals are treated with a test compound. Animals are humanely killed at the end of experiment; the number of follicles are counted to determine if the compound induces changes in ovarian follicle count. A reduction in follicle count would be an indication of destruction of reproductive capacity. In a dominant lethal assay, male mice are treated with a suspect mutagen, and then are mated with females. In addition to the incidences of deaths/resorptions and malformations, the number of implantations and number of corpora lutea are also an important index for measuring developmental toxicity effects. The distribution of the number of implants or the number of corpora lutea has commonly been assumed to be approximately normal. But count data are generally modeled under a Poisson assumption (e.g., Frome et al., 1973). Rai and Van Ryzin (1985) had used a Poisson distribution to model the distribution of implantations.

Let n_{ij} be an observed count from the jth animal in the ith group $1 < i < g$ and $1 < j < m_i$. If n_{ij} has the Poisson distribution

$$p(n_{ij}) = \frac{\mu_i^{n_{ij}} e^{-\mu_i}}{n_{ij}!}, n_{ij} = 0,1,2 \ldots$$

the mean and variance of n_{ij} are

$$E(n_{ij}) = \text{Var}(n_{ij}) = \mu_i$$

In the Poisson model, the mean function is often modeled by a log-linear function,

$$\log(\mu_i \mid z_{ij}) = z_{ij}\beta$$

The dose–response model to test for trend is

$$\mu_i = \exp(\beta_0 + \beta_1 d_i)$$

A common complication in the analysis of count data is that the observed variation often exceed or falls behind the variation that is predicted from a Poisson model. The conventional approach to the extra-variation is to assume that the mean of the Poisson has a gamma distribution that leads to a negative binomial (gamma-Poisson) distribution for the observed data (e.g., Margolin et al., 1981; Lawless, 1987). Other parametric models such as Poisson-lognormal (e.g., Hinde, 1982) and Poisson-inverse-gaussian (e.g., Dean et al., 1989) have also been proposed. Breslow (1984) proposed a quasi-likelihood method as an alternative to the parametric models. This section describes the negative binomial model and quasi-likelihood approach to analyzing the count data.

A. Negative Binomial Model

Assume that n_{ij} is a Poisson with mean λ_i, and λ_i itself is also a random variable with mean μ_i and variance of the form $\phi_i\mu_i^2$, then the unconditional mean and variance of n_{ij} are

$$E(n_{ij}) = \mu_i$$

and

$$\text{Var}(n_{ij}) = \mu_i + \mu_i^2\phi_i = \mu_i(1 + \phi_i\mu_i)$$

If $\phi_i > 0$, then n_{ij} has an extra-Poisson variation; if $\phi_i < 0$, then n_{ij} has a sub-Poisson variation; if $\phi_i = 0$, then n_{ij} becomes a Poisson. In particular, if λ_i has a gamma-distribution with the shape parameter $1/\phi_i$ and scale parameter $\phi_i\mu_i$, then n_{ij} has a negative binomial distribution,

$$p(n_{ij}) = \frac{\Gamma(n_{ij} + \phi_i^{-1})}{\Gamma(n_{ij} + 1)\Gamma(\phi_i^{-1})}\left(\frac{\phi_i\mu_i}{1 + \phi_i\mu_i}\right)^{n_{ij}}\left(\frac{1}{1 + \phi_i\mu_i}\right)^{1/\phi_i}$$

where $\phi_i > 0$. Ignoring the terms involving only observations, the log-likelihood of a negative binomial is

$$L = \sum_{i=1}^{g} \sum_{j=1}^{m_i} \left[n_{ij}\log(\mu_i) - (n_{ij} + \phi_i^{-1})\log(1 + \phi_i\mu_i) \right.$$
$$\left. + \sum_{k=0}^{n_{ij}-1} \log(1 + k\phi_i) \right]$$

The maximum likelihood estimation of the negative binomial model was described in details by Lawless (1987). The significance of the parameters can be tested using either the likelihood ratio test or Wald test. The negative binomial model can be applied to testing for the extra-Poisson variation (i.e., $\phi_i = 0$ vs. $\phi_i > 0$).

Similar to the beta-binomial model, the maximum likelihood estimation of a negative binomial model may be computationally unstable. But, the main limitation of the parametric approach is in its restriction on $\phi \geq 0$. Unlike the proportions of death/resorption, which often exhibit an overdispersed binomial variation, the number of litter implant or the number of corpora lutea may exhibit a sub-Poisson variation. The quasi-likelihood approach provides a method to model sub-Poisson variation data.

B. Quasi-Likelihood Model

The quasi-likelihood approach assumes the mean and variance of count data are of a negative binomial form,

$$E(n_{ij}) = \mu_i \qquad \text{and} \qquad \text{Var}(n_{ij}) = \mu_i(1 + \phi_i\mu_i)$$

The parameter ϕ_i under the negative binomial (or any other mixed Poisson model) is restricted to be positive, but ϕ_i is not necessarily positive under the quasi-likelihood model. The lower bound for ϕ_i is $-\mu_i^{-1}$.

The coefficients of the β's can be obtained by solving the score equations

$$S(\beta_l) = \sum_{i=1}^{g} \sum_{j=1}^{m_i} z_{ijl} \frac{n_{ij} - \mu_i}{\mu_i + \phi_i \mu_i^2} = 0$$

The parameters are calculated by equating with the mean of Pearson χ^2 statistics,

$$\phi_i = \frac{1}{n_i - p} \sum_{j=1}^{m_i} \frac{(n_{ij} - \mu_i)^2}{\mu_i \phi_i^{-1} + \mu_i^2}$$

where $n_i = \sum_j^{m_i} n_{ij}$. If the intralitter correlation parameters are constant then

$$\phi = \frac{1}{N - p} \sum_{i=1}^{g} \sum_{j=1}^{m_i} \frac{(n_{ij} - \mu_i)^2}{\mu_i \phi_i^{-1} + \mu_i^2}$$

where $N = \sum_i^g \sum_j^{m_i} n_{ij}$. The parameters β's and ϕ are estimated by solving $S(\beta_k) = 0$ and ϕ alternately until convergence.

C. Related Results

In the quasi-likelihood framework, the variance is generally modeled as a function of the mean up to a multiplicative constant. A simple variance function is

$$\text{Var}(n_{ij}) = \mu_i(1 + \gamma_i)$$

The corresponding negative binomial distribution is

$$p(n_{ij}) = \frac{\Gamma\left(n_{ij} + \frac{\mu_i}{\tau_i}\right)}{\Gamma(n_{ij} + 1)\Gamma(\mu_i/\tau_i)} \left(\frac{\tau_i}{1 + \tau_i}\right)^{n_{ij}} \left(\frac{1}{1 + \tau_i}\right)^{\mu_i/\tau_i}$$

The difference between the two variance models is that the variance M1: $\mu_i(1 + \phi_i\mu_i)$ is quadratic in the mean, whereas the variance M2: $\mu_i(1 + \gamma_i)$ is linear.

Chen and Ahn (1996) conducted a simulation investigating the use of the quasi-likelihood, extended quasi-likelihood, and pseudo-likelihood approach to estimating and testing the mean parameters relative to two variance models M1 and M2. They considered four mixed Poisson models, two negative binomials (Poisson–gamma mixtures), Poisson–lognormal, and Poisson–inverse-gaussian. The simulations showed that all methods performed well in terms of bias. The variances of estimates from the extended quasi-likelihood and pseudo-likelihood methods were generally smaller than the variance from the quasi-likelihood. For the two variance models, model 2 was more efficient and stable in computation, but model 1 performed more efficiently in terms of the variance and controls the type I when the variance was misspecified.

D. Examples

Two examples were given. The first example was the hydroxyurea data considered in the previous sections. In this example, the effect of the hydroxyurea exposure on the number of implants was analyzed. Because the exposure occurred after implantation, it was not expected that the numbers of implants would be different among the four groups. The means and variances for the four groups are

$$\hat{\mu}_1 = 10.29(3.72), \quad \hat{\mu}_2 = 10.76(5.19),$$
$$\hat{\mu}_3 = 12.75(3.07), \quad \hat{\mu}_4 = 10.50(3.21)$$

The means are much larger than the variance. The data exhibited sub-Poisson variation. The negative binomial model was not appropriate.

The number of implants were compared using the litter-based analysis, Poisson model, and quasi-likelihood approach. In the litter-based analysis, the numbers of implants were transformed by a square root transformation for data normalization. The quasi-likelihood analysis assumed a constant intralitter correlation model. Table 4 contains the summary of the analyses. The three approaches gave the same results for the paired comparisons and the trend test at the 5% significance level. But in the test of homogeneity, the quasi-likelihood analysis showed the most power because it adjusted for the sub-Poisson variation.

TABLE 4   The Test Statistics for the Parametric, Poisson, and Quasi-Likelihood Approaches Computed Under the Three Null Hypotheses

		Control vs. dose			
Approach	Homogeneity	$\mu_1 = \mu_2$	$\mu_1 = \mu_3$	$\mu_1 = \mu_4$	Trend
Litter-based analysis[a]	2.88	0.616	2.783	0.332	0.844
Poisson[b]	3.39	0.398	1.717	0.198	0.543
Quasi-likelihood[b]	14.03	0.672	3.299	0.328	0.834

[a]The column under homogeneity represents an F value, other columns represent t scores.
[b]The column under homogeneity represents a χ^2 value, other columns represent z scores.

TABLE 5   The Observed Number of Oocytes per Mice from the Exposure to 9-Aminoacridine (9AA)

Control	149.0	74.0	93.0	62.0	104.0	60.0	89.0	131.0	131.0	16.0
	93.0	96.0	66.0	78.0	49.0	123.0	80.0	101.0	121.0	108.0
Treated	65.0	84.0	89.0	86.0	63.0	102.0	71.0	110.0	110.0	67.0
	45.0	72.0	143.0	75.0	58.0	64.0	110.0	71.0	34.0	80.0

The second example was from an ovarian toxicity experiment reported by Heindel et al. (1989). In this study, CD-1 mice were treated with 9-aminoacridine (9AA). At the end of the experiment, animals were humanely killed and ovaries were removed. The number of small, growing, and antral follicles were counted. Table 5 contains the numbers of growing follicles per ovary for control and treated groups. The means and variances for the two groups were

$$\hat{\mu}_c = 91.2(1025.1), \hat{\mu}_t = 80.0(647.4)$$

The data exhibited extra-Poisson variation because variances are much larger than the means in both groups.

Under the Poisson model, the estimate and the maximized log-likelihood were

$$\hat{\mu}_c = 91.2, \quad \text{and } L_c = 6407.8$$
$$\hat{\mu}_t = 80.0, \quad \text{and } L_t = 5406.9$$

Under the negative binomial model, the estimates and the maximized log-likelihood are

$$\hat{\mu}_c = 91.2, \hat{\phi}_c = 0.147, \text{and } L_c = 6491.9$$
$$\hat{\mu}_t = 80.0, \hat{\phi}_t = 0.084, \text{and } L_t = 5452.6$$

The likelihood ratio χ_1^2 statistic for testing extra-Poisson variation was 168.2 for control and was 91.4 for the treated group. Both tests were highly significant with $p < 0.0001$. The follicle counts between the two groups were compared using the negative binomial model and quasi-likelihood approach.

In the negative binomial model, the estimates under the null hypothesis $H_a: \mu_c = \mu_t = \mu$ were

$$\hat{\mu} = 86.6, \hat{\phi}_c = 0.115, \hat{\phi}_t = 0.088, \text{and } L_{\max} = 11,943.4$$

The likelihood ratio z statistic was $-(2 \times 1.1)^{1/2} = -1.48$ ($p > 0.05$). In the quasi-likelihood analysis, the Wald z statistic was -1.242 ($p > 0.05$) under M1 variance model, and was -1.236 ($p > 0.05$) under M2 model.

For comparison purpose, the estimates under the Poisson model were H_a: $\mu_c = \mu_t = \mu$ where

$$\hat{\mu}_t = 85.6, \quad \text{and} \quad L_1 = 11,807.3$$

The z value based on the likelihood ratio Poisson model was $-(2 \times 7.4)^{1/2} = -3.85$ ($p < 0.01$). In this example, the analysis under the Possion model showed a significance treatment effect because it did not adjust for the extra-Poisson variation.

VI. ANALYSIS OF CONTINUOUS RESPONSES

The common developmental endpoints having continuous measures are the fetal weight or fetal length, or behavioral measurements conducted on an offspring following birth. Statistical procedures for the analysis of continuous fetal data have been considered (Healy, 1972; Dempster et al., 1984; Rosenkranz and Uhl, 1991; Tsai and Hsu, 1993; Chen and Allen, 1995). The general approach to modeling continuous response data is based on a normal mixed model with two variance components for pups and dams (e.g., Dempster et al., 1984). The method proposed by Tsai and Hsu (1993) allowed for the possibility of different variances for pups in different treatment groups. This section reviewed the mixed hierarchical linear model with two levels of variance; the litter effect is modeled by a nested random factor and dosage by a fixed factor.

A. Linear Mixed Effects Model

Let y_{ijk} denote the response from the kth fetus of the jth animal in the ith group. A mixed effects model for fetal weight is given by

$$y_{ijk} = \mu_i + \gamma_{ij} + e_{ijk}$$

where μ_i is the mean of the ith group, γ_{ij} is the deviation of the jth litter in the ith group, and e_{ijk} is the random error. The parameter μ_i represents fixed effects and γ_{ij} represents random effects owing to litter effect. It is commonly assumed that the random components γ_{ij} and e_{ijk} are independently normally distributed with

$$E(\gamma_{ij}) = 0, \text{Var}(\gamma_{ij}) = \sigma_f^2$$

and

$$E(e_{ijk}) = 0, \text{Var}(e_{ijk}) = \sigma^2$$

Thus, the mean and variance of y_{ijk} are

$$E(y_{ijk}) = \mu_i, \text{Var}(y_{ijk}) = \sigma_f^2 + \sigma^2$$

The (intralitter) correlation between y_{ijk} and $y_{ijk'}$, for $k \neq k'$ is

$$\phi = \frac{\sigma_f^2}{\sigma^2 + \sigma_f^2}$$

The intralitter correlation is assumed constant across dose groups. Rewrite the fetal weight model in a matrix form:

$$y_{ij} = z_{ij}\beta + \gamma_{ij}\mathbf{1} + e_{ij}$$

where

$y_{ij} = (y_{ij1}, \ldots, y_{ijn_{ij}})'$ is an n_{ij} vector of responses.
z_{ij} is a known $n_{ij} \times p$ design matrix.
$\beta = (\beta_1, \ldots, \beta_p)'$ is a $p \times 1$ vector of fixed effect parameters (dosages).
$\mathbf{1}$ is an n_{ij} vector containing 1s.
$e_{ij} = (e_{ij1}, \ldots, e_{ijn_{ij}})'$ is a vector of random errors.

The mean of y_{ij} is $E(y_{ij}) = z_{ij}\beta$, and the covariance matrix of y_{ij} is

$$\text{Var}(y_{ij}) = V_{ij} = \sigma^2 I + \sigma_f^2 J$$

where J is a $n_{ij} \times n_{ij}$ matrix containing 1s. The likelihood function for the ijth animal is

$$L(y_{ij}) = \frac{1}{(2\pi|V_{ij}|)^{N/2}}\exp\left\{-\frac{1}{2}(y_{ij} - z_{ij}\beta)'V_{ij}^{-1}(y_{ij} - z_{ij}\beta)\right\}$$

The log-likelihood function is

$$LL = C - \frac{N}{2}\sum_{i=1}^{g}\sum_{j=1}^{m_i} \log(|V_{ij}|)$$

$$- \frac{1}{2}\sum_{i=1}^{g}\sum_{j=1}^{m_i} (y_{ij} - z_{ij}\beta)'V_{ij}^{-1}(y_{ij} - z_{ij}\beta)$$

where N is the total number of the dams.

Computation techniques for the maximum likelihood estimation of the parameters of mixed effects models have been proposed by many authors (Harville, 1977; Dempster et al., 1981, 1984; Laird and Ware,

1982; Jennrich and Schluchter, 1986; Lindstrom and Bates, 1988). The general approach is to estimate the variance components σ_f^2 and σ^2 first, and then use the variance estimators to estimate the fixed factor parameters β by the reweighted least squares method. For given values of σ_f^2 and σ^2, the estimate of β is the solution of the estimating equations

$$\sum_{i=1}^{g} \sum_{j=1}^{m_i} z'_{ij} V_{ij}^{-1} z_{ij} \beta = \sum_{i=1}^{g} \sum_{j=1}^{m_i} z'_{ij} y_{ij}$$

When the covariance matrix V_{ij} is known, the estimate $\hat{\beta}$ is the uniformly minimum variance unbiased estimator of β. The variances σ_f^2 and σ^2 are replaced by their variance estimators in the calculation. Detailed descriptions of the maximum likelihood and restricted maximum likelihood estimations under mixed effects model were given by Lindstrom and Bates (1988). The estimates can be obtained using the PROC MIXED procedure of SAS (1994). Alternatively, the generalized estimating equations approach can be used to estimate the fixed effects parameters β. Under the normal model, the likelihood-based and GEE approaches have the same estimating equations for the mean parameters, but unlike the likelihood approach, the GEE uses the method of moments to estimate the variance component parameters.

B. Example: Dexamethasone Pup Weight Data

A study on developmental toxic effects from dexamethasone (DEX) exposure conducted at the National Center for Toxicological Research was used for illustration. In this experiment, pregnant CD rats were administered DEX on gestation days 9 through 14 at either 0, 0.2, 0.4, or 0.8 mg kg^{-1} body weight. The animals were sacrificed at day 20. Table 6 contains the fetal weights per each litter for the four groups.

The full model for tests of homogeneity and comparing with control was

$$y_{ijk} = \beta_0 + \beta_i + \gamma_{ij} + e_{ijk}$$

where $\beta_i = \mu_i - \mu_1$, $i = 2,3,4$. The restricted maximum likelihood estimates of the variance components were

$$\hat{\sigma}_f^2 = 0.0597, \quad \hat{\sigma}^2 = 0.0784$$

The estimates by the GEE were

$$\hat{\sigma}_f^2 = 0.0585, \quad \hat{\sigma}^2 = 0.1252$$

The dose–response trend model was

$$y_{ijk} = \beta_0 + \beta d_i + \gamma_{ij} + e_{ijk}$$

The restricted maximum likelihood estimates of the variance components were

$$\hat{\sigma}_f^2 = 0.0809, \quad \hat{\sigma}^2 = 0.0784.$$

The estimates by the GEE were

$$\hat{\sigma}_f^2 = 0.0818, \quad \hat{\sigma}^2 = 0.1489$$

Table 7 contains the summary of the comparison from the litter-based analysis, restricted likelihood estimation, and quasi-likelihood approach. Note that the fixed effects parameters β's can also be estimated by the GEE approach.

VII. ANALYSIS OF MULTIPLE BINARY OUTCOMES

Statistical procedure for the analysis of multiple types of defect (malformation) has not been widely considered. For example, malformations were generally categorized into the external, visceral, and skeletal. A simple approach was to perform an univariate analysis for each malformation type. However, a common practice was to collapse the three malformation types into a single binary response (that is, a fetus was classified as abnormal [malformation] if at least one of the three malformation types was observed), and then performed an univariate analysis on the binary response. This analysis is the simplest approach for the combined analysis of the three malformation types simultaneously. Recently, Lefkopoulou et al. (1989), Lefkopoulou and Ryan (1994), and Chen and Ahn (1997) have proposed using the generalized, estimating equations approach for the multivariate analysis of multiple binary endpoints simultaneously. This section describes a generalized estimating equations approach to analyzing multiple malformation types.

A. Models for Multivariate Binary Outcomes

Let y_{ijkl} be a binary response indicating presence or absence of the lth malformation type for the kth fetus of the jth animal in the ith group, $i = 1, \ldots, g; j = 1, \ldots, m; k = 1, \ldots, n_{ij};$ and $l = 1, \ldots, L$. Let $y_{ijl} = \Sigma_k^n y_{ijkl}$ denote the total number of responses for the lth malformation type of the ijth animal.

TABLE 6 The Fetal Weight Data from a Dexamethasone Developmental Toxicity Study in CD Rats Administered on Gestation Days 9–14 and Sacrificed at Day 20

Dose	Dam	Fetal weight													
0	169	3.38	3.17	3.49	3.48	3.85	3.7	3.97	3.68	3.76	3.36	3.28	2.29	3.68	3.63
	170	2.77	3.02	3.29	3.39	3.37	3.5	3.34	3.55	3.19	3.57	3.21	2.33	3.6	3.17
	171	3.56	3.76	3.43	4.16	3.73	4.09	3.86	3.91	3.97	4.07	3.8	4.2	4.07	3.56
	172	3.04	3.67	3.97	3.54	3.73	3.5	3.75	3.78	3.95	3.97				
	173	3.5	3.63	3.63	3.18	3.68	3.44	3.65	3.9	3.87	3.71	3.62	3.46	3.62	2.81
	175	3.16	3.18	2.88	4.06	3.4	3.88	3.72	3.77	3.84	3.88	3.74	3.93	3.44	3.57
	176	3.89	3.78	3.76	3.84	3.75	3.53	3.14	3.3	3.65	3.9				
	207	2.9	2.6	3.05	3.28	3.18	3.01	3.12	2.72	2.75	2.73				
	208	2.7	2.65	2.94	3.45	3.13	3.47	3.57	3.15	3.62	3.66	3.45	3.58	3.17	3.25
		3.47	3.13												
	209	3.19	3.28	3.36	3.39	3.68	3.95	3.51	3.35	3.73	3.77	3.63	3.86	3.17	3.52
		3.57	3.09												
	219	3.35	3.68	3.37	3.55	3.63	3.8	3.72	3.84	3.88	3.45	3.72	3.31	3.21	3.42
		3.28	3.02												
0.2	221	3.99	3.81	3.85	3.78	3.59	3.74	3.88	3.99	3.43	3.21	3.36			
	211	2.9	3.37	2.96	3.11	3.57	2.89	3.2	3.39	3.77	3.21	3.7	3.56	2.93	
	212	3.24	2.81	3.53	3.15	3.29	3.44	3.17	3.39	3.1	2.86	3.03	3.19	3.11	3.26
		2.85													
	213	3.16	3.39	3.66	3.67	3.48	3.39	3.78	3.83	3.51	3.77	3.72	3.74	3.25	2.97
		3.18													
	214	3.35	3.76	3.7	3.64	3.73	3.86	3.56	3.44	3.91	3.75	3.8	3.84	3.48	2.88
	223	2.87	3.33	3.33	3.39	3.51	3.49	3.33	3.74						
	224	2.61	2.72	2.85	3.34	3.2	3.21	3.17	3.12	3.3	3.32	2.74	3.12	3.11	

346

225	3.34	2.89	3.06	3	3.3	3.26	3.53	3.43	3.31	2.9	3	3.85	3.45	2.37
	3.18													
226	2.8	3.27	3.43	3.23	3.22	3.92	3.51	3.29	3.31	3.61	3.49	4	3.43	3.56
	3.25	3.39	3.35	3.62										
	3.62													

0.4

177	3.45	2.93	3.38	3.62	3.48	3.43	3.17	3.35	3.07	3.69	3.13			
178	3.35	3.6	3.53	2.98	2.82	3.01	2.58	3.38	3.14					
180	3.04	3.09	2.86	2.87	2.84	3.6	2.99	2.84	3.52	3.12	3.29	3.39	3.26	3.4
	3.26	3.18												
181	3.76	3.08	2.9	3.27	3.49	3.65	3.57	3.67	3.42	3.05	3.95	2.63	3.6	3.29
182	2.89	3.16	3.69	3.17	3.75	3.59	3.48	2.97	3.85	3.37	3.76	3.62	3.56	3.51
	3.15	3.49	3.19	2.89										
	3.63	3.21												
184	3.18	3.12	3.43	3.18	3.15	3.09	2.97	3.35	3.63	3.35	3.37	3.62	3.17	3.13
	2.99	2.82	3.06											
215	2.56	2.87	2.82	3.08	2.4	2.96	3.23	3.22	2.88	2.71	3.03	2.64	3	
216	2.67	3.01	3.47	3.2	3.03	2.66	2.94	2.94	3.02	2.82	2.9	2.75	2.53	
217	3.7	3.22	3.45	3.54	3.43	3.7	3.81	3.95	3.32	2.99	4.12	3.59		
218	3.02	3.41	4.22	3.86	3.46	3.55	3.35	3.46	3.46	3.74	2.75	3.12		
228	2.66	2.63	2.8	2.86	2.64	2.65	2.71	2.45	2.75	2.32	3.09	2.62		
230	2.48	2.58	3.22	3.38	2.9	3.21	3.29	3.23	2.82	3.55			3.44	3.16
	2.64													

0.8

288	2.41	2.36	2.56	2.58	2.24	2.01	2.37	2.44	2.25	2.25	2.26	2.13		
161	2.02	2.39	2.61	2.42	2.2	2.44	2.01	1.85	2.06	2.07				
162	2.66	2.17	2.14	2.04	2.15	1.74	1.97	1.82	1.93	1.96				
164	2.12	1.9	2.89	2.13	1.82	2.16	2.3							
165	1.85	1.93	2.28	1.71										
166	1.62	1.72	1.57											
167	2.24	2.4	2.15	2.26	2.02	2.43	2.31	1.92	2.3	2.79	2.35	2.16		

TABLE 7   The χ^2 Values for the Parametric, beta-Binomial, and
Quasi-Likelihood Approaches Computed Under the Three Null Hypotheses

		Control vs. dose			
Approach	Homogeneity	$\mu_1 = \mu_2$	$\mu_1 = \mu_3$	$\mu_1 = \mu_4$	Trend
Litter-based analysis[a]	40.14	-1.407	-3.360	-10.640	-9.148
Restricted MLE[b]	144.51	-1.456	-3.418	-10.740	-10.816
Quasi-likelihood[b]	165.60	-1.576	-3.901	-12.428	-10.399

[a]The column under homogeneity represents an F value, other columns represent t scores.
[b]The column under homogeneity represents a χ^2, other columns represent z scores.

Assume the mean and variance of y_{ijl} are

$$\mathrm{E}(y_{ijl}) = n_{ij}\mu_{il}$$

and

$$\mathrm{Var}(y_{ijl}) = n_{ij}\mu_{il}(1 - \mu_{il})[1 + (n_{ij} - 1)\rho_l] \tag{2}$$

This variance function allows different types to have different over-dispersion parameters. The ρ_l is constant if a common overdispersion parameter for all malformation types is assumed. The correlation between y_{ijl} and $y_{ijl'}$ ($l \neq l'$) is

$$\mathrm{Corr}(y_{ijl}, y_{ijl'}) = \delta$$

where $\delta \neq 0$. Thus, the covariance of y_{ij} and $y_{ij'}$ is

$$\mathrm{Cov}(y_{ijl}, y_{ijl'}) = \delta[\mathrm{Var}(y_{ijl})\mathrm{Var}(y_{ijl'})]^{1/2}$$

In matrix notation, $y_{ij} = (y_{ij1}, \ldots, y_{ijL})$ and $\mu_i = (\mu_{i1}, \ldots, \mu_{iL})$. The mean of y_{ij} is $\mathrm{E}(y_{ij}) = \mu_i$ and the variance–covariance matrix is

$$\mathrm{Var}(y_{ij}) = V_{ij} = (1 - \delta)C_{ij} + \delta C_{ij}^{1/2}\mathbf{1}\mathbf{1}'C_{ij}^{1/2}$$

where $C_{ij} = \mathrm{diag}\{n_{ij}\mu_{il}(1 - \mu_{il})[1 + (n_{ij} - 1)\rho_l]\}$ and $\mathbf{1}$ is a $J \times 1$ column vector containing 1s.

Each mean μ_{ij} is associated with a set of covariates z_{ij} through a logit link function

$$\mathrm{logit}\ \mu_{ij} = \beta z_{ij}$$

An estimate of the coefficient parameter β can be obtained by solving the estimating equation,

$$\sum_{i=1}^{g} \sum_{j=1}^{m_i} D'_{ij} V_{ij}^{-1} (y_{ij} - \mu_i) = 0$$

where $D'_i = [\partial \mu_i / \partial \beta_j]'$. The estimate $\hat{\beta}$ is approximately normal. The variance of $\hat{\beta}$ is $M_0 = (\sum_{i=1}^{g} \sum_{j=1}^{m_i} D'_{ij} \hat{V}_{ij}^{-1} D_{ij})^{-1}$. Liang and Zeger (1986) proposed the robust estimate $V_R = M_0^{-1} M_1 M_0^{-1}$, where

$$M_1 = \sum_{i=1}^{g} \sum_{j=1}^{m_i} D'_{ij} \hat{V}_{ij}^{-1} (y_{ij} - \hat{\mu}_i) (y_{ij} - \hat{\mu}_i)' \hat{V}_{ij}^{-1} D_{ij}$$

Estimates of the variance–covariance parameters, δ or ρ_l can be obtained by the method of moments. Let $S_i = (y_i - \hat{\mu}_i)(y_i - \hat{\mu}_i)'$ be the residual matrix. The parameters ρ_l and δ are estimated by equating the variance matrix V_{ij} with the residual matrix S_{ij}. An estimate of ρ_l is

$$\hat{\rho}_l = \frac{1}{gm_i} \sum_{i=1}^{g} \sum_{j=1}^{m_i} \frac{(y_{ij} - n_{ij}\hat{\mu}_{ij})^2 - n_{ij}\hat{\mu}_{ij}(1 - \hat{\mu}_{ij})}{n_{ij}(n_{ij} - 1)\hat{\mu}_{ij}(1 - \hat{\mu}_{ij})}$$

and the estimate of δ is

$$\delta = \frac{2}{gm_i(m_i - 1)} \sum_{i=1}^{g} \sum_{j=2}^{m_i} \sum_{l=1}^{m_i-1}$$

$$\frac{(y_{ij} - n_{ij}\hat{\mu}_{ij})(y_{il} - n_{il}\hat{\mu}_{il})}{\sqrt{\{n_{ij}\hat{\mu}_{ij}(1 - \hat{\mu}_{ij})[1 + (n_{ij} - 1)\hat{\rho}]\}\{n_{il}\hat{\mu}_{il}(1 - \hat{\mu}_{il})[1 + (n_{il} - 1)\hat{\rho}]\}}}$$

Under a common intralitter correlation model, the estimate of ρ is

$$\hat{\rho} = \frac{1}{L} \sum_{l=1}^{L} \hat{\rho}_l$$

The dose effect on the L malformation types can be tested using the common dose effect model

$$\text{logit}(\mu_{il}) = \beta_d d_i + \beta_l$$

Lefkopoulou and Ryan (1993) considered the score statistic under this common dose effect model; the test derived under a common dose effect model is sensitive to an one-sided (dose-related) alternative. The assumption of a common dose coefficient is strong and unlikely to be precisely true in practice, but will remain valid under a much broader class of alternatives.

B. Example

The example is the ossification data from a developmental toxicity experiment presented by Lefkopoulou et al. (1989) and Lefkopoulou and Ryan (1993). The experiment was to study the effects of in utero exposure to the anticonvulsant phenytoin. The toxicity endpoints were the level of ossification in the forepaw of the offspring, which provided a measure of the degree of skeletal maturity. The control group had 17 litters containing 124 offspring, and the treated group had 19 litters containing 133 offsprings. The eight middle phalanges of the left forepaw (L2, L3, L4, and L5) and right forepaw (R2, R3, R4, and R5) of each offspring were examined. The overdispersion binomial variable was the number of offspring with ossification for each of the eight digits.

The mean μ_{ijl} was modeled as

$$\text{logit}\mu_{ijl} = \beta_d d_i + \beta_l, \quad l = 1, \ldots, 8$$

where β_d and β_l represented dose and digit factors, respectively. Table 8 contains the coefficient estimates with the model-based and robust standard error estimates using two covariance structures. Models 1 assumed independence between the eight digits (an identity working correlation

TABLE 8 The Estimates of Coefficients with the Model-Based and Robust Standard Errors for Two Covariance Models Fitted to the Ossification Data

		Model 1			Model 2	
Coefficient	Estimate	Model-based	Robust	Estimate	Model-based	Robust
β_d	−1.401	0.166	0.385	−1.288	0.195	0.420
β_1	−3.654	0.580	0.485	−3.657	0.575	0.478
β_2	0.093	0.171	0.331	0.060	0.178	0.342
β_3	−0.813	0.192	0.310	−0.836	0.197	0.322
β_4	−5.058	1.151	0.958	−5.041	1.112	0.909
β_5	−3.935	0.583	0.664	−3.936	0.656	0.559
β_6	0.125	0.171	0.306	0.093	0.178	0.321
β_7	−0.208	0.174	0.311	−0.237	0.181	0.323
β_8	−5.058	1.151	0.958	−5.041	1.123	0.909
δ	0			0.340		
ρ	0.045			0.042		

matrix), Model 2 assumed an equicorrelation structure between the eight digits.

Table 8 shows that the coefficient estimates and the robust standard error estimates are similar between two models, except β_2 and β_6. The z values using the model-based standard error estimates were 8.440 and 6.605, and the z values using the robust standard error estimates were 3.639 and 3.067 for model 1 and model 2, respectively. Both models showed a significant dose-related trend.

The z values based on the univariate analysis that at least one of the eight digits was ossified was 2.872. Thus, the multivariate approach gave higher z values than the univariate analysis.

REFERENCES

Altham PME. Two generalizations of the binomial distribution. Appl Stat 27: 162–167, 1978.

Armitage P. Tests for linear trends in proportions and frequencies. Biometrics 11:375–386, 1955.

Barr M Jr, Jensh RP, Brent RL. Fetal weight and intrauterine position in rats. Teratology 2:241–246, 1969.

Bahadur RR. A representation of the joint distribution of responses to n dichotomous items. In: Solomon H, ed. Studies in Item Analysis and Prediction. Stanford, CA: Stanford University Press, 1961.

Bieler GS, Williams RL. Cluster sampling techniques in quantal response teratology and developmental toxicity studies. Biometrics 51:764–776, 1995.

Bowman D, George EO. A saturated model for analysis exchangeable binary data: applications to clinical and developmental toxicity studies. J Am Stat Assoc 90:871–879, 1995.

Bowman D, Chen JJ, George EO. Estimating variance functions in developmental toxicity studies. Biometrics 51:1174–1176, 1995.

Breslow NE. Extra-Poisson variation in log-linear model. Appl Stat 33:38–44, 1984.

Brooks RJ. Approximate likelihood ratio tests in the analysis of beta-binomial data. Appl Stat 33:285–289, 1984.

Carr RJ, Portier C. An evaluation of some methods for fitting dose–response models to quantal response data. Biometrics 49:779–791, 1993.

Carroll RJ, Ruppert D. Robust estimation in heteroscedastic linear models. Ann Stat 10:429–441, 1982.

Catalano PJ, Ryan LM. Bivariate latent variable models for clustered discrete and continuous outcomes. J Am Stat Assoc 87:651–658, 1992.

Chen JJ. Trend test for overdispersed proportions. Biometr J 35:949–958, 1993a.

Chen JJ. A malformation incidence dose response model incorporating fetal weight and/or litter size as covariates. Risk Anal 13:559–564, 1993b.

Chen JJ, Ahn H. Fitting mixed Poisson regression models using quasi-likelihood methods. Biometr J 38:81–96, 1996.

Chen JJ and Ahn H. Marginal models with multiplicative variance components for over-dispersed binomial data. Journal of Agricultural, Biological and Environmental Statistics. (to appear) 1997.

Chen JJ, Allen RR. Analysis of developmental toxicity studies. Testing principles in clinical and preclinical trials. In: Vollmar J, ed. *Biometrie in der chemisch-pharmazeutischen Industrie, V6, Testing Principles in Clinical and Preclinical Trials.* New York: Gustav Fisher Verlag, 1995, pp 101–114.

Chen JJ, Gaylor DW. Correlations of developmental end points observed after 2,4,5-trichlorophenoxyacetic acid exposure in mice. Teratology 45:241–246, 1992.

Chen JJ, Kodell RL. Quantitative risk assessment for teratological effects. J Am Stat Assoc 84:966–971, 1989.

Chen JJ, Li L-A. Evaluation of statistical models for analysis of trinomial responses from reproductive and developmental toxicity experiments. Biometr J 34:231–241, 1992.

Chen JJ, Li L-A. Dose-response modeling of trinomial responses from developmental experiments. Stat Sin 4:265–274, 1994.

Chen JJ, Kodell RL, Howe RB, Gaylor DW. Analysis of trinomial responses from reproductive and developmental toxicity experiments. Biometrics 47:1049–1058, 1991.

Chen JJ, Ahn H, Cheng KF. Comparison of some homogeneity tests in analysis of proportions in teratologic studies. Environ Ecol Stat 1:315–324, 1994.

Cochran WG. Some methods for strengthening the common 2 tests. Biometrics 12:417–451, 1954.

Cornwall GA, Carter MW, Bradshaw WS. The relationship between prenatal lethality or fatal weight and intrauterine position in rats exposed to diethylstilbestrol, zeranol, 3,4,3′,4′-tetrachlorobiphenyl, or cadmium. Teratology 30:341–349, 1984.

Cox DR. The regression analysis of binary sequences (with discussion). J R Stat Assoc B 20:215–242, 1958.

Crowder MJ. beta-Binomial ANOVA for proportions. Appl Stat 27:34–37, 1978.

Davidian M, Carroll RJ. Variance function estimation. J Am Stat Assoc 82:1079–1091, 1987.

Dean CB, Lawless JF, Willmot GE. A mixed Poisson–inverse-gaussian regression model. Can J Stat 17:171–181, 1989.

Dempster AP, Rubin DB, Tsutakawa RK. Estimation in covariance components models. J Am Stat Assoc 76:341–353, 1981.

Dempster AP, Selwyn MR, Patel CM, Roth AJ. Statistical and computational aspects of mixed model analysis. Appl Stat 33:203–214, 1984.

Donnor A, Eliasziw M, Klar N. A comparison of methods for testing homogeneity of proportions in teratologic studies. Stat Med 13:1253-1264, 1994.

Environmental Protection Agency. Guidelines for developmental toxicity risk assessment. Federal Register 56:63797-63826, 1991.

Fitzmaurice GM, Laird NM. Regression models for a bivariate discrete and continuous outcome with clustering. J Am Stat Assoc 90:845-852, 1995.

Freeman MF, Tukey JW. Transformations related to the angular and the square root. J Am Stat Assoc 21:607-611, 1950.

Frome EL, Kutner MH, Beauchamp JJ. Regression analysis of Poisson distributed data. J Am Stat Assoc 68:935-940, 1973.

Fung KY, Krewski D, Rao JNK, Scott AJ. Tests for trend in developmental toxicity experiments with correlated binary data. Risk Anal 14:621-630, 1994.

Gaylor DW, Chen JJ. Dose-response models for developmental malformations. Teratology 47:291-297, 1993.

Gladen B. The use of jackknife to estimate proportions from toxicological data in the presence of litter effects. J Am Stat Assoc 74:1049-1058, 1979.

Harville DA. Maximum likelihood approaches to variance component estimation and to related problems. J Am Stat Assoc 72:320-340, 1977.

Haseman JK, Hogan MD. Selection of the experimental unit in teratology studies. Teratology 12:165-172, 1975.

Haseman JK, Kupper LL. Analysis of dichotomous response data from certain toxicological experiments. Biometrics 35:281-293, 1979.

Heindel JJ, Thomford PH, Mattison DT. Histological assessment of ovarian follicle number in mice as a screen for ovarian toxicity. In: Hirshfiled AN, ed. Growth Factors and the Ovary. New York: Plenum, 1980, pp 421-426.

Healy MJR. Animal litters as experimental units. Appl Stat 21:155-159, 1972.

Hinde J. Compound Poisson regressions. In: Gilchrist R, ed. GLIM 82: Proceedings International Conference of Generalized Linear Models. Berlin: Springer-Verlag, 1982, pp 109-121.

Jennrich RI, Schluchter MD. Unbalanced repeated measures models with structural covariance matrices. Biometrics 42:805-820, 1986.

Jensh RP, Brent RL, Barr M Jr. The litter effect as a variable in teratologic studies of the albino rat. Am J Anat 128:185-192, 1970.

Kimmel CA, Gaylor DW. Issues in qualitative and quantitative risk analysis for developmental toxicology. Risk Anal 8:15-19, 1988.

Krewski D, Zhu Y. Applications of multinomial dose-response models in developmental toxicity risk assessment. Risk Anal 14:595-609, 1994.

Kupper LL, Haseman JK. The use of a correlated binomial model for the analysis of data from certain toxicological experiments. Biometrics 34:69-76, 1978.

Kupper LL, Portier C, Hogan MD, Yamamoto E. The impact of litter effects on dose-response modeling in teratology. Biometrics 42:85-89, 1986.

Laird NM, Ware JH. Random-effects models for longitudinal data. Biometrics 38:963–974, 1982.

Lawless JF. Negative binomial and mixed Poisson regression. Can J Stat 15:209–225, 1987.

Lefkopoulou M, Moore D, Ryan LM. The analysis of multiple correlated binary outcomes: application to rodent teratology experiments. J Am Stat Assoc 84:810–815, 1989.

Lefkopoulou M, Ryan LM. Global tests for multiple binary outcomes. Biometrics 49:975–988, 1993.

Liang KY, Hanfelt J. On the use of the quasi-likelihood method in teratological experiments. Biometrics 50:872–880, 1994.

Liang KY, Zeger SL. Longitudinal data analysis using generalized linear models. Biometrika 73:13–32, 1986.

Liang K-Y, McCullagh P. Case studies in binary dispersion. Biometrics 49:623–630, 1993.

Lindstrom MJ, Bates DM. Newton–Raphson and EM algorithms for linear mixed-effects models for repeated measures data. J Am Stat Assoc 83:1014–1022, 1988.

McCullagh P, Nelder JA. Generalized Linear Model, 2nd ed. London: Chapman & Hall, 1989.

Margolin BH, Kaplan N, Zeiger E. Statistical analysis of the Ames *Salmonella/* microsome test. Pro Nat Acad Sci USA 76:3779–3783, 1981.

Moore DF, Tsiatis A. Robust estimation of variance in moment methods for extra-binomial and extra-Poisson variation. Biometrics 47:383–401, 1991.

Nelder JA, Pregibon D. An extended quasi-likelihood function. Biometrika 74:221–232, 1987.

Ochi Y, Prentice RL. Likelihood inference in a correlated probit regression model. Biometrika 71:531–543, 1984.

Pack SE. Hypothesis testing for proportions with overdispersion. Biometrics 42:967–972, 1986.

Paul SR. Analysis of proportions of affected foetuses in teratological experiments. Biometrics 38:361–370, 1982.

Paul SR. On the beta-correlated binomial distribution – a three parameter generalization of binomial distribution. Commun Stat Theory Methods 16:1473–1478, 1987.

Paul SR, Islam AS. C(α) tests for homogeneity of proportions in toxicology in presence of beta-binomial over-dispersion. In: Williams D, ed. Statistics in Toxicology. New York: Oxford University Press, 1995.

Rai K, Van Ryzin J. A dose–response model for teratological experiments involving quantal responses. Biometrics 41:1–9, 1985.

Rao JNK, Scott AJ. A simple method for the analysis of correlated binary data. Biometrics 48:577–586, 1992.

Rosenkranz G, Uhl R. Statistical evaluation of offspring parameters in embryotoxicity studies. In: Hothorn L, ed. Lecture Notes in Medical Informatics 43, Statistical Methods in Toxicology. New York: Springer-Verlag, 1991.

Ryan LM. Quantitative risk assessment for developmental toxicity. Biometrics 48:163–174, 1992.

Ryan LM. Using historical controls in the analysis of developmental toxicity data. Biometrics 49:1126–1135, 1993.

Ryan LM, Catalano PJ, Kimmel CA, Kimmel GL. On the relationship between fetal weight and malformation in developmental toxicity studies. Teratology 44:215–223, 1991.

SAS Institute, Inc. Getting Started with PROC MIXED. Cary, NC: SAS Institute Inc., 1994.

Soper KA, Clark RL. Data-based scores improve power and robustness of exact trend tests of embryonal rat survival. Unpublished manuscript, 1991.

Smyth GK. Generalized linear models with varying dispersion. J R Stat Assoc B 51:47–60, 1989.

Tarone RE, Gart JJ. On the robustness of combined tests for trends in proportions. J Am Stat Assoc 75:110–116, 1980.

Tsai RE, Hsu JJ. Estimation of treatment effects in animal reproductive toxicology studies. American Statistical Association 1993 Proceedings of Biopharmaceutical Section; ASA, Alexandria, VA, 1993.

Wedderburn RWM. Quasi-likelihood functions, generalized linear models, and Gauss–Newton method. Biometrika 61:439–447, 1974.

Williams DA. The analysis of binary responses from toxicological experiments involving reproduction and teratogenicity. Biometrics 31:949–952, 1975.

Williams DA. Extra-binomial variation in logistic linear models. Appl Stat 31:144–148, 1982.

Williams DA. Dose–response models for teratology experiments. Biometrics 43:1013–1016, 1987.

Williams DA. Estimation bias using beta-binomial distribution in teratology. Biometrics 44:305–308, 1988.

Zeger SL, Liang KY. Longitudinal data for discrete and continuous outcomes. Biometrics 42:121–130, 1986.

Zeger SL, Liang K-Y, Albert PS. Models for longitudinal data: a generalized estimating equation approach. Biometrics 44:1049–1060, 1988.

Zhu Y, Krewski D, Ross WH. Dose–response model for correlated multinomial data from developmental toxicity studies. Appl Stat 48:583–598, 1994.

11

The In Vitro Ames Tests

WHERLY P. HOFFMAN
Eli Lilly and Company, Greenfield, Indiana

I. INTRODUCTION

Genetic toxicological tests are among the early animal studies designed to establish a safety profile for a compound. Of a battery of short-term genetic assays, the *Salmonella typhimurium*-microsome test developed by Ames and associates (1,2), is the most commonly used genotoxicity test. The design, statistical analyses, and the interpretation of the results will be discussed in this chapter. Section II includes the background for the relevance of Ames tests to the toxicological safety profile. Section III describes the designs of the Ames tests. Section IV provides a review of some statistical methods employed for the evaluation of the mutagenicity of a compound. In Section V, we discuss the methods reviewed and some important issues in the evaluation of mutagenicity based on Ames assay results, and in Section VI, we draw concluding remarks to summarize this chapter.

II. BACKGROUND

In this section, a brief summary is presented of why the Ames assay was developed and how this assay is conducted. The procedure of conducting the Ames test is described without too much detail. This section is not intended to give readers enough information to conduct the assay after reading it; it is intended to provide readers with a general understanding of how the responses are obtained and thus leads naturally into the following sections on the design and statistical methods employed for statistical analysis.

A. Why the Ames Assay

When developing a potentially beneficial compound, one has to establish its safety profile. Animal in vivo and in vitro tests are designed to serve this purpose. In general, the testing includes acute toxicity tests in rodents, genetic toxicity tests, developmental toxicity tests, 30-day up to 1-year general animal toxicity tests, and carcinogenicity tests in rodents. Of these general tests that are needed to demonstrate the safety of a compound and gain future success for its registration worldwide, the most costly test is the carcinogenesis assay in rodents. Therefore, bacterial test systems designed to identify the mutagenic potential of a compound are employed as predictive tests of potential carcinogenicity. McCann and associates (3) examined the relation between carcinogenesis and mutagenesis, and they indicated that further efforts were needed to design a battery of genetic short-term tests for the prediction of carcinogenicity. Among the genetic short-term tests that are conducted in practice, Purchase (4) concluded that the Ames test is the only established test for the prediction of carcinogenicity. Although, the Ames assay alone is not enough to predict the carcinogenicity of a compound, it is the most used genetics test and warrants a full discussion.

B. The Ames Assay

The Ames assay is an in vitro assay in that it does not use live animals; instead, it uses bacterial cells. Typically, the bacterial strains used in the Ames assays are *Salmonella typhimurium* strains, TA1535, TA1537, TA98, and TA100, plus an additional *Escherichia coli* strain, WP2urvA. Although WP2uvrA was added to the bacterial test system after the Ames assay was developed, it is the same as the four *S. typhimurium* strains in all aspects for the conduct and analysis of the experiment. Therefore, in this chapter, Ames assay will refer to the assay of the four *S. typhimurium* strains: TA1535, TA1537, TA98, and TA100, and the *E. coli* strain, WP2urvA. For each strain of the bacteria, a mixture of proper amounts of three ingredients is first prepared in a tube. The three ingredients are (a) about 10 or 100 million bacterial cells; (b) a test article, which can be a compound, negative control, or positive control; and (c) the Ames solution, which includes histidine, tryptophan, and biotin. The mixture is then poured into a plate for the growth of revertant colonies. Because in vivo, a metabolized test article may induce different effects from a nonmetabolized test article, to mimic an in vivo system, it is usually tested both with and without metabolic activation by rat liver enzymes (S9 mix).

Histidine is an essential substance for the growth of *S. typhimurium* bacterial cells. Bacterial cells can be classified into two types by their ability to generate histidine: (a) the wild-type (prototrophs), normal cells that can grow in the absence of supplemental histidine because they are capable of generating their own; and (b) the auxotrophs, mutated cells that can not grow without supplemental histidine. A trace amount of histidine is provided at the start of the experiment to sustain the bacterial cells at the beginning and thus allow the possible expression of back mutation later. After a 48-h incubation period for the bacterial colonies to grow, back-mutated cells will form visible colonies, and one can count these colonies in the plate. Auxotrophs can mutate back to wild-type as a result of the mutagenic effects of a test article and these back-mutated colonies are called *revertant colonies*. Because reverse mutation may occur spontaneously without any compound, a negative control is always included in the assay to account for spontaneous reverse mutation. If a compound is not a mutagen, then one would not expect a large increase in revertant colonies over the spontaneous revertant colonies in the negative control. Therefore, the number of revertant colonies is the response for evaluation of the mutagenic effect of a test article. A significant increase in revertant colonies in the compound-treated plates is an indication of a positive response for bacterial mutation.

III. DESIGN

The Ames assay is typically conducted both with and without metabolic activation for each of the five bacterial strains. For each bacterial strain, five or more concentration levels of a compound and proper concentration levels for the negative and positive controls are determined by scientists. A positive control is required for the validity of the assay, but it is not included in the evaluation of the mutagenicity of a compound. A negative control is needed to account for spontaneous reverse mutation in the evaluation of the compound's effects. Historical control data are useful for further evaluation of positive effects associated with a compound. Each dose level is tested in triplicate, and each of the triplicate plates is prepared independently. Therefore, if five concentrations are selected for each bacterial strain, then a total of 50 sets of triplicate data from the compound (five concentrations, two types of activation, and five strains of bacteria) and ten sets of triplicate data from each of the negative control and positive control are the results of the assay.

The purpose of the Ames assay is to evaluate the mutagenic effects of a compound. A suitable selection of the concentration levels of a compound for testing is essential. Logarithmically spaced concentration levels are determined by scientists in an attempt to capture an increasing trend in the response. However, if the concentration of the compound is too high, then one would expect a downturn in the number of revertant colonies as a result of the toxicity. For determination of the concentration levels for the Ames assay, a compound is assayed at a wide range of concentration levels up to 5000 μg per plate for each bacterial strain. Based on the preliminary results, five to seven concentration levels are then selected using a top concentration of 5000 μg per plate, adjusted for toxicity. The highest concentration may be very close to the toxic level. Although there is variation in the design of the Ames assay among laboratories in the pharmaceutical industry, based on guidance published in *Federal Register* 61(80), on April 24, 1996, the design discussed here is a representative of designs commonly used in the pharmaceutical industry.

IV. STATISTICAL METHODS FOR AMES TEST DATA

Proper statistical analysis should account for various sources of variability in the response. Therefore, one needs to identify different sources of variability in the assay data before considering the analysis. From the variability and some assumptions, we discuss various statistical and nonstatistical methods for the analysis of revertant colonies obtained from the Ames assay. Elder (5) and Mahon and associates (6) gave a good overview of statistical methods for the Ames *Salmonella* assay. Here we will begin the discussion with some basic information on data in Section IV.A. Then, selected methods will be discussed to bring about different approaches for the analysis of Ames assay data. The methods discussed are modified two- and threefold rules in Section IV.B, nonparametric methods in Section IV.C, and parametric methods in Section IV.D.

A. Understanding Data

What is the distribution of the number of revertants from the Ames test? Before suggesting an answer, let us understand the data first and try to identify various sources of variability in it. For each replicate plate, a separate mixture of the selected strain of bacterial cells, the test article, and a solution of histidine, tryptophan, and biotin is made in a tube. Therefore, the numbers of revertants from the triplicate plates are independent. Because auxotrophs need to grow in a histidine-sufficient environment, a small amount of histidine is supplied at the beginning of the assay. For each strain of bacteria, variability in the number of revertants can be a result of the number of bacterial cells that are plated at the beginning of the assay, amount of histidine provided initially, concentration of the test article, contents of the Ames solution, amount of S9 mix, duration of the incubation time, or others. In a laboratory, attempts are made to control all factors so that changes in the revertant counts would reflect the effect of the compound through the concentration levels.

To demonstrate that a compound is not mutagenic, one has to test it at high enough concentrations and rule out doubts that cells may not have been challenged enough. Pilot runs are usually conducted first to select proper concentration levels for each strain of bacteria. The final selection often includes concentration levels that are very close to the toxicity threshold of the bacterial cells. Consequently, one may observe a downturn in the number of revertants when some of the concentration levels of a compound are higher than the toxicity threshold of the bacterial cells.

Because the number of bacterial cells initially plated is large (about 10^7) and the probability of a cell mutating back from auxotrophic to prototrophic is small, the resulting revertant counts of such rare events may have a Poisson distribution. Does the number of revertants X follow a Poisson distribution $p(X = x, \lambda)$ where

$$p(X = x, \lambda) = \frac{\lambda^x e^{-\lambda}}{x!} \text{ for } x = 0, 1, 2, \ldots \qquad (1)$$

and λ is the mean rate of back mutation? One can examine this either graphically or by performing a statistical test. To obtain a good assessment of the distribution assumption, both approaches require more data than what is generally available from one assay. When a sufficient amount of data is available, one can check this Poisson assumption by plotting the sample variance against the sample mean on a logarithmic scale. A linear relation with slope near 1 is an indication of Poisson distribution. Or one can perform Fisher's dispersion test (7) for a sample of n counts, $x_1, x_2, \ldots, x_n$, which compares the test statistic

$$\frac{\left[\sum_{i=1}^{n} (x_i - \bar{x})^2\right]}{\bar{x}} \tag{2}$$

to a χ^2 distribution with $n - 1$ degrees of freedom, where $\bar{x}$ is the average of the n revertant counts. Stead and associates (8) reported no overdispersion in their experience, whereas Vollmar (9) and Margolin and associates (10) observed overdispersion. Because each laboratory may have its unique features in conducting the assay and controlling the assay environment, an assessment of overdispersion should be performed based on its own historical data, and reevaluation should be performed periodically.

If the rate of back mutation λ from replicate to replicate is not a constant, then the excess of variability in replicates over the mean would suggest that the revertant counts are a random sample from a mixture of Poisson distributions. For ease of further references in later sections, we will follow the parameterization of Margolin and associates (10). If λ is a random variable with a gamma distribution, then the revertant counts are a mixture of Poisson model with a negative binomial distribution

$$p(X = x|\mu,c) = \binom{x + c^{-1} - 1}{x}\left[\frac{\mu}{(\mu + c^{-1})}\right]^x\left[\frac{c^{-1}}{(\mu + c^{-1})}\right]^{c^{-1}} \tag{3}$$

$$\text{for } x = 0, 1, 2, \ldots$$

where $c \geq 0$ and $\mu > 0$. The mean of this mixture of Poisson counts is μ and the variance is $\mu(1 + c\mu)$. The extra variability in the Poisson counts is reflected by the dispersion parameter c. Large values of c indicate inadequacy of modeling without accounting for the extra variability in the sampling.

B. Modified Two- and Threefold Rules

The two- and threefold rules declare a given test article to have induced a positive response if a concentration-related increase in the number of revertant colonies is at least twice the control count for strains TA98, TA100, and WP2urvA, or three times the control count for strains

TA1353 and TA1537. The comparison is based on the average number of revertants from the replicates for the control and each concentration level. The treated averages are compared with the control average. In the event that there is a downturn in the number of revertants owing to toxicity, the evaluation criteria are applied to only the results up to the nontoxic level. The modified two- and threefold rules specify that the increases must be observed in at least two consecutive concentrations or in the last nontoxic concentration level.

C. Nonparametric Methods

Vollmar (9) examined the results from the European Collaborative Ames-Test Study 1977–1978, and the plots of log-range versus log-mean indicated that the number of revertants did not follow a Poisson distribution. Overdispersion was evident between laboratories as well as within each laboratory. It was recommended that nonparametric methods be applied to the Ames assay results. Two rank-based tests were considered: the Jonckheere test (11) for monotonic concentration effects and the Kruskal–Wallis test (12) for other effects, including a downturn at the toxic levels. Given 713 Ames test results, the Jonckheere test was superior to the Kruskal–Wallis test and was recommended as the routine statistical method for qualitative evaluations. Vollmar pointed out that, in general, three to five replicate samples were necessary for achieving a statistical significance level of 0.05.

Wahrendorf and associates (13) proposed a nonparametric approach to the analysis of Ames assay data. Assume that there are K concentration levels with n_k replicates at the kth level and the total number of replicates is N. In their approach, the concentration levels were arranged in K increasing levels with $K = 1$ for the control. For a given j, $1 \leq j \leq K$, the revertant counts from all K concentration levels are assigned to one of the two categories: (a) the "below" category for levels 1 to j, and (b) the "above" category for levels $j = 1$ to K. The revertant counts are ranked from low to high. If there are no concentration-related effects, then the sum of the ranks L_j from the below category should be the product of the midrank, $(N + 1)/2$, and the number of observations in the below category. Define L as the sum of the below categories corresponding to j for $1 \leq j \leq K - 1$. If a compound does induce a positive trend in the number of revertants, then the ranks in the above category would be relatively higher than those in the below category. Therefore, positive trends are associated with smaller values of L and a test statistic for positive trends is L. Wahrendorf and associates provided critical values for L based on Monte Carlo simulations for standard designs in their paper. Incorporating the expectation, $E_0(L)$, and variance, $Var_0(L)$, of L under the null hypothesis of no concentration-related effects, the resulting standardized test T for the alternative hypothesis of an increasing trend is a one-sided test

$$T = \frac{E_0(L) - L}{\sqrt{Var_0(L)}}, \tag{4}$$

where $E_0(L)$ and $Var_0(L)$ are defined (11) by the total sample N and s_j, the number of observations in the below category for a given j as follows,

$$E_0(L) = \frac{N + 1}{2} \sum_{j=1}^{K-1} s_j \tag{5}$$

$$Var_0(L) = \frac{N + 1}{2} \left[\sum_{j=1}^{K-1} s_j(N - s_j) + 2 \sum_{j=1}^{K-2} \sum_{k=j+1}^{K-1} s_j(N - s_k) \right] \tag{6}$$

The T statistic is approximated by a normal distribution. In addition to the test proposed in the foregoing, Wahrendorf and associates also provided a calculation for the probability $\hat{q}_j$ that a revertant count from the below category is smaller than that from the above category for a given j. Under the null hypothesis of no concentration-related effects, $\hat{q}_j$ is expected to have a value of 0.5. This probability gives insight to the change of trends in the revertant counts and is helpful for further understanding the type and strength of the trends.

D. Parametric Modeling

Parametric methods include regression on transformed data assumed to be normally distributed (14) in the next section, nonlinear regression on data assumed to be Poisson distributed either with or without extra variation, using a full likelihood or quasi-likelihood approach in Section IV.D.2, and biologically based models incorporating extra-Poisson variation (9,15,16) in Section IV.D.3.

1. Linear Regression on Logarithmically Transformed Revertant Counts

Chu and associates (14) at the In Vitro Program of the National Cancer Institute (NCI)/National Toxicology Program (NTP) evaluated the statistical methods for Ames assay data, based on results from 2362 tests performed in four laboratories on 17 test articles. In defining the screening criteria for adequate data, they defined *toxic dose level* as

> any dose level which was greater than the dose eliciting the highest average response and which had every response less than the lowest single response in the highest average response dose level.

Evidence of toxicity is a decrease in the number of revertants after reaching the toxic level. Therefore, when a downturn is present in the revertant counts and the peak mean revertant count occurs at concentration level c_i, then the toxic levels are those concentration levels, c_j, for $j > i$, that have all revertant counts smaller than the lowest revertant count at concentration level c_i.

Once the toxic concentration levels are identified, evaluation of the mutagenic effects will be based on data obtained in the nontoxic concentration range. One approach to the statistical evaluation of the mutagenic effects is regressing the logarithmically transformed revertant count on the logarithmically transformed concentration level (14). Because the control concentration level is 0 and the log transformation of 0 does not exist, the recommendation was to increase all concentration levels by 1. The validity of this regression approach lies in the appropriateness of the normality assumption resulting from the log transformation on the revertant counts. Mutagenicity is established by a statistically significant positive slope of the regression line. Chu and associates required a test to have at least five concentration levels, including a negative control, and each with a minimum of two replicates. For instance, when concentration levels are approximately equally spaced, instead of adding 1 to all concentration levels to allow for the log transformation on the 0 concentration level, an alternative was recommended by Margolin and associates (17). The concentration level of the negative control is selected so that all concentration levels are equally spaced on the logarithmic scale.

2. *Nonlinear Regression on Revertant Counts*

Although rare events are often modeled by Poisson models, and it seems reasonable to consider the small number of revertants in about 10 million bacterial cells a Poisson random variable, there are statistical concerns in the assumption of simple Poisson distribution. Evidence of extra-Poisson variation was observed by some, but not all. Because replicates are required at each concentration level, accumulating historical control data for examination of the adequacy of the Poisson assumption is essential. Under the Poisson assumption, the revertant counts can be modeled by a generalized linear model (18) with Poisson distribution and logarithmic link. Positive trends in the treated groups can be tested in a sequential fashion by a trend test (19) if identifying the concentration level associated with no-observable-effect is of interest. For laboratories that exhibit extra-Poisson variation in the historical control data, the generalized linear model can be adjusted using a quasi-likelihood method for the extra-Poisson variation. The extra-Poisson variation is accounted for by including an extra factor in the variance of the model. The extra factor can be estimated by the square root of Pearsons χ^2 divided by the degrees of freedom. This analysis can be carried out using PROC GENMOD in SAS 6.11 (20).

If the mean rate for back mutation λ, in Eq. (1) is a random variable with gamma distribution, then the posterior distribution of the revertant counts is a negative binomial distribution as in Eq. (3). Thus, the extra-Poisson variation can be incorporated in the modeling and evaluation of the mutagenicity of a compound using a full-likelihood approach.

3. *Biologically Based Models*

Nonmonotonicity observed as a downturn in the revertant counts is not uncommon in practice. Bacterial cells subject to toxicity are inhibited from full expression of mutagenicity. Once a definition of a toxic concentration level is established, then one can eliminate the toxic concentration levels and model the mutagenic effects of a compound using the remaining data. An alternative to this two-step modeling approach is to model both mutagenicity and toxicity of a compound simultaneously. Margolin and associates (9) developed biologically based models for modeling the mutagenicity and toxicity while accounting for the extra variation in the Poisson distribution in the revertant counts from the Ames assay. The choice of their models depends on the number of generations the bacterial cells have for their histidine supply, the number of generations the compound is mutagenic, and the number of generations the compound is toxic. Two basic assumptions of the biologically based models are that mutagenic and toxic effects are independent, and the durations of bacterial cells being mutagenic and toxic are not affected by the concentration of the compound. The mean μ of the negative binomial distribution, is related to the number of bacterial cells exposed to the test object N_0, and the probability of resulting a revertant colony when exposed to the compound at concentration level d, $P(d)$, as

$$\mu = N_0 P(d) \tag{7}$$

We will discuss the two simplest cases when the bacterial cells have enough histidine supply for just one generation and the compound is mutagenic for one generation, but toxic for either one or infinitely many generations. If a compound is toxic for only one generation, then $P(d)$ is

$$P(d) = (1 - e^{-\alpha + \beta d}) \cdot e^{-\gamma d} \tag{8}$$

where α and β are positive and γ is nonnegative. However, if the compound has long-lasting toxicity, then $P(d)$ is

$$P(d) = (1 - e^{-\alpha + \beta d}) \cdot [2 - e^{-\gamma d}]_+ \tag{9}$$

where $[y]_+ = \max(y, 0)$. The spontaneous back mutation rate, mutagenicity, and toxicity are modeled through parameters α, β, and γ. The evaluation of the Ames data is based on models (8) and (9) in combination with Eq. (7) and the negative binomial distribution in Eq. (3) through parameters α, β, γ, and c. If there is no toxicity, then $\gamma = 0$, and models (8) and (9) are identical. Mutagenicity of a compound is evaluated by testing the null hypothesis of $H_0: \beta = 0$ against the alternative of $H_a: \beta > 0$. Margolin and associates (9) approximated the distribution of the ratio of the maximum likelihood estimate of β, $\hat{\beta}$, and its standard error, se $(\hat{\beta})$, by a standard normal distribution. The se $(\hat{\beta})$ was obtained based on the Fisher information matrix evaluated at the maximum likelihood estimates of α, β, γ, and c. However, further research by Margolin and associates (15) identified problems with the two models. Inflated type I error rates were reported for both models. Their proposal to contain the type I error rates was performing a pretest on $\gamma = 0$ to identify the presence of toxicity. The pretest of $H_0: \gamma = 0$ against $H_a: \gamma > 0$ is a likelihood ratio test

$$\lambda_\gamma = 2[L(\alpha, \beta, \gamma; c) - L(\alpha, \beta, 0; c)] \tag{10}$$

where $L(\alpha, \beta, \gamma; c)$ is the maximum of the log-likelihood of the data. If the toxicity is not supported by the data, then the mutagenicity parameter β will be tested by the likelihood ratio test in Eq. (10) constrained on $\gamma = 0$,

$$\lambda_\gamma = 2[L(\alpha, \beta, 0; c) - L(\alpha, 0, 0; c)] \tag{11}$$

Otherwise, the mutagenicity parameter β will be tested by

$$\lambda_\gamma = 2[L(\alpha, \beta, \gamma; c) - L(\alpha, 0, \gamma; c)] \tag{12}$$

Histidine is necessary for the growth of auxotrophic cells. In the biologically based models described in the foregoing, histidine diffusion was not considered, and each cell will have a local supply of histidine. However, if histidine does diffuse through the agar plate, then the revertant counts should be a function of the amount of histidine as well. Krewski and associates (16) proposed generalization of the biologically based models by Margolin and associates (9) to allow for diffusion of histidine in an agar plate.

V. DISCUSSION

The original and modified two- or threefold rules are simple to use and have been compared with other methods (14,21). Chu and associates reported favorable performance of the modified twofold rule based on results from 2362 tests performed in four laboratories on 17 test articles.
Define the false positive and false negative as follows:

False positive = negative tests determined by consensus of microbiologists that is concluded positive using the decision rule.
False negative = positive tests determined by consensus of microbiologists that is concluded negative using the decision rule.

Among the methods that gave higher false-positive conclusions than false-negative conclusions are the modified twofold rule which gave 4.1% false-positive and 1.8% false-negative results and the positive linear trend test described in Section IV.D.1, which gave 20.0% false-positive and 0.4% false negative results. If the modified twofold rule is supplemented with a modified threefold rule, one would expect the proportion of false-positive results to decrease further.

For situations when there is no convincing evidence for the assumptions of Poisson distribution, overdispersion in the Poisson distribution, and the normality distribution of the transformed data, the nonparametric methods discussed in Section IV.C – namely, the Jonkeere test and the method proposed by Wahrendorf and associates – seem plausible. The latter also provides a descriptive quantity for assessment of the types of increasing trends and the possibility of downturn owing to toxicity. An example of revertant counts of strain TA100 in triplicate of (66, 82, 64), (66, 73, 87), (89, 84, 86), (76, 83, 87), (87, 103, 91), and (89, 98, 82) corresponding to the concentration levels of 0, 10, 30, 50, 100, and 300 μg per plate, respectively, was taken from Stead and associates (8). The nonparametric method by Wahrendorf concluded a highly significant mutagenic effect with p-value = 0.0028, based on normal approximation and p = 0.0016 based on critical values established by Monte Carlo simulations. If the modified twofold rule were applied to the data, no mutagenic effects would be concluded.

Parametric methods with the assumptions of Poisson distribution with or without extra variation and negative binomial distribution of the revertant counts use statistical tools in modeling the counts for mutagenicity, toxicity, and dispersion. Whereas the modified twofold rule only calls for simple averages of the revertant counts. While the modified twofold rule demonstrated good agreement with the consensus of the microbiologists in the NCI/NTP study (14), it was considered too conservative by statisticians in general. It is clear that if the statistical methods were adopted, be it parametric or nonparametric, then there will be many more statistically significant findings than when using the modified twofold and threefold rules. To address the differences in the mutagenicity of compounds using statistical evaluation and biological evaluation, several issues merit further discussion here. They are

1. The use of historical control data
2. The toxicity threshold of a bacterial cell to a test article
3. Extra-Poisson variation in the revertant counts
4. The amount of histidine provided
5. The relation between statistical significance and biological significance

Clearly, these issues are all interrelated and, therefore, the discussion may not be in the order listed. Because in practice, most laboratories conducted Ames assays in triplicate, it is difficult to identify if extra-Poisson variation is present in the revertant counts within each experiment. A historical database for negative control data should be a must for examining the assumption of excessive variation in the revertant counts. In addition, a historical database can provide a base range for the evaluation of compounds that may yield statistical significance that is not biologically important. Because there may be variations among various laboratories, it is best for each laboratory to establish its own database for the historical negative control.

The toxicity threshold of a bacterial cell to a test article may be determined using the rule described by Chu and associates or by 50–90% lethality. In other words, the number of revertants in the treated plates have to be reasonably low to indicate a toxic effect. Statistical methods can then be applied without modeling the toxic effects. However, if the rules are not accepted by the regulatory agencies, statistical modeling may be the best way to determine the presence of the toxic effects.

Biologically based models for different combinations of mutagenicity and toxicity lead to different models. How one determines the number of generations that the histidine supply will last, the number of generations the compound will be mutagenic, and the number of generations the compound will be toxic is unclear.

VI. CONCLUSIONS

At this point, no consensus has been reached on statistical methods for analyzing and interpreting the Ames. This is reflected in the ICH guideline for genetoxicity (22) which does not mention any statistical methods for the evaluation of the test results. Considering the small set of numbers that the Ames assay provides for each bacterial strain, statistical methods designed to evaluate the mutagenic effects should reflect the biological significance to be of any help to microbiologists. Statistical methods that find biologically small increases statistically significant with a small p-value are not desirable and may slow down the development of a compound unnecessarily. Any statistical methods recommended for the routine data analysis for the Ames assay should be validated by a collection of compounds with known mutagenicity. A historical database is a must in the evaluation of the mutagenicity of the compounds and should be established in each laboratory. When a historical database is unavailable, nonparametric approaches may be a better choice than parametric methods. Statistical methods should support microbiologists' findings when the effects, mutagenic or nonmutagenic, are clear, and should guide scientists when the effects are unclear. Because the modified twofold and threefold rules seem to agree well with the consensus of microbiologists (14), further work in this area is needed to compare various proposed statistical methods with the modified twofold and threefold rules based on known compounds.

ACKNOWLEDGMENTS

The author would like to thank Marcia Rexroat for many helpful discussions.

REFERENCES

1. Ames BN, Lee FD, Durston WE. An improved bacterial test system for the detection and classification of mutagens and carcinogens. Proc Natl Acad Sci USA 70:782–786, 1973.

2. Ames BN, McCann J, Yamasaki E. Methods for detecting carcinogens and mutagens with the *Salmonella*/microsome mutagenicity test. Mutat Res 31: 347, 1975.

3. McCann J, Gold LS, Horn L, McGill R, Graedel TE, Kaldor J. Statistical analysis of *Salmonella* test data and comparison to results of animal cancer tests. Mutat Res 205:183, 1988.

4. Purchase IFH. An appraisal of predictive tests for carcinogenicity. Mutat Res 99:53, 1982.

5. Edler L. Statistical methods for short-term tests in genetic toxicology: the first fifteen years. Mutat Res 277:11, 1992.

6. Mahon GAT, Middleton B, Robinson WD, Green MHL, Mitchell I, Tweats DJ. Analysis of data from microbial count assays. In: Kirkland DJ, ed. Statistical Evaluation of Mutagenicity Test Data. Cambridge: Cambridge University Press, 1989, p 26.

7. Fisher RA. The significance of deviations from expectation in a Poisson series. Biometrics 6:17, 1950.

8. Stead AG, Hasselblad JP, Greason JP, Claxton L. Modelling the Ames test. Mutat Res 85:13, 1981.

9. Vollmar J. Statistical problems in the Ames test. In: Kappas A, ed. Progress in Mutation Research, vol 2. Amsterdam: Elsevier/North-Holland Biomedical Press, 1981, p 179.

10. Margolin BH, Kaplan N, Zeiger E. Statistical analysis of the Ames *Salmonella*/microsome test. Proc Natl Acad Sci USA 78:3779, 1981.

11. Jonckheere AR. A distribution-free *k*-sample test against ordered alternative. Biometrika 41:133, 1954.

12. Kruskal WH, Wallis WA. Use of ranks in one-criterion variance analysis. J Am Stat Assoc 47:583, 1952.

13. Wahrendorf J. A nonparametric approach to the statistical analysis of mutagenicity data. Mutat Res 147:5, 1985.

14. Chu KC, Patel KM, Lin AH, Tarone RE, Linhart MS, Dunkel VC. Evaluating statistical analyses and reproducibility of microbial mutagenicity assays. Mutat Res 85:119, 1981.

15. Margolin BH, Kim BS, Risko KJ. The Ames *Salmonella*/microsome mutagenicity assay: issues of inference and validation. J Am Stat Assoc 84:651, 1989.

16. Krewski D, Leroux BG, Bleuer SR, Broekhoven LH. Modeling the Ames *Salmonella*/microsome assay. Biometrics 49:499, 1993.

17. Margolin BH, Resnick MA, Rimpo JY, Archer P, Galloway SM, Bloom

AD, Zeiger E. Statistical analysis for in vitro cytogenetic assays using Chinese hamster ovary cells. Environ Mutat 8:183, 1986.

18. McCullagh P, Nelder JA. Generalized Linear Models, 2nd ed. London: Chapman & Hall, 1989, p 198.

19. Tukey JW, Ciminera JL, Heyse JF. Testing the statistical certainty of a response to increasing doses of a drug. Biometrics 41:295, 1985.

20. SAS/STAT software: changes and enhancements, through release 6.11. Cary, NC: SAS Institute Inc, 1996, p 231.

21. Margolin BH. Statistical studies in genetic toxicology: a perspective from the US National Toxicology Program. Environ Health Perspective 63:187, 1985.

22. ICH Harmonised Tripartite Guideline. Guidance on specific aspects of regulatory genotoxicity tests for pharmaceuticals, 1995.

12

The In Vitro Chinese Hamster Ovary Cell Mutagenesis Studies

JEN-PEI LIU

National Cheng-Kung University, Tainan, Taiwan

SHEIN-CHUNG CHOW

Covance Inc., Princeton, New Jersey

I. INTRODUCTION

In vitro mutagenesis tests are genetic toxicological studies, at the early drug development, to provide initial assessment of the safety profile of potential and promising pharmaceutical entities. Short-term assays using mammalian Chinese hamster ovary (CHO) cells for identification of mutagens and potential carcinogens include the hypoxanthine–guanine phosphoribosyl transferase (CHO/HGPRT) mutagenesis assay, sister chromatid exchange (SCE), and chromosome aberration cytogenetic assays. The response variables of these in vitro assays are counts. The count data from the CHO/HGPRT test, as shown in Snee and Irr (1981), do not follow a Poisson distribution whereas, as demonstrated by Margolin et al. (1986), the Poisson distribution fits the SCE counts quite satisfactorily. The design and statistical methods for analysis of the counts data from CHO/HGPRT assays and SCE tests based on CHO cells will be introduced and discussed. Section II provides the background and a brief description of the experimental procedure for a

CHO/HGPRT assay. Statistical designs and rationale for the transformation recommended by Snee and Irr (1981) will be given in Section III. The background and a short introduction to the in vitro cytogenetic sister chromatid exchange and chromosome aberration using Chinese hamster ovary cells will be provided in Section IV. Section V presents the statistical design and rationale of the recommended statistical methods for analysis of SCE counts by Margolin et al. (1986). Final remarks and discussion will be given in Section V.

II. BACKGROUND OF THE CHO/HGPRT ASSAY

Hsie et al. (1975) showed that the clones resistant to 6-thioguanine (6-TG) are developed from a mutation occurring at the hypoxanthine-guanine phosphoribosyl transferase (HGPRT) locus of cultured Chinese hamster ovary cells (CHO). Consequently, the CHO/HGPRT assay, based on demonstration of induction of 6-TG-resistant mutation in CHO cells, developed by Hsie at Oak Ridge National Laboratory, has proved to be a reliable and sensitive qualitative method to evaluate mutagenic potential of pharmaceutical entities. Snee and Irr (1981) gave a brief description of the procedure for the CHO/HGPRT assay, which is given in the following:

   To control variability among different experiments, the same subclone of the original CHO cells, isolated by Hsie et al. (1975) should be used in all experiments. The cells were cultured in hypoxanthine-deficient Ham's F12 medium which contains 10% heat-inactivated dialyzed fetal calf serum in 5% CO_2, at 95% relative humidity, and 37°C. The procedures recommended by O'Neill et al. (1977) for culturing, expression passage, toxicity testing, and mutant selection can also be applied to the CHO/HGPRT assay. These cells were treated with the pharmaceutical entities for 18 h. After 5 h the treatment was stopped, the celled were then allowed to recover in fresh medium overnight. The mutagenesis studies used HGPRT-deficient cells with medium containing hypoxanthine, aminopterin, and thimidine (HAT). Because of phenotypic lag, a period called expression time was required to propagate mutagen-treated cells in F12 medium before selection for 6-TG-resistance. It usually takes 8 days after the addition of the pharmaceutical entities, which require three transfers, on the same day, day 3 or 4, and on day 6. In general, the subsequent culture used only 10^6 cells and 20–90% of the cells were subcultured at each transfer and at the selection steps. The rest of the cells were discarded. The response variable of the CHO/HGPRT assay at a particular dose level or control is called the mutation frequency, which is referred to as the mutants per 10^6 surviving cells computed by correcting the absolute number of mutants in the sample for plating efficiency (the number of colony-forming units) of the sample.

III. DESIGN AND STATISTICAL METHODS FOR THE CHO/HGPRT ASSAYS

A. Design for the CHO/HGPRT Assays

The basic design for a typical CHO/HGPRT assay is a completely randomized design (CRD), which consists of a negative (or solvent) control, a positive control, and three to four dose levels of the pharmaceutical compound under investigation. Two replicates are usually included at each dose level, including the controls. For a full assessment of mutagenic potential of the test pharmaceutical, the CHO/HGPRT assay is performed in duplicated trials as shown in Table 1 to evaluate whether similar results can be reproduced; in other words, to test the presence of the trial-by-dose interaction. The dose levels are chosen to be equally

TABLE 1   Design for the CHO/HGPRT Mutagenesis Assay

Group	Trial	
	1	2
1	Negative control	Negative control
	Rep 1	Rep 1
	Rep 2	Rep 2
2	Positive control	Positive control
	Rep 1	Rep 1
	Rep 2	Rep 2
3	Dose level 1	Dose level 1
	Rep 1	Rep 1
	Rep 2	Rep 2
.	.	.
.	.	.
.	.	.
t	Dose level $K - 1$	Dose level $K - 1$
	Rep 1	Rep 1
	Rep 2	Rep 2

spaced either on the original or on a logarithmic scale. Table 2 presents a data set given in Snee and Irr (1981) for an experiment with a negative control and four dose levels to evaluate mutagenic potential of 5-bromodeoxyuridine (BUDR).

B. Analysis for the CHO/HGPRT Assays

It is quite clear from Tables 1 and 2, that the objectives of the CHO/HGPRT assay include (a) to investigate and characterize the dose–response relation, (b) to identify the dose level beyond which the test pharmaceutical is mutagenic, and (c) to verify whether a similar conclusion can be reproduced by test of the trial-by-dose interaction. As a result, an approach to achieve the three objectives is to apply the traditional parametric method, with the following model to X_{ijk}, the mutation frequency observed at replicate k at dose level j of trial i:

$$X_{ijk} = \mu + T_i + D_j + TD_{ij} + e_{ijk} \tag{1}$$

where μ is the overall mean ST_i is the fixed effect of trial i, and D_j is the fixed effect of dose j, TD_{ij} is the interaction between trial i and dose j, and e_{ijk}, is the experiment error associated with X_{ijk}, $k = 1,2$; $j = 1$, . . . , K; $i = 1,2$.

TABLE 2 Mutation Frequencies of the CHO/HGPRT Assay for BUDR

Dose (μg ml^{-1})	Trial 1	Trial 2	Average Original	Average Transformed
0	5.6 13.0	26.1 6.0	10.8[a]	1.4480[b]
25	1.8 0.0	1.8 28.2	3.4	1.2482
50	33.9 26.1	42.7 7.3	23.9	1.6200
100	198.7 224.8	185.6 121.9	179.0	2.1792
125	241.2 274.8	353.5 269.7	282.4	2.3327

[a]Average based on the inverse transformation $X = y^{(1/0.15)} - 1$.
[b]Average based on the transformation of $Y = (X + 1)^{0.15}$.
Source: Snee and Irr, 1981.

The experiment errors e_{ijk} are assumed to be independently and identically distributed (iid) as a normal distribution with mean 0 and variance σ^2; that is,

$$e_{ijk} \overset{iid}{\sim} N(0, \sigma^2).\tag{2}$$

Although each experiment for CHO/HGPRT is performed as a CRD design, the duplicated trial can be viewed as a full two-factor factorial experiment with trial and dose as factors. Hence, analysis for mutation frequencies from CHO/HGPRT assays is quite straightforward if the assumptions for the experimental errors are satisfied. Denote $\overline{X}_{...}$, $\overline{X}_{i..}$, $\overline{X}_{.j.}$, and $\overline{X}_{ij.}$ as the observed overall mean, the observed treatment means of trial i, of dose j, and of treatment combinations of trial i and dose j, respectively:

$$\overline{X}_{...} = (1/4K)\Sigma\Sigma\Sigma\, X_{ijk}$$
$$\overline{X}_{i..} = (1/2K)\Sigma\Sigma\, X_{ijk}, i = 1, 2$$
$$\overline{X}_{.j.} = (1/4)\Sigma\Sigma\, X_{ijk}, j = 1, \ldots, K$$

and

$$\overline{X}_{ij.} = (1/2)\Sigma\Sigma\, X_{ijk}, i = 1, 2, \text{ and } j = 1, \ldots, K$$

Let SST, SSt, SStr, SSD, SSTD, SSE be total sum of squares, treatment sum of squares, trial sum of squares, dose treatment sum of squares, the sum of squares for trial-by-dose interaction, and error sum of squares, respectively, which are given as follows:

$$\text{SST} = \Sigma\Sigma\Sigma\, (X_{ijk} - \overline{X}_{...})^2$$
$$\text{SSt} = \Sigma\Sigma 2(\overline{X}_{ij.} - \overline{X}_{...})^2$$
$$\text{SStr} = \Sigma\Sigma 2K(\overline{X}_{i..} - \overline{X}_{...})^2$$
$$\text{SSD} = \Sigma\Sigma 4(\overline{X}_{.j.} - \overline{X}_{...})^2$$
$$\text{SSTD} = \text{SSt} - \text{SStr} - \text{SSD}$$
$$\text{SSE} = \text{SST} - \text{SSt}$$

The corresponding analysis of variance (ANOVA) is given in Table 3. If assumption (2) is true, then the mean square error is an unbiased estimator for σ^2. The presence of trial-by-dose interaction is then concluded if

$$F_{TD} = \frac{\text{MSTD}}{\text{MSE}} > F(\alpha, K - 1, 2K)\tag{3}$$

TABLE 3 The Analysis of Variance Table for the Design
in Table 1 of the CHO/HGPRT Assay

Source of variation	df	Sum of squares		Mean square	
Trial	1	SStr		MStr	
Dose	$K - 1$	SSD		MSD	
Linear	1		SSL		MSL
Quadratic	1		SSQ		MSW
Higher order	$K - 3$		SSHO		MSHO
$T \times D$ interaction	$K - 1$	SSTD		MSTD	
Error	$2K$	SSE		MSE	
Total	$4K - 1$	SST			

where MSTD is the mean square for trial-by-dose interaction, and MSE
is the mean square error, $F(\alpha, df_1, df_2)$ is the upper αth quantile of a
central F distribution with degrees of freedom df_1 and df_2.

If F_{TD} is not statistically significant at the prescribed nominal level,
one can proceed to test the main effect of dose levels. The response
at dose levels are concluded statistically significantly different at the α
significance level if

$$F_D = \frac{\text{MSD}}{\text{MSE}} > F(\alpha, K - 1, 2K) \tag{4}$$

where MSD is the mean square for the drug effects.

After a statistically significant dose effect is concluded by (4), we
need to characterize the dose–response relation and to identify the dose
beyond which the test pharmaceutical is mutagenic. Characterization of
the dose–response relation can be accomplished by partition of dose sum
of squares into $K - 1$ individual sums of squares with single degree of
freedom for linear or quadratic relation between the responses and dose
levels through the technique of linear contrasts. A linear contrast of dose
means is a linear combination of the treatment means for dose in which
sum of the coefficients in the linear combination is zero; that is,

$$L = \Sigma c_j \overline{X}_{.j.}$$

where $\Sigma c_j = 0$.

Two linear contrasts L_1 and L_2 are said to be orthogonal to each
other if the sum of the cross-products of their coefficients is also zero.

Relative to the structure of the design for CHO/HGPRT design, the sum of squares for linear contrasts can be computed as

$$\text{SS}(L_h) = \frac{(\Sigma c_{h_j} \overline{X}_{.j.})^2}{d_h}, h = 1, \ldots, K - 1;$$ (5)

where $d_h = \Sigma C_{hj}^2/4$.

A statistically significant relation determined by the linear contrast L_h is concluded at the α significance level if

$$F_h = \frac{\text{SS}(L_h)}{\text{MSE}} > F(\alpha, 1, 2K), h = 1, \ldots, K - 1$$ (6)

The coefficients of the linear contrasts for identification of linear, quadratic, cubic dose relation for various number of dose levels are given in Table 4.

Suppose that there is no trial-by-dose interaction, then a dose level is declared to be mutagenic if

$$t = \frac{(\overline{X}_{.j.} - \overline{X}_{.1.})}{\sqrt{\text{MSE}/2}} > t(\alpha, 2K), j = 2, \ldots, K$$ (7)

TABLE 4   Coefficients of Orthogonal Linear Contrasts for Equal-Dose Levels

No. of dose levels	Dose level	Linear	Quadratic	Cubic
3	1	−1	1	
	2	0	−2	
	3	1	1	
4	1	−3	1	−1
	2	−1	−1	3
	3	1	−1	−3
	4	3	1	1
5	1	−2	2	−1
	2	−1	−1	2
	3	0	−2	0
	4	1	−1	−2
	5	2	2	1

where $t(\alpha, 2K)$ is the upper αth quantile of a central t distribution with degrees of freedom $2K$.

C. Distribution of Mutation Frequencies and Transformation

The foregoing statistical methods for analyses of the mutation frequency from CHO/HGPRT assays are based on the crucial assumption that the experiment errors are iid normal with mean 0 and variance σ^2. In addition, this assumption also implies that the variance is homogeneous among all dose levels, including the negative and positive controls. However, the assumptions have to be verified by the data. The response variable of the CHO/HGPRT is the count of the number of the mutants per 10^6 surviving cells. As a result, the distribution of the mutation frequencies is more likely to follow a discrete distribution, rather than a continuous distribution, such as the normal distribution. Snee and Irr (1981) used the data of a series of experiments conducted at laboratories of du Pont de Nemours and Co. to determine the distribution of the mutation frequency and the nature of the experimental variability. This data set consists of a total of 760 observations obtained from a series of experiments conducted over an 18-month period with 29 chemicals of known mutagenic potential. Each individual experiment contained at least one negative control.

Snee and Irr (1981) reported that a large variability was exhibited in the frequency of spontaneous mutants observed in the negative controls of the experiments. They compared the results of the 90 negative controls from 45 experiments with 11 different compounds and found no statistically significant difference among these negative controls of the 45 experiments. As a result, the data of mutants observed in these different negative controls can be pooled together as a single sample. The distribution of the mutation frequency is skewed to the right with a very long tail. The mean, median, and standard deviation are respectively, 13.9, 10.6, and 13.8. If the mutation frequency follows a Poisson distribution, the mean and variance should be approximately equal; and a plot of variance versus mean should be a 45° straight-line through the origin. However, the ratio of variance to mean for this data set is 13.8, which indicates the data of mutation frequency cannot come from a Poisson distribution. In addition, they also reported that the data from the accumulation of spontaneous mutation frequencies and the ethyl methanesulfonate-induced mutation frequencies with time did not follow a Poisson distribution either, as shown in Table 5.

TABLE 5 Frequency of 6-Thioguanine-Resistant Mutant Clones from the Same Culture of CHO Cells

Sample number	Spontaneous mutants	Mutants induced by EMS
1	0	500
2	0	433
3	3.9	471
4	5	371
5	2.7	491
6	2.7	510
7	1.2	381
8	16.8	348
9	0	388
10	2.5	495
Mean	3.5	439
Variance	24.8	3837
Variance/mean	7.1	8.7

Source: Snee and Irr, 1981.

To determine the nature of the experiment variability, Snee and Irr (1981) fitted (1) without the trial-by-dose interaction to the data from each of 29 chemicals. The estimated overall mean and the square root of the mean square error were obtained for each of 29 chemicals. There was a very strong positive relation between the square roots of mean square errors and the estimated overall means. In other words, the homogeneous variance assumption is violated by the raw data. The plot of the residuals versus the predicted values also provided the evidence for such violation. In addition the normal probability plot of the residuals (Fig. 1) also suggested that the data did not follow a normal distribution.

To overcome these deficiencies exhibited by the data of mutation frequencies to satisfy the assumptions of the parametric methods described in the foregoing, Snee and Irr (1981) derived a transformation formula for the raw data so that the residuals have a normal distribution through the Box–Cox power transformation (Box and Cox, 1964), which has the following form:

$$Y = (X + A)^{\lambda} \tag{8}$$

where A and λ are some constants.

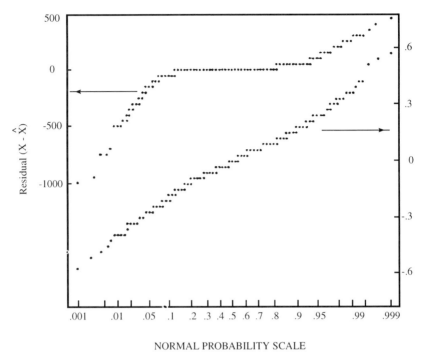

FIGURE 1   Normal probability plot. (From Snee and Irr, 1981.)

The constant A for the data of mutation frequency is recommended as 1 to avoid mathematical inconvenience when the zero frequency occurs. However, the value of λ must be estimated from the data by selecting it to minimize the error sum of square calculated from the residuals of the assumed model. The model used by Snee and Irr (1981) for estimation of λ is given as

$$Y_{hij} = \mu + C_h + T_{i(h)} + D_{j(h)} + e_{hij} \qquad (9)$$

where Y_{hij} is the transformed mutation frequency for chemical h, trial I and dose level j; μ is the overall mean; C_h is the fixed effect of chemical h; $T_{i(h)}$ is the fixed effect of trial i of chemical h; $D_{j(h)}$ is the fixed effect of dose j of chemical h; and e_{hij} is the experimental error associated with Y_{hij}; $h = 1, \ldots, H; I = 1, \ldots, 2, j = 1, \ldots, K$. With a complete set of 760 observations from 29 chemicals, Snee and Irr (1981) found that a value of 0.15 for λ minimizes the error sum of squares with 95% confidence intervals from 0.12 to 0.18. As a result, the transformation formula for the mutation frequencies was recommended by them is given as

$$Y = (X + 1)^{0.15} \tag{10}$$

Before the parametric statistical methods introduced in the foregoing can be applied to the transformed mutation frequencies, the homogeneous variance assumption and normality assumption must first be verified. Figure 1 gives the normal probability plot of the residuals of the data transformed by (9), which reveals no large departure from the normality assumption for the transformed residuals. In addition, contrary to the raw data, there is no correlation between the observed overall means and standard deviations calculated for 29 chemicals. Figure 2

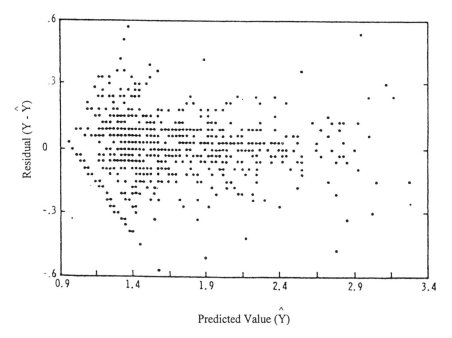

FIGURE 2 Plot of transformed predicted values versus residuals. (From Snee and Irr, 1981.)

provides the plot of the residuals versus the predicted values computed for the transformed data with $\lambda = 0.15$. The complete randomness demonstrated by Fig. 2 and lack of correlation between the observed overall means and standard deviations strongly indicate that the variance computed from the data transformed by Eq. (9) is indeed homogeneous. Figure 3 displays the histograms of the untransformed and transformed mutation frequencies, which also indicate that the distribution of the transformed data can be approximated quite satisfactorily by a normal distribution.

As a result, the analysis should be performed on the transformed mutation frequencies by replacing X_{ijk} in (1) with

$$Y_{ijk} = (X_{ijk} + 1)^{0.15}$$

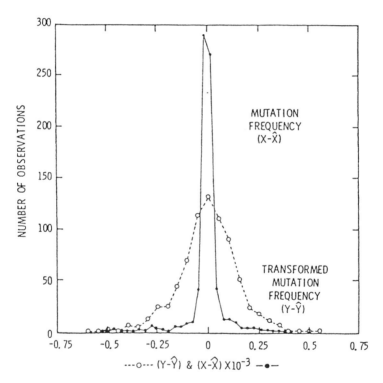

FIGURE 3 Histograms of untransformed and transformed residuals. (From Snee and Irr, 1981.)

TABLE 6 The Analysis of Variance Table for the Data[a] Given in Table 2

Source of variation	df	Sum of squares	Mean square	F
Trial	1	0.0138	0.0138	
Dose	4	3.5294		
Linear	1	3.1508	3.1508	110.28[b]
Quadratic	1	0.1251	0.1251	4.38
Higher order	2	0.2535	0.1267	4.43[c]
$T \times D$	4	0.1285	0.0321	1.12
Error	10	0.2587	0.0286	
Total	19	3.9575		

[a]Based on the transformation $Y = (X + 1)^{0.15}$.
[b]P-value is smaller than 0.01.
[c]P-value is smaller than 0.05.
Source: Snee and Irr, 1981.

The ANOVA table based on (1) and Table 2 for the transformed data is given in Table 6. From Table 6, an unbiased estimate for the variance of the experimental error is given as 0.0286. First, the trial-by-dose interaction was not statistically significant at the 5% nominal level (p-value > 0.05). As a result, the results for the two trials are similar and reproducible; hence, they can be pooled together for inference of the dose effects. Next, the dose effect is statistically significant at the 5% nominal level. Further partition of dose sum of squares based on linear contrasts described earlier reveals a statistically significant linear (p-value < 0.01) and higher-order (p-value < 0.05) dose–response relation. One possible explanation for detection of both linear and higher-order relations is that the response at the lower-dose levels (<50 μg·mL^{-1}) is actually a plateau, but the mutation frequency grew exponentially when dose level goes beyond 50 μg·mL^{-1}. Additional t-tests comparing individual dose levels versus the negative control using (7) showed that the mutation frequencies at the two higher-dose levels are significantly larger statistically than that of the negative control (p-value < 0.01). On the other hand, there is no statistical significant difference in the mutation frequency between the lower two dose levels and the negative control (p-value > 0.05).

IV. BACKGROUND OF IN VITRO CYTOGENETIC ASSAYS USING CHO CELLS

In vitro cytogenetic assays for chromosome alteration have been recognized as sensitive tests for identification of mutagens and potential carcinogens. In addition they can serve as complementary assays to the in vitro Ames *Salmonella* tests discussed in Chapter 11 (Ashby et al., 1985). On the other hand, the cytogenetic endpoint; such as sister chromatid exchanges (SCEs), is positively correlated with mutagenicity and carcinogenicity data. As a result, the induction of SCE is recommended as a short-term screening assay for detection of potential mutagens and carcinogens. However, because of differences in various techniques, there is extreme variability among laboratories in the results of cytogenetic assays with SCE as the endpoint. In 1985, Galloway et al. (1985) proposed a standard protocol for in vitro cytogenetic assays with CHO cells as a short-term, routine screening assay that generates reproducible results among different laboratories.

The medium used by Galloway et al. (1985) in their experiments was McCoy's 5A medium, supplemented with 10% fetal calf serum and L-glutamine (2 mM), in which CHO cells were grown at 37°C in a humidified atmosphere of 5% CO_2 in air. The day before treatment, cultures were prepared at a uniform cell density for exponentially growing cultures of CHO cells at approximately 1×10^6 cells per 75-cm^2 flask. Cultures were handled under gold lights to prevent photolysis of DNA containing bromodeoxyuridine (BRDU). Only cells and culture medium were contained in the negative controls. In addition, the same concentration of solvent as that in the test cultures was included in the solvent controls. A total of 17 compounds were tested under a common protocol at both Litton Bionetics and Columbia University in a blinded manner. The results of SCEs and chromosome aberrations were comparable between the two laboratories. See Galloway et al. (1985) for more details about metabolic activation system (S-9), test chemicals and controls, dose selection, and methods for scoring sister chromatid exchanges and chromosome aberrations.

V. DESIGN AND STATISTICAL METHODS FOR COUNTS FROM SISTER CHROMATID EXCHANGES

The design for SCE from in vitro cytogenetic assays using CHO cells is also a completely randomized design, with a setup similar to that described for CHO/HGPRT assays and in Table 1. In general, with the negative control, a total of four to ten dose levels, probably logarithmically spaced, are usually tested in an experiment. At each dose level, the number of sister chromatid exchanges per cell are scored for each of 50 cells from a single 75-cm² flask. Sometimes, it is not uncommon that replicate 25-cm² flasks are used, in each of which 25 cells were scored for SCE. Because, an in vitro cytogenetic assay may require several days to complete all dose levels, it is imperative that the same individual perform all scoring work for SCEs on the same day.

Let Y_{hijk} represent the SCE counts for cell k of replicate j on day h at dose i, $k = 1, \ldots, k_{hij}$; $j = 1, \ldots, n_{hi}$; $i = 1, \ldots, I$; and $h = 1, \ldots, H$. The data structure for SCE counts on day h is illustrated in Table 7 for $k_{hij} = K$ and $n_{hi} = n$. Under the postulate that occurrence of

TABLE 7 Data Structure of Sister Chromatid Exchange Counts

Day	Dose	Replicate			
		1	2	j	n
1	1	Y_{1111}	$Y_{1121} \cdots$	$Y_{11j1} \cdots$	Y_{11n1}
		.	. $\cdots$	. $\cdots$	.
		.	. $\cdots$	. $\cdots$	.
		.	. $\cdots$	. $\cdots$	.
		Y_{111K}	$Y_{112K} \cdots$	$Y_{11jK} \cdots$	Y_{11nK}
		.	. $\cdots$	. $\cdots$	.
		.	. $\cdots$	. $\cdots$	.
h	i	Y_{hi11}	$Y_{hi21} \cdots$	$Y_{hij1} \cdots$	Y_{hin1}
		.	. $\cdots$	. $\cdots$	.
		.	. $\cdots$	. $\cdots$	.
		Y_{hi1K}	$Y_{hi2K} \cdots$	$Y_{hijK} \cdots$	Y_{hinK}
		.	. $\cdots$	. $\cdots$	.
		.	. $\cdots$	. $\cdots$	.
H	I	Y_{HI11}	$Y_{HI21} \cdots$	$Y_{HIj1} \cdots$	Y_{HIn1}
		.	. $\cdots$	. $\cdots$	.
		.	. $\cdots$	. $\cdots$	.
		Y_{HI1K}	$Y_{HI2K} \cdots$	$Y_{HIjK} \cdots$	Y_{HInK}

sister chromatid exchanges is a rare event, the distribution of the SCE counts per cell should be adequately described by a Poisson model. Margolin et al. (1986) gave the following four assumptions to justify the use of a Poisson distribution for the SCE counts:

1. All cells in the flask experienced the same environment.
2. For a small length of any chromosome in a given cell, the probability of occurrence of an SCE is essentially proportionally to that length, regardless of the identity of the chromosome or location of the length on the chromosome.
3. The probability of occurrence of more than one SCE in a small length of chromosome is negligible.
4. The occurrence of SCEs in nonoverlapping lengths of a chromosome are stochastically independent.

The last three assumptions are the usual assumption for a Poisson process, whereas the first assumption assures that the average of SCE counts is a constant from cell-to-cell in a uniform environment provided by the same flask. From the description of the experiment and scoring mechanism, three sources of variability in SCE counts can probably be identified: the variability between cells within the same flask, the variability between replicated flasks on the same day, the variability between days. They are referred to, respectively, as intercellular intraflask variability, intraday interflask variability, and interday variability.

To verify whether the variability of the SCE counts per cell within the same flask can be reasonably explained by a Poisson distribution, one quick method is to check whether the ratio of variance to mean, computed from the SCE counts per cell, is approximately equal to 1. For a formal test for the SCE counts per cell from replicate j at given dose i on day h, $(Y_{hij1}, \ldots, Y_{hijK})$, Margolin et al. (1986) suggested application of the following dispersion test, $j = 1, \ldots, n_{hi}$; $i = 1, \ldots, I$; and $h = 1, \ldots, H$:

$$T_1 = \frac{\Sigma(Y_{hijk} - \overline{Y}_{hij.})^2}{\overline{Y}_{hij.}} \tag{11}$$

where $\overline{Y}_{hij.} = (1/K)\Sigma Y_{hijk}$ is the mean count over K cells, and K is usually 50 cells or 25 cells for SCE counts.

The assumption of a Poisson model for description of SCE counts per cell in a common flask is rejected at the α significance level if

$$T_1 > \chi^2(\alpha, K - 1) \tag{12}$$

where $\chi^2(\alpha, K - 1)$ is the upper αth quantile of a central χ^2 distribution with $K - 1$ degrees of freedom.

Margolin et al. (1986) has shown that a Poisson model satisfactorily describes the intraflask SCE control counts from Galloway et al. (1985). If the SCE counts per cell within the same flask follows a Poisson distribution, then the sum of SCE counts over all cells from the same flask also follows a Poisson distribution with the mean parameter being the number of cells times the mean parameter per cell. The next step is then to verify whether the cumulative SCE counts of replicated flasks on the same day can also be fitted adequately by a Poisson distribution. Denote $Y_{hij.}$ as the cumulative SCE counts over K cells for replicate j at given dose i on day h; that is,

$$Y_{hij.} = \Sigma Y_{hijk}, j = 1, \ldots, n_{hi};$$
$$i = 1, \ldots, I; \text{and } h = 1, \ldots, H$$

Then the dispersion test in Eq. (11) can be easily extended to test whether, given that the day means are approximately constant, $Y_{hij.}$ observed from replicated flasks on the same days follow a Poisson distribution. The null hypothesis that a Poisson process can satisfactorily describe the cumulative interflask SCE counts for dose i on day h is rejected at the α significance level if

$$T_2 = \frac{\Sigma(\overline{Y}_{hij.} - \overline{Y}_{hi..})^2}{\overline{Y}_{hi..}} > \chi^2(\alpha, df_2) \tag{13}$$

where $\overline{Y}_{hi..} = (1/n_{hi})\Sigma Y_{hij.}$ is the mean cumulative count over n_{hi} replicated flasks and $df_2 = n_{hi} - 1, i = 1, \ldots, I; h = 1, \ldots, H$.

Data from Galloway et al. (1985), as demonstrated by Margolin et al. (1986), indicated that the cumulative SCE control counts from replicated flasks on the same day can be satisfactorily described by a Poisson distribution. However, a Poisson model cannot adequately fit the cumulative SCE control counts from all replicated flasks over several days. As a result, it seems that the interday variability can not be explained by a Poisson random sampling mechanism. Let $Y_{hi..}$ be the cumulative SCE counts over all replicated flasks and m_{2j} be the total number of cells scored for dose i on day h, $i = 1, \ldots, I; h = 1, \ldots, H$. The null hypothesis of a Poisson distribution for $Y_{hi..}$ is rejected at the α significance level if

$$T_3 = \frac{\Sigma(Y_{hi..} - m_{hi}\overline{Y}_{.i..})^2}{m_{hi}\overline{Y}_{.i..}} > \chi^2(\alpha, H - 1), \tag{14}$$

where $\overline{Y}_{.i.} = \Sigma Y_{hi.}/(\Sigma m_{hi})$ is the overall mean cumulative count from the entire laboratory at dose i.

Margolin et al. (1986) concluded that the interday variability cannot be explained by a Poisson distribution for the SCE control data obtained from both Columbia University and Litton Bionetics. One possible explanation is that different individuals performed scoring of the SCE counts. From the foregoing discussion, both distributions of the SCE counts per cell and the cumulative SCE counts per flasks, observed on the same day, can be adequately described by Poisson models. As a result, in vitro cytogenetic assays for SCE counts should be performed for all dose levels on the same day. Given the empirical evidence provided by Margolin et al. (1986), the SCE counts at dose i can be added over all cells from replicated flasks for examination of a possible trend between the cumulative SCE counts and dose levels. Because all assays should be performed on the same day, the subscript for day is dropped in the subsequent discussion. Denote the cumulative SCE counts at dose i by $Y_{i..}$, where

$$Y_{i..} = \Sigma \Sigma Y_{ijk}, i = 1, \ldots, I$$

Margolin et al. (1986) suggested the use of Cochran–Armitage test (Cochran, 1954; Armitage, 1955) to investigate whether a possible linear trend exists between SCE counts and dose levels $x_0, x_1, \ldots, x_r, r = I - 1$. Define the overall mean for the entire experiment as

$$\overline{Y} = \frac{\Sigma \Sigma \Sigma Y_{ijk}}{(\Sigma \Sigma k_{ij})}$$

and the number of total cells at dose i as

$$k_i = \Sigma k_{ij}, I = 1, \ldots, I$$

and

$$SS(x) = \Sigma k_i (x_i - \overline{x})^2$$

where $\overline{x}$ is the arithmetic mean of the dose levels.

Then a statistically significant linear trend is concluded at the α significant level by the Cochran–Armitage test statistic if

$$T_4 = \frac{\Sigma x_i (Y_{i..} - k_i \overline{Y})^2}{[\overline{Y} SS(x)]} > \chi^2(\alpha, 1) \tag{15}$$

The actual dose levels, $d_0, d_1, \ldots, d_r$, employed in an in vitro cytogenetic assay using CHO cells are usually logarithmically spaced. As a result, if the true dose levels are used in (15), then the Cochran-Armitage test would be a test for comparison of the response at the highest dose level with the weighted average response from all other dose levels, because extreme weight will be given to the response at the highest dose level. Therefore, Margolin et al. (1986) recommended the following transformation of the original dose levels as

$$x_i = \begin{cases} \log_{10}(d_i), & \text{if } i = 1, \ldots, r \\ x_1 - [(x_r - x_1)/(r - 1)], & \text{if } i = 0 \end{cases}$$

VI. DISCUSSION

The mutation frequency from the CHO/HGPRT test and the numbers of SCE from the in vitro cytogenetic assay are counts. Extra-Poisson variability exists for the mutation frequency, whereas the data of the SCE counts observed on the same day are quite adequately explained by a Poisson model. However, the objectives of the assays are to investigate whether promising pharmaceuticals are also possible mutagens and potential carcinogens, to examine and characterize the dose–response relation, and to identify the dose level beyond which they become mutagenic. Snee and Irr (1981) recommended the transformation of the original mutation frequency by (9) before application of (1) to analysis of the transformed data. On the other hand, Margolin et al. (1986) suggested the use of the Cochran–Armitage test for detection of a trend between the SCE counts and dose levels.

The value of 0.15 for λ is based on the empirical evidence from 760 observations in the CHO/HGPRT assays performed on 29 chemicals over a period of 18 months. It is unknown whether λ still remains constant over all these years. In addition, it seems that selection of 0.15 for λ lacks some biological justification or explanation. On the other hand, after the analysis is performed on the transformed data of the mutation frequency, the results may need to be presented on the original scale by the inverse transformation for a better interpretation, as shown in Table 2. However, because the Box–Cox power transformation is not linear, the average mutation frequency on the original scale at a particular dose level obtained from the inverse transformation of the average of the transformed data is biased. The direction and magnitude of this bias require thorough investigation.

The Cochran–Armitage test recommended by Margolin et al. (1986) provides sufficient power to detect a linear trend between the SCE counts and dose levels, as shown by their simulation results. However, when the dose–response relation is in other forms, such as quadratic or cubic, the Cochran–Armitage test might not be powerful. In addition, the trend test does not allow an individual comparison between dose levels and the negative control to identify the dose levels beyond which the test pharmaceutical is mutagenic or carcinogenic. Both the theory of and the experience for applications with generalized linear models (McCullagh and Nelder, 1989) have become quite mature and sophisticated. As a result, the data of mutation frequency and SCE counts can be directly analyzed on the original scale through a regression framework provided by the generalized linear models. More empirical experience is urgently required on the comparison between the methods suggested in this chapter and the approaches through generalized linear models.

Galloway et al. (1985) suggested categorization of chromosome aberrations into three types: simple, complex, and total. The simple category includes aberrations such as breaks and terminal deletions, and complex aberrations include exchanges and rearrangements, whereas total group represents an amalgamation of all types of structural aberrations. Margolin et al. (1986) found that a binomial model seems to adequately fit the data from chromosome aberrations. They also suggested use of the Cochran–Armitage test for a linear trend between the response and dose levels. The simulation study performed by Margolin et al. (1986) showed that a sample size of 50 cells per dose per design will provide adequate power to detect a linear trend for the SCE counts by the Cochran–Armitage test. However, owing to the low spontaneous occurrence rate of aberrant cells, Margolin et al. (1986) recommended that for the standard protocol developed by Galloway et al. (1985) at least 200 cells per dose per design be used to provide sufficient power for detection of a linear trend between chromosome aberrations and dose levels.

REFERENCES

Armitage P. Test for linear trends in proportions and frequencies. Biometrics 11: 375–386, 1955.

Ashby J, de Serres FJ, Draper M, Ishidate M Jr, Margolin BH, Matter BE, Shelby MD, eds. Evaluation of Short-Term Tests for Carcinogens: Report of the International Programme on Chemical Safety Collaborative Study on In Vitro Assays. Amsterdam: Elsevier/North Holland, 1985.

Box GEP, Cox DR. An analysis of transformation (with discussion). J R Stat Assoc B 26:211–256, 1964.

Cochran WG. Some methods for strengthening the common χ^2 tests. Biometrics 10:417–451, 1954.

Galloway SM, Bloom AD, Resnick M, Margolin BH, Nakamura F, Archer P, Zeiger E. Development of a standard protocol for in vitro cytogenetic testing with Chinese hamster ovary cells: comparison of results for 22 compounds in two laboratories. Environ Mutagen 7:1–51, 1985.

Hsie AW, Brimer PA, Mitchell TJ, Gosslee DG. The dose–response relationship for ethyl methanesulfonate-induced mutations at the hypoxanthine–guanine phosphoribosyl transferase locus of cultured Chinese hamster ovary cells. Som Cell Genet 1:247–161, 1975.

Margolin BH, Resnick MA, Rimpo JY, Archer P, Galloway SM, Bloom AD, Zeiger E. Statistical analyses for in vitro cytogenetic assays using Chinese hamster ovary cells. Environ Mutagen 8:183–204, 1986.

McCullagh P, Nelder JA. Generalized Linear Models, 2nd ed. London: Chapman & Hall, 1989.

O'Neill JP, Brimer PA, Machanoff R, Hirsch GP, Hsie AW. A quantitative assay of mutation induction at the hypoxanthine–guanine phosphoribosyl transferase locus of cultured Chinese hamster ovary cells (CHO/HGPRT system): Development and definition of the system. Mutat Res 45:91–101, 1977.

Snee RD, Irr JD. Design of a statistical method for the analysis of mutagenesis at the hypoxanthine–guanine phosphoribosyl transferase locus of cultured Chinese hamster ovary cells. Mutat Res 85:77–93, 1981.

Index